THE CAUSE OF AUTISM

Concepts and Misconceptions

Gary Steinman, MD,PhD[1,2]
Editor-in-Chief

With Associate Editors:
Roberta Zuckerman, BA
David Mankuta, MD,MPH[3]
Frank Gray, EdD[1]

1 – Touro College of Osteopathic Medicine, New York, NY
2 - Long Island Jewish Medical Center, New Hyde Park, NY
3 - Hadassah-Hebrew University School of Medicine, Jerusalem, Israel

THE CAUSE OF AUTISM: Concepts and Misconceptions

Editor-in-Chief: Gary Steinman

Associate Editors: Roberta Zuckerman

David Mankuta

Frank Gray

ISBN: 978-0-9665105-3-9

Library of Congress Control Number: 2014948882

Published by:
Baffin Books Publishing
19918 Epsom Course
Hollis, New York 11423

First printing: 2014
Page layout: Theodore Thompson
Cover design: CoverDesignStudio/Gimp 2.8.10®
Printed by: CreateSpace®
Printed in the United States of America
E-mail: baffinbookspublishing@aol.com

CONTRIBUTORS

Cindy	Agu	Nicole	McGill
Nimrah	Ahmed	Jonathon	Marshall
Jemima	Akinsanya	Erica	Mirigliani
Kessiena	Aya	Mina	Mosaad
Ruslan	Banai	Samantha	Mucha
Oyewale	Bello	Maryan	Nasralah
Marissa	Botwinick	Rohit	Navlani
Julia	Brothers	Marissa	Opilas
Tatiana	Carrillo	Christa	Patrick
Tova	Chein	Victoria	Pham
Dimple	Chhatlani	Lidianny	Polanco
Cynthia	Clark	Brian	Pritchard
Shelley	Co	Thomas	Quinn
Nicholas	Daprano	Katherine	Redford
Elina	Davydov	Paola	Reveco
Corina	Din-Lovinescu	Matthew	Rosner
John	Farag	Andrew	Ross
Matthew	Fasullo	Gabrielle	Rozenberg
Mario	Flores	Andrew	Rudin
Marlee	Forte	Szymon	Rus
Jeffrey	Gardere	Alexis	Sandoval
Daniel	Herzog	Snaha	Sanghvi
Victor	Hoang	Laura	Schiraldi
Ekaterina	Hossny	Brett	Schupack
Qiuying	Huang	Renata	Segal
Sebastian	Jofre	Christopher	Shackles
Joslyn	Joseph	Araj	Sidki
Mary	Joseph	Karolina	Siniakowicz
Karen	Justiniano	Benyamin	Steinman
Bethlehem	Kassaye	Venus	Steinman
Milena	Kaufman	Nathaniel	Strock
Marina	Kishlyansky	Kseniya	Svyatets
Susan	Ko	Kenneth	Swanson
Bina	Kviatkovsky	Kari	Tabag
Margaret	Kwan	Brian	Temple
Daniel	Lefkowitz	Katherine	Triplett
Jean-Paul	Leva	Katherine	Williams
Yifan	Li	Marta	Wronska
Dana	Libov	Clover	Youn
Aldo	Manresa	James	Yu
Cassandre	Marseille	Sina	Zomorrodian

The Cause of Autism

- Concepts and Misconceptions -

Chapter 5: Nutrition

Chapter 6: Maternal infection; neurogenic disorders

Chapter 7: Inoculation

Chapter 8: Genetics; redox

Chapter 9: Therapy

PROLOGUE

Correlation versus *Causation*

"My first-born child, Mikey, was fine during his first 18 months of infancy. He was growing normally and was cheerful within a loving, attentive home environment. Mikey played nicely with his toys and liked to share them with playmates. However, nearing his second birthday, we began to notice that he was not developing socially similar to other children his age. He now tended to avoid interaction with other children and seemed to prefer playing by himself. Mikey would spend hours arranging his blocks in a row, disassembling them, and then repeating the same action over and over again. We expected him to be speaking single words and two-word phrases by this time, but he only babbled incoherently without answering us when we called him by name. He acted as though we were not in the same room with him.

When our pediatrician was approached about this situation, he suggested that our son should be evaluated by a neuropsychologist. I told the specialist that I had no medical difficulties before or during my pregnancy with Mikey. None of the children in our extended families had problems comparable to what we were witnessing with our son. We lived in a comfortable, middle-class neighborhood. Mikey weighed 7 pounds at his 40-week birth and cried soon after delivery, following an 8-hour, uncomplicated labor. My husband and I were both 28 years old at the time of Mikey's birth.

After a detailed evaluation, the doctor concluded that our son was autistic."
Signed, Anonymous

Definition of autism

Autism is a highly variable neurodevelopmental disorder marked by deficiencies in social interaction, communication, outside interests, and behavior. The general term of Autism Spectrum Disorder (ASD) includes classical autism, Asperger syndrome, and pervasive development disorder (PDD - not otherwise specified). Asperger syndrome is a high-functioning form of ASD with no derangement in communication. The designation of PDD is applied when all the criteria for Asperger and/or autism are not met. These problems typically become apparent in early childhood between 6 months and 3 years of age. Since the general definition and characterization of autism by the American psychiatrist, Leo Kanner, as a unique psychopathologic entity appeared in the early 1940s, little attention was paid to it by the general public until the last 15-20 years. It is now an increasingly common subject of medical research.

This book represents a comprehensive endeavor to examine the multiple etiologies that have been proposed to explain the cause of autism. Some confusion has arisen in defining exactly what are the specific criteria to be applied in diagnosing this disorder, to distinguish it from other neuropathologic conditions (chapter 1D). In recent years, the issue of autism has reached major levels of concern and attention among scientific and general audiences.

Although much research effort and substantial funding amounts have been devoted to uncovering the cause of autism, little is currently known with certainty about its etiology(ies). Much like other unsolved medical mysteries, autism is believed to result from an environmental trigger interacting with a genetic propensity. As a result of the public alarm that has justifiably developed, numerous hypotheses have been generated without sufficient research evidence to identify the main pathologic process(es) causing autism. No one explanation has sufficient supporting data to claim a clear, comprehensive cause-and-effect relationship. Unfortunately, quite a few of these unverified proposals have persisted for various reasons (chapter 1A).

Some of these proposals, such as a purported link with vaccination, are still believed to be valid by the general public, in spite of numerous studies negating or refuting them. A major source of this confusion has resulted from the tendency of the popular press to overemphasize the meaning of "breakthrough" scientific discoveries, many of which are repetitions of previously discarded or discredited claims. The public is often uncertain and ill-informed about what issues are well-founded and deserve additional attention and credible support (chapter 2B). Hence, the primary goal of this book is to separate fact from fiction for ultimately elucidating the true etiology(ies) of autism. In this process, unsubstantiated therapies will be questioned.

Contemporary view of the genesis of autism:
GENETIC PROPENSITY + ENVIRONMENTAL TRIGGER →AUTISM

GENETICS = genomic proclivity to be translated into
neuropathologic characteristics mediated by
appropriate promoters (triggers).

TRIGGERS = heavy metals, oxidative stress, viruses, hypoxia,
pesticides, inflammation.

- *IN OTHER WORDS* -

To develop autism, a fetus/infant would typically:
1) possess a specific genetic modification, and
2) be exposed to one or more environmental triggers.

The authors of this book have 3 main objectives:
1) to describe the key hypotheses and observations put forward;
2) to analyze pertinence and credibilty in each case; and
3) to distinguish between correlations and cause-and-effect associations.

Confusion often results if a distinction is not clearly made between correlation and causation. For example: *It has been proven by repeated experimentation that if during an eclipse you beat on drums, the eclipse always goes away*! Coincidence or association does not necessarily imply causation. In analyzing and relating the possible claim of a cause-and-effect relationship of research data, it is important to question such terms as "appears to be", "implicated in", "associated with", "linked to", and "suggesting." This conveys as much meaningful information as "etc., etc." at the end of a series of items. The weakest of all such mental exercises is unsubstantiated intuition. This is especially risky if an emotional overtone is subjectively implanted in the analysis of research findings.

If a particular phenomenon is coincident in time with or preceding a distinct outcome, it cannot necessarily be implied *a priori* that one event causes the other. Uncorroborated claims advanced before a specific outcome is realized are similarly suspect. Coincident effects should not always be taken as representing a common cause. Correlation and causation may be associated characteristics, but may not necessarily be related functionally in every instance. As a result, caution must be used in claiming the specific etiology of a complex medical condition such as autism. As the title of this book connotes, finding the fundamental cause of autism is a major undertaking of medical research which has resulted in new findings as well as deadends, but may not have reached its ultimate goal of cure or prevention as yet.

Cause-and-effect

In 1883, Robert Koch proposed three essential requirements to define the basis of particular infections. In light of modern medical advances and the specific factors characteristic of autism, these postulates can now be broadened and modified for the issue at hand in this book as follows:

1. The suspected causal factors must be constantly associated with the disease.
2. The suspected causal dysfunction must be identified within an affected individual.
3. When a susceptible host is genetically modified appropriately (e.g., silencing of a specific gene), the same symptoms of the spontaneous disease must develop in the test case as when occurring naturally.

Especially with the third postulate, a differentiation would be made between a simple coexistence and a definitive causation. For example, in chapter 7A it is emphasized that rigorous studies have failed to identify a cause-and-effect relationship between autism and vaccination. The numerous studies which followed the original claim of an association between the two have convincingly eliminated causation in this argument. On the other hand, the appearance of autism-like behavior in mice bred to have specific genes deleted or inactivated tends to satisfy this postulate (chapters 6C,8A). If elevated levels of an environmental toxin (e.g., mercury, lead) are often found in individuals with neurologic dysfunctions, it does not necessarily follow that autism would automatically be included within this group of affected subjects (chapters 4A,4B,5D).

A variation of these criteria would be an ailment marked by the deficiency of a key metabolite or hormone. If the condition is ameliorated by replacement or augmentation of the inadequate factor, the satisfaction of Koch's causation requirements would be met. If a deficiency of this factor can be determined at birth, it could also serve as a prospective biomarker to anticipate the subsequent development of autism. If this, in fact, is the central etiologic key to autism, replacement in the deficient neonate could reduce or eliminate the pathologic processes otherwise leading to the overt disease. By design, this explanation is simplistic since it ignores heterogeneity, multifactoriality, and potential unrelatedness between affected autistic patients. The final resolution of this enigma and design of an effective therapeutic approach will have to take into account idiosyncratic variations among individuals as well.

If particular areas of the brain are known to direct certain peripheral actions and such areas are typically identified as affected in autism, an operational relationship can be proposed (chapters 3B-3D).

It was recently reported that mothers of autistic children exhibit anti-brain antibodies four times as often as randomly selected mothers (10.5 versus 2.6%) (1). It was concluded from these data that autoimmunity is correlated with the genesis of autism. In only 10% (and not 100%) of the cases, the two "correlates" appeared together. At this stage of research, it is unfounded to speculate that maternal autoimmunity is the cause of autism. Rather, it may well be that the two phenomena (maternal autoimmunity and infantile autism) originate together in only some cases as a consequence of a third, independent causative factor, yet to be determined.

Environmental variability

Careful selection of experimental conditions is necessary to isolate one issue from many concurrent ones in order to identify causation. This is one of the reasons why identical (monozygotic) twins who live together are often recruited for medical research studies (chapter 1C,8A). In contradistinction, with a study of a large heterogeneous population living under different social or ecological conditions, it is more difficult to identify a potential, unique cause if extraneous factors, such as diet or weather, may play a controlling or modifying role as well.

As underscored in chapter 1C, the occurrence of autism is believed to be determined by both genetic and environmental conditions. Apparent geographic and sociologic variations of occurrence of autism spectrum disorder (ASD) have been identified (chapter 1B). If the intrauterine environment with monozygotic twin gestations has some inequalities (such as local variability in intrauterine conditions during gestation), the chance of exhibiting autistic behavior may not be the same for both babies. This might account for why autism does not occur in both members of all such sets 100% of the time, whether monozygotic or dizygotic (chapter 8A). As an example, one study considered the fingerprints of normal monozygotic quadruplets (2). These physical characteristics are primarily established by the pattern of fingertip volar pads genetically determined and expressed by the eighteenth week of fetal life. However, local intrauterine environmental variations might modify the resultant prints of each. This agrees with the generalization that no two people have the same set of fingerprints.

A second publication reports on discordant anomalies in monochorionic twins (3). The structural/functional errors in one of the two fetuses in each set affect the central nervous, cardiovascular, and genitourinary systems in particular. This would suggest a non-genetic etiologic departure from the norm in the environment of one twin as distinct from the other.

Autism concordance in twin sets was found in one study to be 31% for dizygotic and 88% for monozygotic twins (4). This twin survey supported the contention that the etiology of autism has a genetic component. Concurrent medical conditions, such as Fragile X Syndrome and tuberous sclerosis, are typically found in only 10% or less of ASD cases, whereas a combination of environmental and genetic factors is believed to be the basis of classical autism (5).

Among many modified associated genes which could be cited here as examples, *Engrailed 2* and *Serotonin Transporter Engrailed 2*, which encode for a protein affecting development of the cerebellum, are often (but not always) found coexistent with autism (6). It is proposed that the common forms of ASD are the result of multiple malformed genes (7). The variability found between individual cases of autism may be due to a panoply of effecting genes or an assortment of environmental modifiers. However, no single version of such genetic abnormalities has been found in most or all cases of autism.

Application of findings

Raising an autistic child represents a major social, emotional, and financial stress on the parents and other siblings in the home (chapters 2A-2C). Many approaches have been attempted to rehabilitate the affected child. A number involve medical and psychological therapies of limited value (chapters 3I,4A,8B). Others concentrate on skills which the child may use to make some positive contributions to his life and the atmosphere in the family home (chapters 2A-2C). Because of the neurologic infirmity characteristic of this disease, the prospect of reversal of nerve tissue damage is minimal with the present state of knowledge (chapter 6A), although recent discoveries with stem cell therapy may hold out hope of some functional improvement in the future (chapter 9B).

In this fashion, credible and unfounded beliefs that have arisen will be identified, without absolute partiality given to any particular one. In addition, the benefits from the broad, up-to-date examination of the field, rather than an investigation concentrating on just one or a few aspects, makes this book informative for the general public and practitioner. The responsibility of the scientist/physician to honestly uncover the true cause of conditions such as autism is clear (chapters 1A,2B). What is still uncertain is if the reason for the recent apparent statisical rise in cases of autism is due to changing diagnostic criteria (chapter 1D), analytical acumen (chapter 1C), true clinical rise in the incidence of the disease, monetary investment in expanded surveillance (chapter 1B), or a combination of reasons .

Overall objectives and conclusions

Since the year 2000, the number of research reports published annually in the scientific literature dealing with this subject has quadrupled. Although autism has also received a great deal of attention recently in the popular press and is currently the subject of many advanced research projects throughout the world, little is known about the etiology of this condition. As noted above, many hypotheses have been proposed to explain what factors or agents may induce this problem; none has led to the gathering of sufficient supporting data to claim convincing insight into the cause. Some of the hypotheses reviewed in this book have been disproven or abandoned because of unsupportive research or abandoned findings, but are included here for completeness and historical significance. It is generally believed that autism arises because of a genetic predisposition, coupled with an environmental trigger (Conclusions and Prospectus).

Maternal exposure to certain pharmaceuticals and environmental (industrial) pollutants during pregnancy has been correlated with the appearance of autistic behavior in the offspring (chapters 4A-4F). Whether this represents a cause-and-effect relationship or merely an interesting coincidence is uncertain. However, the rate of autism diagnosis continues to rise, in spite of efforts to avoid these teratogenic agents, such as valproic acid, during gestation.

Research into cause and treatment of any medical condition is regulated by ethical standards (chapter 1A). For example, if a new antibiotic were known to also increase the possibility of an infant developing autism, it would be unacceptable to do a double-blind prospective microbiological study without the parents being advised of this potential disadvantage. On the other hand, if the antibiotic were also known to diminish the chance of autism, such a study could prove beneficial in treating infections as well.

It is not an objective of this book to review and critique all of the various treatment modalities that have been instituted to "cure" or ameliorate the manifestations of autism in affected children. Autism is currently incurable, in contrast to recent claims in the media to the contrary. Many "therapists" have made assertions that the techniques they use (e.g., chelation for heavy metal removal) diminish the signs and symptoms of the disease. However, there is little concrete, objective evidence that the aberrant neurologic processes evoking autistic behavior in particular are modified by such methods (e.g., lead chelation – chapter 4B). On the other hand, rehabilitation and remediation of behavioral traits have their place in enhancing the quality of life of autistic children and adults. Although difficult to implement, certain modalities, such as speech and occupational therapy, have aided affected children to more constructively and productively integrate into general society (chapters 2A-2C).

Several correlations will be described in this book, showing associated co-morbidities which may or may not be the result of a common etiologic process also inducing autistic behavior in the same individuals. Ascertaining cause with high probability is difficult, especially in neuropsychiatric conditions. Therefore, with a thorough search of the pertinent scientific literature, a list of the key subjects dealing with the cause of autism was assembled. Each subject considers the physiologic/anatomic changes which distinguish autism from normal neurologic functions (chapters 3B-3F), or discussed the underlying mechanisms which are believed to promote these abnormalities (chapters 3G,3H,4A-4F,6A-6D,8C).

The Table of Contents of this book lists most, but not all, of the subjects that have been considered in this regard. Many are based on recent scientific discoveries which have been explored specifically for their possible application in the autism search:

1) Changing DSM definitions.

2) Genetic mutations.

3) Psychologic/familial environmental dynamics.

4) Brain pathology – both communications within the brain and neural connections to various parts of the body.

5) Neural dysfunction and dysmyelination.

6) Heavy metal toxicity (e.g., mercury, lead).

7) Teratogenic drugs.

8) Pesticides and environmental pollutants.

9) Perinatal hypoxia.

10) Oxidative stress.

11) Hyperglycemia/obesity.

12) Viral infection.

13) Insulin-like growth factor.

14) Vaccination.

Although claims now appear in the research literature that significant advances have been achieved recently in understanding and treating autism, in reality not much meaningful progress in comprehending the actual cause of this disorder has been made in the last two decades. One of the big problems with autism research is that most hypotheses have reached a dead end or are stuck for lack of positive proof. As a result, no means for reducing or preventing the malady in the first place have emerged. However, in the frustration researchers have felt, the same ideas keep being resurrected in the literature, thereby hindering progress forward. On the other hand, it is hoped that medical student-authors bring forth fresh, new ideas and insight which help make this book an innovation in the field. For the reader, a careful study and comprehension of the information conveyed in this book will give an overview of the topics central to an appreciation of the complexity of this field.

It is generally believed that, given enough time and money, ANY medical enigma can be resolved expeditiously. On average, there are about 125 new cases of autism identified in the US daily (8). Currently, the estimated total annual cost of caring for autistic children and adults in the United States amounts to $126 billion, largely covered by custodial family members themselves. In 1997, at the request of Congress, the National Institutes of Health created its Autism Coordinating Committee (NIH/ACC). The purpose of this effort was to increase the funding and stimulation of research to elucidate the cause of autism. In 2007/2008, NIH established funding for 11 Autism Centers of Excellence throughout the country to study autism-associated biomarkers and related genes, as well as environmental risk factors. Since the initiation of that effort, little has been reported by researchers which would give a well-founded, comprehensive insight into the etiology, treatment, and/or cure of the disease.

The general public understands that since researchers are only human, most are well-intentioned but suffer from the same emotional and sociologic limitations as any person. In particular, they are slow to abandon commonly accepted, but inadequately proven, concepts. On the other hand, new viewpoints face a wall of rejection until the older, unproductive approaches are discarded for lack of success. A classic case is that of Gregor Mendel, a quiet Augustinian friar who uncovered in the early 19th century the basic laws of modern day genetics. He had a great deal of difficulty getting his findings published in an obscure scientific journal because it contradicted the accepted dogma of the day. It was not until 50 years after his death that his proposals were acknowledged as being the true basis of genetics.

Many of the proposals discussed in the chapters of this book have turned out to be unfounded. A prime example of this is the refutation of the proposed link between vaccination and autism. As noted in a front page article in the *Wall Street Journal*, dated July 21, 2013, a scientifically refuted proposal that related autism to MMR (mumps, measles, rubella) vaccination is still affecting children adversely today (chapter 7A). In particular, the rate of measles is rising rapidly 15 years after the publication of this derelict report which induced parents to avoid vaccinating their children. Perhaps the most surprising realization is that some parents still believe that vaccination and autism are causally related. This is not to say that all disproven hypotheses are potentially harmful, but it does attest to the inertia of removing such ideas from the public psyche to make room for better propositions.

Most chapters in this book are organized around:

HYPOTHESIS (Introduction) – OBSERVATIONS – CONCLUSIONS.

In the Conclusions section in particular, proposed etiologies of autism are scrutinzed. The purpose of this final review is to determine the apparent value and applicability of the various hypotheses enumerated in that chapter. This allows for a succinct comparison of the relative importance of each such idea in promoting the general goal of solving the autism enigma. To aid the reader in locating related discussions in other parts of this book, notations of "**chapter xx**" are added to the text.

For the most part, discussions of the various treatments of patients already diagnosed with autism have been avoided here. On the other hand, each of the chapters in this book reviews one or more of the proposed etiologies of autism and ends with a Conclusion section. The purpose of that analysis is to determine the possible value of the hypothesis reviewed in that chapter. This allows for a succinct comparison of relative importance of each such idea in promoting the general goal of uncovering the cause of autism.

Emphasis has been given in distinguishing causation from correlation in the reported observations related to elucidating the origin of autism with each hypothesis. To comprehend the cause of autism and thus be able to foretell its subsequent appearance in the child, it would be necessary to determine the presence of unique biomarkers as predictive signs of the disorder before symptoms can be detected overtly. Such a thorough prospective study of many children remains to be carried out with any of the proposed etiologies of autism discussed here before or soon after birth to potentially arrest the development or progression of the disease.

"Grant me the strength, time and opportunity always to correct what I have acquired, always to extend its domain; for knowledge is immense and the spirit of man can extend indefinitely to enrich itself daily with new requirements. Today he can discover his errors of yesterday and tomorrow he can obtain a new light on what he thinks himself sure of today."

Oath of Maimonides (1135-1204)

Literary/medical education innovation

Nearly all of the chapters in this book were researched and analyzed by current medical students of Touro College of Osteopathic Medicine in New York City. When the idea for this book was first conceived by the editors, an announcement was sent to all students to survey their interest in any of the key subjects related to the etiology of autism. Those attracted to this undertaking followed up with a formal proposal. Approximately 85 students were finally selected for participation in this literary project (see list of Contributors), which apparently has never been attempted to this extent in any medical school before.

Under the supervision and direction of senior faculty/editors, draft chapters were written and refined. The students were given orientation in evaluating the scientific merit of research publications and approaches to be taken in evolving a meaningful presentation.

The student-authors applied principles and knowledge learned in the classroom and at the bedside in a scholarly presentation of relevant issues and consequences in this subject. This promoted the expression of fresh, new ideas and insights in this important subject as well. Special attention was given to landmark discoveries, clarity practicable for the general as well as professional reader, avoidance of unsubstatiated claims, statistically supported conclusions, and integration of chapters to uniformly convey the message of the book. Examples of the pre-medical school backgrounds of some of these student-authors are:

"... worked as a CPA ... business operations consulting."

"... duties included resolving practice management issues..."

"... training the new lab members."

"... Project Coordinator... Autism Birth Cohort study (NIH/NINDs funded)"

"... science research ... nine scientific publications."

"... Research Technician ... Integrative Cancers Research at MIT."

"... worked on and became published with ... inheritable mutation causing leukemia."

"... Scientific Program Analyst – National Human Genome Research Institute, NIH."

"... trained Special Olympic athletes ... majority were autistic."

"... research in pursuit of treatments for HIV-1 ..."

"...identifying molecular factors involved in physiological and pathological angiogenesis."

"... investigated the metabolic demands of cancer cells ..."

"... behavioral therapist, specializing in autism."

Disclaimer

In no way is this book intended to function as an exhaustive, detailed medical reference or primary source. Before making medical decisions, the reader must consult with knowledgeable experts and authoritative sources for more complete, targeted explanations and advice as needed. This text is designed to provide an overview of relevant, solid information on the subject matter covered. The editors, authors, and publisher do not intend for this book to serve as a sole, primary source of advice for making independent medical decisions to institute or discontinue any mode of related therapy.

Since the intended emphasis of the book is a search for the etiology of autism, treatment modalities of already affected children are largely not discussed here.

The chapters of this book were carefully reviewed and modified, as needed, by the four editors for scientific accuracy and clarity, although no guarantee can be given that no unintended errors in the text have persisted. Every effort has been devoted to making this book as thorough, objective, concise, reliable, and up-to-date as possible. Errors related to typographical and technical matters may have entered the manuscript unintentionally. Since medical science can be expected to advance subsequent to the publication of this book, the most current findings and opinions should be obtained from appropriate professionals and reputable scientific journals firsthand. This educational text should only be used as a general guide and not as an ultimate source for making personal medical decisions. No portion of this book may be copied or reproduced without the written permission of the Editor-in-Chief or the publisher.

Therefore, the authors, consultants, editors, and publisher of this book shall have neither liability nor responsibility to any person or entity with respect to any loss or damage caused, or alleged to be caused, directly or indirectly, by the information contained in this book. It is not the intention of the publisher, editors, or authors of this book to advocate for or against any particular therapeutic approach to dealing with autism. It is more appropriate for parents of plausibly or actually affected children to seek out the advice of recognized experts and medical specialists for this purpose who refrain from making unrealistic or baseless promises of cure. Care must be taken to consider critically questionable therapeutic approaches or exaggerated claims of potential cure or improvement unfounded on credible scientific proofs and observations. The intensive emotional strain experienced by such loving, concerned, well-intentioned parents must be counterbalanced by rational review and evaluation.

INTRODUCTION;BACKGROUND

Chapter 1A - Scientific Credibility

Margaret Kwan

[The dissemination of scientific findings can be hampered by human nature which sometimes obstructs progress through overemphasis of weakly based findings, compromised standards, altered findings, and unnecessary repetition of previously dispelled hypotheses – Ed.]

Hypothesis

In an age where scientific information is very accessible, the public finds itself inundated with all the current science trends. The question is, how do researchers and scientists decide what should be publicized as truth? Additionally, how should someone in the general public, who has little or no technical background, evaluate scientific research and the claims that are being made? To echo the French philosopher Voltaire, with great knowledge comes great power, and, in turn, even greater responsibility.

This introductory chapter of the book will look critically at how researchers conduct their projects, conclude, and publish the results of their studies. Furthermore, it will be questioned how the popular press reports these findings for public consumperion, with their accompanying claims as though the results are new, novel, and superior to prior studies. Of greatest importance to the message of this book is the distinction between what findings are descriptions of bio-phenomena which, by chance or by common etiology, coexist with autism, in contradistinction to well-elucidated causative factors.

Topics to be discussed here include biostatistics that go into scientific study validation, what organizations fund research projects and why, and what modes of research are being used. This is with the objective of analyzing our current models of and approaches to basic research, and whether or not these models produce valid results and substantiated claims:

1) Media influences of public opinion;
2) Funding;
3) Research methods;
5) Comprehension of research reports;
6) Believable solutions for the scientific layman;
7) Improvement of the overall health of the general population; and
8) Publication credibility, validity, and originality.

Observations

The Scientific Approach is heralded as being purely objective and infallible. The power to identify facts based on unbiased data and the nature of being purely objective and evidence-based give the Scientific Approach credibility. These qualities, however, are dependent on the person who is conducting the study. The qualities that give the Scientific Approach credibility are also the same qualities that render the public vulnerable to potential harm when a study publishes false information since patient healthcare protocols are based on published research. A study tainted by bias, financial motives, media over-exaggeration, or fabricated evidence does not have the best interest of the public. The Wakefield autism study is an example of how even one publication can adversely affect people's healthcare decisions (chapter 7A). By publicizing erroneous information using manipulated data, one doctor seem to have prioritized his own prestige over the well-being of the general public.

American society today is largely conditioned to expect instant knowledge in rapid broadcasts of information. Medical problems brought to the attention of the public by the media require answers within a short timeframe—months, weeks, or even minutes. This creates incredible pressure on scientists to provide, at the least, explanations for the medical problem of interest. Scientific research, however, is usually a lengthy process that involves data collection, experimentation, and much trial-and-error. The route to collect the needed materials/subjects and to execute an appropriate experiment can take months, even years. Then, once the results and data have been assembled, additional time must be spent drafting the results of the experiment into a research article which then must be submitted and approved for publication by scientific journals using a peer review procedure. Recent development of online publishing has expedited this phase somewhat, but it has also exacerbated public demand for immediate scientific discovery. While instant media coverage of scientific discoveries in the making is an important part in keeping the general public informed, once a study that is not supported by sufficient data has been publicized, the idea is difficult to redact. Years after the Wakefield study was discredited, scientists and physicians still meet parental resistance to child vaccinations—an issue that has tragically resulted in outbreaks of measles and pertussis, potentially deadly diseases that could have been prevented (1).

The success of media professionals, however, is largely contingent on which organization can broadcast the newest, and often most shocking, trends. Consequently, the media has no time to wait for researchers to examine a claim thoroughly enough to meet the standards of the scientific community. Media will, therefore, often seize on a scientific claim in its early, preliminary stages of investigation: observation. The scientific method starts with observation, from which a general hypothesis is made about a phenomenon and its plausible causation. There are many stringent criteria that a research study must achieve in order to become accepted knowledge by the scientific community. The time and effort needed to adequately investigate a scientific claim can take years to complete, yet the general public and media may be completely unaware of the length of time many research studies require in order to be thorough and definitive.

Hypothesis formulation is often aided by meta-analyses of several similar reported studies on the subject in question. For example, if drinking coffee is proposed to increase a medical student's grades, studies of coffee consumed versus percentage scored on medical school exams will be plotted against each other, and a correlation coefficient will be calculated.

Depending on how strong the correlation is, a researcher can decide to pursue the relationship further. In the age of technology, these data are easy to access and the potential to propose plausible correlations is limitless. Due to the need for constant material to construct headlines, the media will often pick up the latest trend in scientific propositions at this point.

The problem with premature publication of scientific hypotheses or early findings, however, is they are only preliminary ideas and not thoroughly investigated proof of causation. The correlation observed may be strongly indicative of causality. Premature conclusion of true causation, however, is precarious because there is always the possibility that the observed association is mere coincidence. For example, an observation is made that students who scored in the top third of their medical school class also had the highest granola bar consumption rate. A hypothesis can then be proposed that the ingredients in the bars contribute to a student's success in medical school. There may indeed be a positive relationship between the numbers of granola bars consumed versus medical school class rank, but the correlation could be due to a multitude of factors. To name a few, granola bars do not require cooking time so a student can spend more time studying instead of cooking, or perhaps the vending machines outside of the school library only sell granola bars. Ultimately, the correlation between granola bars and class rank may be apparent, but one cannot infer that eating granola bars will lead to success in medical school. A research study would have to demonstrate that eating oats causes higher brain functioning by using a scientific method to quantify a change in brain functioning, such as brain imaging or an increase in biochemical brain enzyme usage. Not only must this mechanism be proven at a molecular level, the data must be reproducible, in order to prove that the data were not acquired by luck. Publicizing this claim without sufficient evidence may lead to readers erroneously believing that they should consume more granola bars to be academically successful, which can be high in sugar and detrimental to one's health if consumed in excess. Until the mechanism of an observed scientific phenomenon has been undisputedly proven, by conducting a prospective study in which the effects of other possible variables are neutralized, causation cannot be confirmed.

Broadcasting scientific claims that have not been validated is dangerous. Many people take these tenuous claims seriously and will alter their lifestyles to include or exclude the topic of the study. This is risky because if an item is vilified, people may exclude the object from their lives even if it is necessary to maintain health such as a vaccine or carbohydrates from their diet. On the other hand, if an object is hailed as a miracle remedy, people will go to extraordinary lengths to include the item in their lives even if it is in an excess that is detrimental to one's health, such as vitamins or herbal supplements. Most of the public, however, does not have the education or experience to recognize that these actions based on unsubstantiated, weak health claims are potentially harmful. Experts in the field should be aware that collaborating with media to publicize health claims may produce severe repercussions when people start following such advice in excess. Thus, scientists and healthcare providers must actively warn the general public on potential dangers of unsupported health claims.

Fabricated evidence is a consequence of how research via the scientific method can be disseminated. There is tremendous pressure on the researchers to achieve results that support the tested hypothesis. Such emphasis has, in part, been responsible for the recent rise in unacceptable plagiarism and the increase in retracted publications (2). According to the World Association of Medical Editors, literary plagiarism is defined as the copy of 6 words or more in order, without proper referencing (3). Computer programs are now available to screen whole books, such as this one, in a matter of minutes by comparing the text to a large population of previously published books and manuscripts.

Supporting parties have little interest in funding studies that yield inconclusive results; they want to ensure that whatever they underwrite leads to a favorable return for their investment. In this context, a scientific investment is favorable if the research results support the initial hypothesis that the funding organization anticipates.

It is now common practice to specify from the start what areas of interest Government and private funding agencies want to be considered, in contradistinction to pathfinding new approaches which may or may not lead to positive results. Such a *modus operandi* discourages new thinking in old problems, like autism. This dichotomy may present a biased conflict of interest in the way research subjects are selected. Goal-specific funding can influence *a priori* what specific topics are approved for scientific investigation. As a consequence, new insights may be delayed. For example, a coffee company pays a research team to investigate whether drinking coffee leads to getting accepted into medical school. There is a strong motive to support that hypothesis because the company can use the results as a marketing claim. If the media hints that drinking coffee is a common theme amongst people who get accepted into medical school—a lucrative career requiring intelligence and hard work—the public can be convinced that buying coffee will lead to success. Thus, news media are often utilized at this time during ongoing research to publicize a new common headline: "Early studies show possible link." Financial and publicity motives can pressure research teams to find any evidence supporting these claims. If, however, the evidence does not corroborate the claim that drinking coffee leads to personal success, the coffee company has no incentive to publicize these data; it could negatively impact the sales of coffee. In this way, many research studies that cannot support a claim are overshadowed by other studies that can provide "conclusive" scientific reports. What remains of the inconclusive studies are unsubstantiated claims that have been circulated within the public. Furthermore, the pressure to prove a scientific claim may compel researchers to unethically distort data to "prove" that a hypothesis is substantiated.

Financial motives play a major part in furthering claims yet to be supported by scientific research, whether creating a market for a drug, vilifying a vaccine competitor, or enticing citizens to follow your news channel. Ultimately, research projects must be supported somehow, because there is not enough funding from unbiased organizations to cover the majority of the innovative scientific research proposed today. For example, the US National Institutes of Health approves less than 10% of the common fund grant applications submitted via the RPG/Direct source (4). Thus, vulnerable research institutions must accept grants from organizations that may have clear conflicts of interests concerning the objectivity of a study. In essence, the fund manager becomes the unspoken supervisor of the researchers, who in turn are contracted to find evidence supporting the manager's theory. This schema offers an explanation for the apparent lack of data refuting publicized health claims. If the data collected by the researchers do not complement the sponsor's agenda, the donor (such as pharmaceutical firms) can determine whether or not the results are acceptable. Even more alarming is the possibility that the data could be manipulated by the researchers in order to appease investors and gain a publication.

Ideally, funding for financially unbiased research should be readily available from impartial organizations. The reality of scientific research in general, however, is that funding from impartial organizations is limited; many research groups accept funding from any organization that offers money to cover salaries and expenses.

To protect against unethical biases in research, there are guidelines in place that require researchers to disclose the source of funding and any conflicts of interest associated with it. There is, however, little regulation that monitors how often researchers reveal their funding sources; it is at the researcher's sole discretion to disclose any potential conflict of interest. However, public health claims have the power to influence consumer activity. Thus, not only should researchers take it upon themselves to self-police what they publish, but they should also maintain a high standard of integrity in their studies. Data withheld or tailored to fit the financial gains of an organization can distort the truth, lead to erroneous health advice, and ultimately harm people.

For readers who do not have the learning or training required to be an expert on a subject, there are several steps that should be taken to evaluate a scientific study. One simple way to assess a study is to look at the sample size, which is usually denoted by the letter "n" and is reported in the conclusion section of a research article. Whether or not the sample size was appropriate, based on the known population, is a good method to evaluate if the study is relevant. A study size that only comprises <1% of a population being studied could be an inaccurate representation, because inferring data from such a small sample size could lead to many errors. The test group is just not large enough to be an accurate representation of the population in question. The number of test subjects needed to be relevant, however, can vary greatly depending on ther overall examined population. For example, if a study wants to assess the amount of satisfaction in Americans who own spider monkeys as pets, the sample size might be n = 5, which is a small number. If, however, only 10 Americans in the United States own spider monkeys, then 5 would be illustrative of 50% the total population - rendering n = 5 as a fairly representative sampling. The validity of a research study's sample size requires knowledge of the population being studied. Therefore, this information should be sought out by the researchers, media personnel, or readers and evaluated against the current study.

Additionally, there are two values provided in every research publication that can further aid readers in assessing a scientific study: Power or Probability (P), and Confidence Interval (CI). Power is a statistical representation of how likely the study's data were acquired by coincidence, given the sample size studied; the lower the P value, the better. In general, a study is considered valid only if the P value is less than 0.05, which means there is less than a 5% chance the data are a result of coincidence. The Confidence Interval is a statistical measure of how relevant the results are to the general population. Most research studies do not accept a CI value of less than 95%; if the researchers did a random sample of a group of people, 95% of the people studied would fall within a certain numeric interval. For example, if a study published that an average American medical student drinks 3 cups of coffee a day with a 95% CI of 1-5 cups, meaning that the researchers conducting the study are 95% confident that medical students, as a whole, drink between 1-5 cups of coffee a day. Consequently, a study that reports a 95% CI interval of 1-5 cups of coffee will have a different implication than a study that reports researchers are 95% confident medical students drink between 1-100 cups of coffee per day; the larger the interval the more vague the results. Therefore, by assessing the size of the CI interval, the reader can gain a sense of how specific a study's results are. The P and CI values of any study are valuable numbers to know when gauging the validity of a research study. Any study that does not fall within the parameters of conventionally accepted P and CI values should be questioned in terms of relevance to the general population.

Readers should also note the date of the research study. Research data are now collected at an incredible rate, which means that our knowledge of scientific concepts is being revised constantly. Until causation has been undeniably proven, an outdated study may support an incorrect hypothesis. Therefore, when a journalist cites research studies for publications, he/she could potentially find an older study that will support even an erroneous claim. Older references may contain outdated knowledge, especially if more current studies were conducted on the topic. Other studies may be too expensive to conduct on a yearly basis and are thus current even if the information was collected more than a decade ago. Thus, validity based on date is a subjective value. If the subject in question is not a widely accepted scientific fact, readers should always check if the references used are current. While many components are important in evaluating a research article, reviewing the sample size, confidence interval, and date can give readers the ability to quickly evaluate the integrity of a research study. The validity of a study should be assessed by readers every time in order to protect themselves against misleading scientific claims.

Ultimately, researchers should maintain the highest standards of ethics when conducting and publishing their studies, because anything less has the potential to seriously harm people. In Alabama in 1932, an experiment was launched by the Public Health Service to study the effects of untreated syphilis (5). The study, titled the "Tuskegee Study of Untreated Syphilis in the Negro Male," recruited African-American males as the test subjects, in exchange for free food and medical care. The researchers hoped to solidify their knowledge of how syphilis ravages the body, which could yield clinically useful information about how to diagnose and treat this debilitating disease. Perhaps this would be justifiable because syphilis first manifests as relatively painless genital sores; if left untreated, it will eventually cripple the afflicted individual with paralysis, extremely painful skin lesions, and death. The men involved in the study, however, were never informed that they would be withheld treatment even if it proved to be effective at treating syphilis. Easily transferred, the disease spread quickly from the men in the Tuskegee control group to their wives and family, many of whom died painful deaths.

In theory, the Tuskegee study aimed to protect future patients from the crippling effects of syphilis by studying its natural disease course. In practice, however, the investigation harmed the participants who did not receive treatment. When human lives become involved in scientific research, it is ethically wrong to withhold treatment and to conceal portions of the features of the experiment. Ultimately, the study was identified as immoral because the participants and some of the participants' families suffered from a disease that could have been treated.

Scientific research has the potential to uncover the cause of disease, manufacture a cure, and heal people. On the other hand, great harm can be done in the name of science, such as with the Tuskegee Syphilis Study. Of more recent concern was the experimentation on Jewish prisoners of Nazi concentration camps without prior consent during World War II. Studies by the Nazis included investigating infectious disease immunization, antibiotic trials, and the physiology behind twins, to name a few. When the Nazis conducted their experiments, however, the methods they used were appalling. They inoculated prisoners without agreement or explanation with infectious organisms, such as tuberculosis, in order to study the prevention and treatment of these diseases. They tested the efficacy of sulfa drugs on prisoners that were mutilated by the experimenters, with the goal of giving the test subjects gangrene. They also experimented on pairs of twins: recruited children had their limbs amputated, or given lethal injections in order to dissect and study them (6). Although they sought to discover answers to pressing scientific questions, the experiments performed by the Nazi doctors were cruel, causing mutilation, excruciating pain, and death to the prisoners that were used. As a result, in 1974, the United States implemented Title 45 Code of Regulations Part 46 which stipulated that research on humans requires fully informed, safe, and voluntary participation by prospective test subjects before the initiation of the study. In addition, the question remains if such results should be subsequently applied after the War if they had potential value and cannot be derived by alternative, more benign means.

Today, there are strict guidelines that must be followed by researchers in order to conduct a study, especially when the study involves humans. These guidelines state that participants must be fully informed of, and consent to, the entire nature of the study and if there are any known side effects possible. A study may not be conducted if there is an increased risk of death associated with its administration. Many clinical trials today also use "double blind" studies to decrease the possibility of bias, in which the participants and the researchers do not know which group gets the treatment under consideration and which gets a placebo. Additionally, if research shows that a treatment is beneficial to the diseased participants at any time during the study, all afflicted participants must be offered the treatment. In the event that a treatment is shown to be beneficial, its mechanism of action may not always be known once administered to the entire study group, yet it would be unethical to withhold treatment from the other participants. Many of these research guidelines limit the advancement of scientific knowledge, but they are in place to prevent experiments from risking the lives and health of the study participants.

The ability of the scientific method to lead to medical breakthroughs and cure debilitating diseases is a powerful and wonderful motivator to pursue clinical research. I, too, held this unwavering view of science, until I came across a study that caused me to question the subjectivity of scientific research. I was in my last class of the day, an upper division undergraduate class that reviewed published research articles about free radical biochemistry. It was cutting-edge research, with science so obscure I had little knowledge of the majority of hypotheses prior to this class. Yet, my classmates, professors, and I sat in disbelief when we discovered that one of the articles was based on doctored evidence. That day we reviewed a journal article investigating the French Paradox. A student transferred the images into the computer for presentation. In the context of a printed journal, the SDS gels would have been innocuous. However, when the images were enlarged at projector-size, it was obvious that the gel bands had been digitally manipulated in a way that supported the hypothesis of the study. The entire classroom realized that this published scientific article, which concluded that the chemical compound of red wine provided cardiovascular protection, was based on fabicated evidence. The manipulated proof was a serious breach in professional accountability because it presented a potential danger to the unenlighted public as a whole if scientific claims are made based on false evidence. Many similar studies are often cited to support major public health broadcasts. If scientific knowledge has the capacity to cure disease, however, there also remains the ability to cause a proportional amount of harm if not carefully controlled. The day I witnessed blatant fabrication of evidence deeply affected me, because I realized how easily scientists could fabricate data and make claims based on false data.

Misleading data may harm people, such as in the Wakefield vaccine publication (chapter 7A). An investigation done in 2011 discovered that Andrew Wakefield had manipulated his data by reporting that the patients in his study first exhibited autism symptoms after they received the vaccine, when in fact many of the patient's parents reported symptoms much earlier. The skewed timeframe of the patient's symptoms gave Wakefield results that supported his hypothesis, when in actuality there was no correlation.

Wakefield is not the only scientist to have manipulated data in order to gain favorable results. In January, 2014, Japanese researchers at the Riken Center for Developmental Biology published two scientific papers demonstrating that normal cells could acquire the ability to become stem cells when stimulated by certain triggers. The results from the study, however, could not be replicated in other laboratories and an investigation months later found the studies to have errors suggesting the data had been manipulated and that images from the study did not match images published in the paper (7). By July, 2014, both papers were retracted from the journal *Nature* and one of the main participants subsequently committed suicide.

In October, 2013, Dong-Pyou Han, a researcher at the Iowa State University was also found guilty of tampering with his samples in a way that made his vaccine for HIV appear to successfully eradicate the virus. In December, 2013, Dr. Han lost his grants and resigned for falsifying his research studies (8).

While the amount of fabricated data IS in the minority, the Wakefield study demonstrated how catastrophic even one fabricated study can be. When the healthcare of patients depends on vital studies regarding issues such as the HIV vaccine, stem cells, or deadly viruses, even one fabricated study is an egregious event. Additionally, not only does a dishonest study adversely affect patient healthcare, it puts the Scientific Approach in a questionable position which creates a barrier between the general public and professionals that is difficult for scientists to overcome. Once broken, the trust of the general public can be difficult to regain.

We must always remind ourselves that human life is sacred and the quest to discover and publish new knowledge has the ability to affect people negatively as well. Such events could mislead subsequent scientific undertakings and delay resolution of the true cause-and-effect question. It took many decades of experience and lack of therapeutic success to convince the medical community that gastric ulcers were not caused by stress. Prior scientific studies, in which ulcers were induced in rats by subjecting them to stressful situations and then treating the symptoms of the ulcers with antacids, linked ulcers in rats to stress. However, these studies did not assess for the presence of hidden causative factors, termed "confounding factors," with double-blinded studies. As a result of the misconception that ulcers are caused by stress, many gastroenterologists treated their patients who had ulcers with antacids and advised them to drink dairy products to soothe the stomach. This treatment regimen, however, only exacerbated the disease and often caused the stomach lining to perforate and bleed, or develop cancer. After such disease progression, the patient often needed a partial or full stomach resection and many patients never regained full health. Although Barry Marshall, an internal medicine doctor, published evidence that increasingly supported his theory that gastric ulcers were caused by the bacteria, *Helicobacter pylori*, many experts in the field of gastrointestinal diseases—namely, the gastroenterologists and scientists—refused to accept Marshall's theory (9). Because the gastroenterologists failed to accept the theory that gastric ulcers were caused by a bacterium, these physicians failed to provide antibiotics for their patients with gastric ulcers. Ultimately, the patients that had not received correct treatment of antibiotics suffered. While the current treatment protocol includes antibiotics and medications that reduce the amount of acid produced by the stomach, the use of acid-regulating medication is mostly for symptomatic relief of stomach irritation by acid; it does not treat the culprit that causes gastric ulcers.

Conclusions

The scientific community must always pursue the high standards of unadulterated truth and pure lucidity, whether they relate to the participants, data collection, financial support, or publication of the research study. By demanding truth, honesty, and clarity from scientific research, we can protect ourselves against the potential harm incurred from imprudent announcements of "breakthrough" scientific discoveries.

In the case of autism research in particular, too much emphasis has been and is still being placed on perpetuating and repeating secure projects of marginal innovation and trail-blazing. Research modalities that happen to be currently in vogue are pressed to elucidate previously unobserved phenomena, even though they may have little to do with the question at hand. New paths of thinking and investigation are deferred or discarded in the interest of showing benefactors that SOMETHING is being accomplished, even though it may be repetitive and fails to make groundbreaking inroads into solving the autism enigma. Many of the hypotheses to be discussed in this book have been disproven repeatedly, but remain in the professional and lay psyche because of the unrelenting need to do something of questionable achievement rather than chancing negative results. The computer age has rapidly introduced major discoveries which advance complex technological applications within short periods; the same should be possible with autism research.

Chapter 1B - Geographic Trends

Kenneth Swanson

[The search for a geographic parameter which might give some insight into the cause of autism surprisingly revealed that economic and educational factors correlated to some degree with the incidence. In particular, familial economic status and parental academic achievement suggested that accessing proper medical attention might be the key to this observation – Ed.]

Hypothesis

The diagnosis of autism spectrum disorders (ASD) appears to occur more often in some locations than it does in others. Nearly every state or state grouping, known as a division, has a distinct childhood prevalence of ASD diagnosis defined as cases per one hundred children below age 18. The criteria to label a child as autistic are currently in a state of flux due to changing diagnostic definitions (chapter 1D). The purpose of this chapter is to examine why these geographic prevalence differences occur (1,2). A distinction probably exists between *actual* autism occurrence and *apparent* autism diagnosis.

The fifty states of the American Union are used for comparison here because small scale data such as by neighborhood, by ethnic grouping, or by family are not yet available. "Divisions" are employed to illustrate the trend on a larger scale. When these are considered, the general distribution of autism diagnosis becomes more apparent by averaging out special local characteristics and idiosyncrasies.

The US Census Bureau partitions the Country into arbitrary divisions for the sake of presenting data. Divisions are regions arbitrarily chosen by proximity of bordering states and thereby draw a convenient larger scale depiction for demonstrating trends. The United States is comprised of nine divisions: New England, Mid-Atlantic, East North Central, West North Central, South Atlantic, East South Central, West South Central, Mountain, and Pacific (3,4).

It appears that broad-based attributes of the residents of these divisions influence the number of autism cases diagnosed. Actual autism case prevalence will not be known until the bias due to these traits is eliminated. The characteristics examined in this chapter are median income, percent of the population holding BA/BS and advanced academic degrees, population density, and total population. These characteristics were chosen because they are illustrated by objective, numerical data that could very easily impact a person's likelihood to seek medical care.

Two hypotheses are investigated here:

1)   The first is that States with higher mean income and achieved educational levels have higher rates of autism diagnosis. It is presumed that a population that has spent more time in academia would be more astute in having their children examined, because they are more aware of pertinent information. In general, it is believed that people with more resources available would be less hesitant to spend it on specialized health evaluations.

2)   The second hypothesis is that total population and population density will also show a lesser, but still positive, trend. This is may be due to specialized healthcare being more readily available in larger cities.

About the data

Median income, population density, and total population data from 2010 (3,5) are considered here, while the most recent educational attainment figures from 2009 are utilized (4). Data on gross numbers of autistic children which were divided by the total childhood population are also from 2010 (1). All statistical analysis presented in this chapter are performed by the author, but all data are obtained from the US Department of Education and the US Census Bureau. The US Department of Education monitors the raw number of diagnoses in children of all ages under the Individuals with Disabilities Education Act (IDEA) definition:

"Autism means a developmental disability significantly affecting verbal and nonverbal communication and social interaction, generally evident before age three that adversely affects a child's educational performance. Other characteristics often associated with autism are engagement in repetitive activities and stereotyped movements, resistance to environmental change or change in daily routines, and unusual responses to sensory experiences"(1).

For the sake of this chapter, "autism" and "autistic spectrum disorders" are used interchangeably because the data collected by the US Department of Education do not differentiate the two upon presentation.

Observations

Firstly, the table below shows each state ranked in order of its autism diagnosis per population under 18 years old. Minnesota is found to have the most diagnoses of autism, while Iowa has the least amount of diagnoses.

4

27

Rank	State	% population under 18 diagnosed with autism	Rank	State	% population under 18 diagnosed with autism
1	Minnesota	1.049	26	Idaho	0.444
2	Maine	0.928	27	Wyoming	0.443
3	Oregon	0.89	28	Arizona	0.437
4	Massachusettes	0.798	29	Delaware	0.433
5	Rhode Island	0.745	30	Nebraska	0.426
6	Connecticut	0.719	31	Georgia	0.423
7	Pennsylvania	0.715	31	Utah	0.423
8	Indiana	0.686	33	Alaska	0.41
9	California	0.668	34	Hawai'i	0.402
10	New Jersey	0.603	35	Arkansas	0.388
11	Maryland	0.599	36	Tennessee	0.377
12	Vermont	0.597	37	Alabama	0.366
13	Virginia	0.591	38	Kentucky	0.363
14	Michigan	0.584	39	North Dakota	0.355
15	Wisconsin	0.579	40	South Carolina	0.337
16	Ohio	0.557	41	West Virginia	0.336
17	New Hampshire	0.55	42	South Dakota	0.334
18	Nevada	0.532	42	Kansas	0.334
19	Washington	0.503	44	Oklahoma	0.314
20	New York	0.495	45	Mississippi	0.296
21	North Carolina	0.493	46	Louisiana	0.289
22	Illinois	0.485	47	Colorado	0.287
23	Missouri	0.483	48	New Mexico	0.282
24	Florida	0.456	49	Montana	0.27
25	Texas	0.451	50	Iowa	0.099

All five of the parameters mentioned previously show a positive correlation with autism diagnosis. The magnitude of the trends varies, but not by a very significant amount.

Starting on a broader scale, the trends by division very positive when relating autism to divisional average median income (r = 0.85), bachelor's degrees (r = 0.86), advanced degrees (r = 0.87), and population density (r = 0.72). [The value, r, is the correlation coefficient; the higher the r, the closer is the correlation – see chapter 1A.] Conversely, total population is weakly correlated (r = 0.2) to the rate of autism diagnosis. To emphasize this distinction, autism diagnosis versus median income bydivision is presented below (1-5).

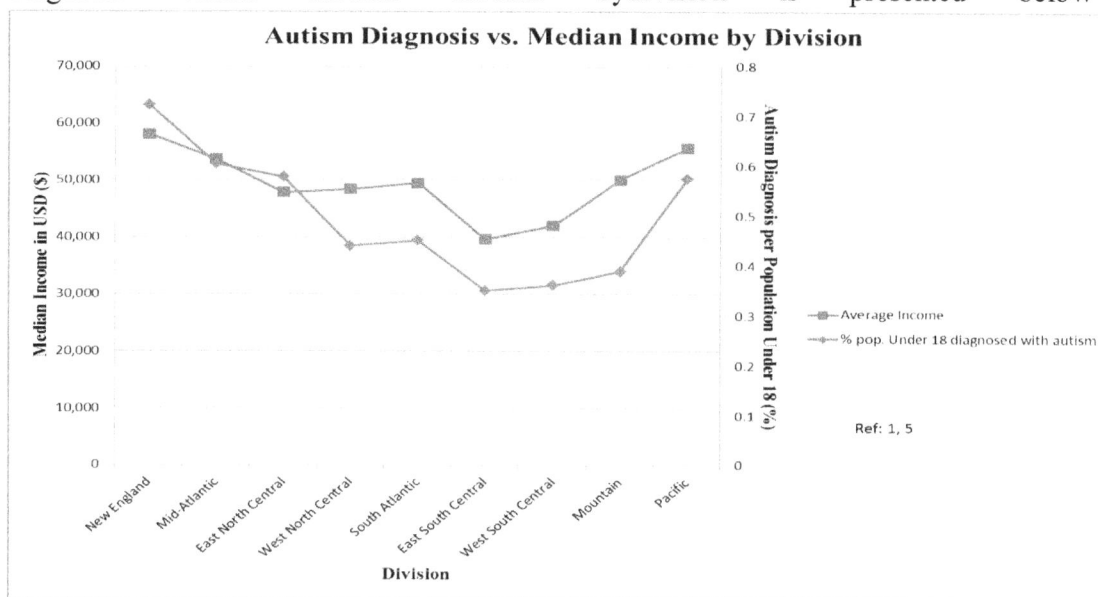

Autism Diagnosis vs. Median Income by Division

The New England Division has the highest average rates of diagnosed autism, median income, bachelor's degrees, advanced degrees, and total population, but is second to the mid-Atlantic in population density. The East South Central division has the lowest average autism diagnosis rates, income, bachelor's degrees, and advanced degrees; however,it does not have the lowest population density or total population.

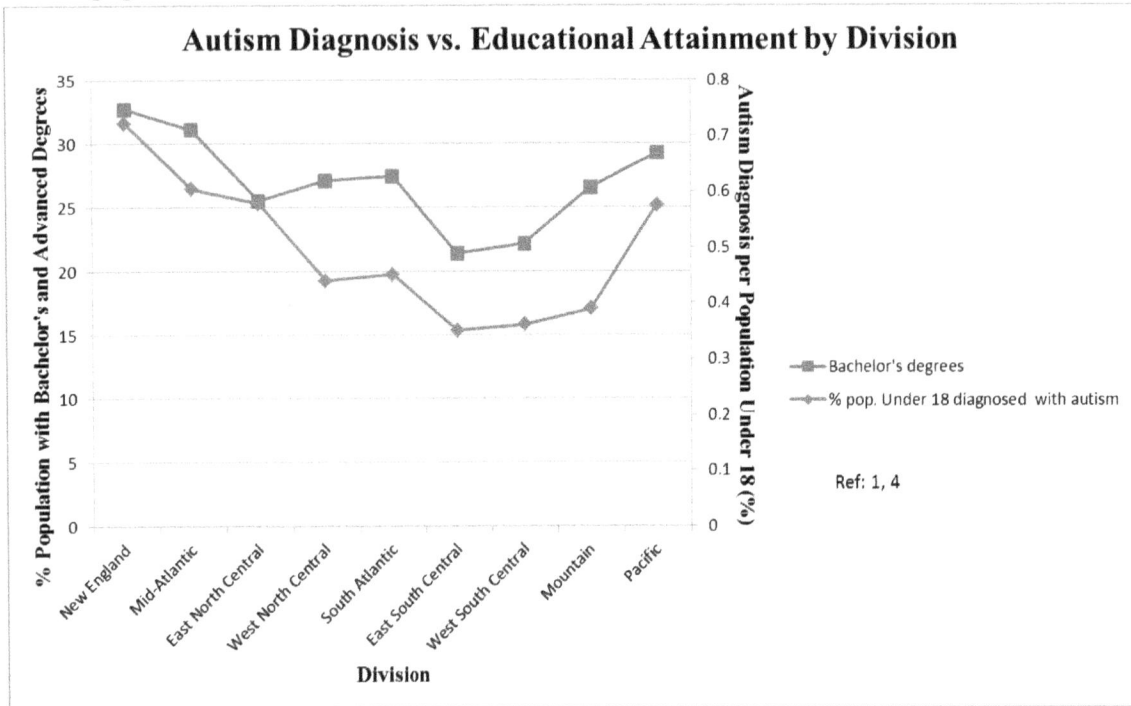

On a more specific scale, a direct relationship exists between median income and autism diagnosis per childhood population ($r = 0.41$). States with a higher median income are more likely to have a higher ASD diagnosis rate. This suggests that the more money parents make, the more likely they are to have a child that is suspected of having ASD appropriately studied (1,3).

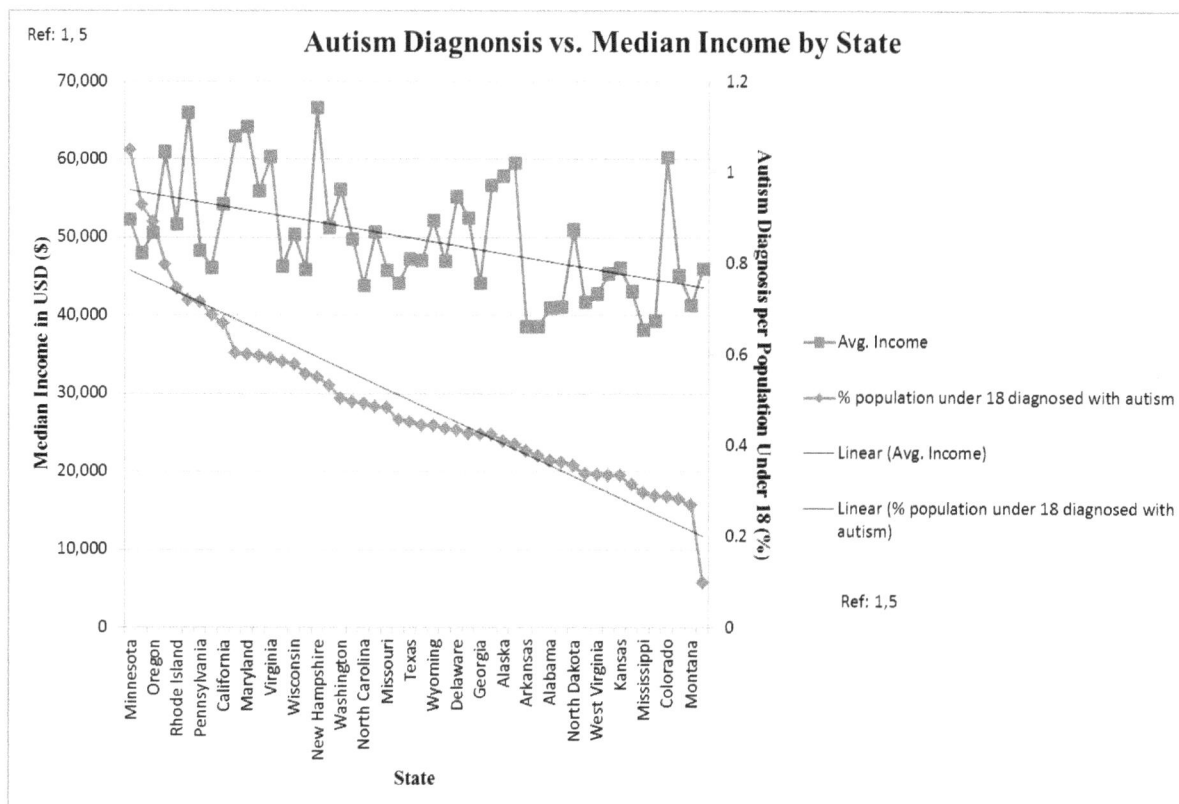

Autism Diagnonsis vs. Median Income by State

Ref: 1, 5

A direct relationship also exists between autism diagnosis per capita under age 18 and population with bachelor's degrees ($r = 0.45$) and advanced degrees ($r = 0.48$). State populations with more educational attainment are likely to have a higher ASD diagnosis rate, suggesting that parents who have gone to college and graduate school are more likely to have children that are diagnosed with ASD (1,4).

That the incidence of autism is directly a function of family income or parental academic achievement seems unlikely, but that parental awareness is higher is probably more appropriate. The last two trends (median income and educational attainment) clearly show that public awareness of autism suffers greatly and an alternative method is needed to reach people of all educational levels. If formal education is the only way that people are adequately informed of autism, then under-diagnosis will not improve.

Lastly, total population ($r = 0.18$) is not as strongly correlated with autism diagnosis as income and educational attainment. However, population density ($r = 0.38$) does correlate similarly with income and must not be discounted. This suggests that although density is often related to improved availability of health care, larger state populations do not necessarily have more awareness or resources; but more people closer together do seem to increase diagnosis numbers (1-3).

Conclusions

Improvements must be made to provide all families the resources to have their autistic children *diagnosed* and to receive proper care. Income, educational attainment, total population, and population density are not evenly distributed (2,5). On the one hand, two studies done in California confirmed a correlation between maternal educational level, family income, and autism incidence. In contradistinction, such a relationship to socioeconomic factors was not found in European subjects, especially where access to healthcare was universal (6,7).

Wealth by itself probably has little, if any, direct impact on the actual tendency to develop autism, but whether or not a child is diagnosed expeditiously as such does. A financially secure family with a child exhibiting abnormal behavior will more likely possess the means to have their child examined than a family without the same fiscal capacity. It is doubtful that familial intellectual abilities alone have a direct impact on the actual occurrence of autism in their offspring. Parents with more education are, in all probability, more likely to recognize and be attuned to childhood developmental delays. It can be hypothesized that populations possessing fewer academic degrees as well as inferior access to health facilities are less likely to seek proper analysis of aberrant childhood behavior. Furthermore, the correlation is even more positive for advanced degrees than it is for bachelor's degrees. However, over-diagnosis among the highly educated is also a possibility.

If these parameters (wealth and parental education) influence the rate of diagnosis of autism as much as they appear to, then knowledge of these conditions seems to be more common in those with sufficient finances, education, and proximity than in the general population. Information and resources must reach people with lower median income and educational attainment, as well as those in more sparsely-populated areas. The evidence shown here suggests that American society in particular must reconsider how it views and deals with recognition of autism.

Chapter 1C – Occurrence Rate
Marina Kishlyansky, Marta Wronska

[It is uncertain if the recently reported apparent rise in occurrence of autism is due to increasing pathogenesis or to change in diagnostic criteria of those identifying such cases. These studies support the contention that autism is due, in part, to an inherited tendency. – Ed.]

Hypothesis

When discussing epidemiological findings, an important distinction should be drawn between incidence (rate of occurrence) and prevalence. Incidence refers to the number of new cases of a disorder in a specific population within a specified period of time; prevalence refers to the total number of individuals affected with a disorder in a given population (1,2) (chapter 1B).

Over the past few decades, reports have announced an apparent increase in the estimated rates of autism spectrum disorder (ASD) (1,2). Such upward trends, known in the popular media as the "autism epidemic," have prompted numerous studies that have yielded a myriad of statistical data and have expanded our appreciation of the vastness of this condition. The reasons for the apparent increase in autism figures remain unclear. In this chapter, we attempt to clarify part of the current misconceptions in this field by providing a review of recent epidemiological evidence. In particular, we include data pertaining to the general prevalence of diagnosed autism in the United States and worldwide, a commentary discussing the nature of the apparent upward trend, and a review of current methodological limitations in data collection. Additionally, we appraise recurrence rates of ASD among twin pairs and siblings, and discuss cross-cultural contrasts and the influence of immigration status on reported rates of this condition.

Observations

The Center for Disease Control and Prevention (CDC) provides statistics and data on ASD figures in the United States. As of March, 2014, surveys published by the CDC, collected from 11 sites in United States reported that 14.7 per 1000 children, which is one in 68 children, of 8 years of age, have ASD (1,3). These data demonstrate a 29% increase in rates of autism occurrence when compared to studies from 2008, 64% increase when compared to 2006 values, and a 123% increase compared to data collected in 2002. The highest and lowest estimated rates were collected from sites in New Jersey (21.9 per 1000) and Alabama (5.7 per 1000), respectively (1) (chapter 1B). Evidently, these findings suggest a continued upward trend in diagnosed ASD cases overall.

The newest data demonstrate that the median age at diagnosis varies by subtypes of ASD (chapter 1D). With all diagnostic subtypes combined, the median age at first diagnosis is 53 months (1). With respect to sex differences, it is estimated that 1 out of every 42 boys and 1 out of every 189 girls have ASD (Conclusions and Prospectus). Therefore, males are about four to five times more likely than females to be diagnosed with this condition, a ratio which has remained relatively constant throughout the years (4). However, as emphasized by the CDC, the above statistics are not based on a national homogenous sample population. Therefore, they cannot be generalized to the United States population as a whole (1).

There is an ongoing debate in the field of ASD research about the nature of the reported "autism epidemic". Some evidence in the literature suggests that higher prevalence figures may not be due to a true increase in the number of new cases, but rather, due to other various artifacts. The complex nature of autism, lack of diagnostic biologic markers, modifications in diagnostic criteria, increased availability of services and special education programs, and improved awareness of ASD among the general public, child caretakers, and teachers could be responsible for the reported apparent upward trend (1,2,4) (chapters 1D,2A).

An important issue to consider when analyzing statistics in the field of autism is the lack of standardized data collection methods and screening techniques in surveys of prevalence rates (2). Since no reliable biomarker for ASD is currently available, proper diagnosis requires a team of professionals who have clinical experience and training in this field. However, access to reliable diagnostic resources varies across different sites in the United States as well as in other countries. This may result in diagnostic tools being used by individuals who have personal objective bias or are not sufficiently trained, thereby introducing inaccuracies into the diagnostic process, which may affect estimated rates (4). As such, studies that rely solely on parent-filled questionnaires considered to have lower reliability and validity than those which include a professional input.

Another aspect of methodology that could skew prevalence proportions is sample size used and whether retrospective or prospective analysis was performed. In general, studies examining smaller sample size or studies using retrospective analysis report lower figures compared to prospective studies or studies with larger sample sizes (1,5) (chapter 1A). Due to the apparent variability between study designs used to survey rates of ASD, combining epidemiological findings by performing a cross-study analysis for the purpose of generalizing to the population as a whole might prove to be challenging. Fombonne compared eight studies conducted within the same year in the US and the UK, and found a substantial variability in estimates of ASD numbers among these reviews. Specifically, there was a 14-fold variation in data gathered by the US studies, and a 6-fold variability in figures from UK surveys. Fombonne concluded that since the data for all studies were collected within the same year, the observed variability could not be attributed to passage of time and was, therefore, a result of methodological differences between these studies (2). Moreover, since studies of prevalence could provide variable values, even when data are collected within the same year, estimates of ASD trends across time should also be treated with caution.

A portion of the ASD data is collected from special education programs across the US. As described by the CDC, a wide variation exists for eligibility criteria used by such programs to screen children for autism (1). For example, in the state of Colorado, depending on the school district, a child with ASD can either be classified under the category of physical disability or autism. In addition, screening protocols for autism used by school systems may differ from those used in primary health care settings, and thus may offer less accurate assessments of ASD. Interestingly, the reported rate of increase in the frequency of autism in US special education programs during the 1990's correlates with rates of decrease in mental retardation diagnosis, a phenomenon known as "diagnostic substitution" (6) (chapter 2C). This means that a greater proportion of children who would have been previously diagnosed with other disabilities were now being identified with autism (2,6). As such, the rising reported trends in such programs could be attributed partly to changes in referral and identification practices, rather than to true increase in ASD prevalence among school-aged children.

One of the biggest diagnostic challenges for professionals in this field is distinguishing between children with autism and those with other developmental disorders. In general, a single analytical tool is not considered sufficient for making a diagnosis and a multidisciplinary evaluation is recommended (4). However, one of the widely used guides for ASD diagnosis is "The Diagnostic and Statistical Manual of Mental Disorders" (DSM) (1,4) (chapter 1D). Various editions of the DSM have been published to date. Differences in autism definitions between older and more recent iterations of the DSM, specifically, broadening the diagnostic boundaries, have been proposed to partially account for the apparent increase in reported prevalence rates of ASD (1,2,4). The newest DSM edition, DSM-5, was released in May, 2013 and includes revised criteria for diagnosis of ASD. Some experts in this field predict that these changes may help create more accurate diagnostic classification for individuals with autism and a decrease in rate of ASD diagnosis(4). However, since the new criteria include substantial modifications of the older editions, these changes are likely to make comparisons with prior estimated prevalence rates challenging.

To date, the extent to which the above-described confounding factors could contribute to the apparent increase in reported rates of ASD remains uncertain (1,2,4). More studies using the same protocols over several years are required in order to improve accuracy of reported data.

Recurrence among siblings

Family and twin studies suggest that ASD is, to a large extent, a heritable condition (1). This observation is based mainly on the large reported differences in concordance rates between monozygotic and dizygotic twins (see below). A concordance rate is a statistical measure which indicates the probability that a pair of individuals will both have a certain trait/disease, given that one of them has the trait/disease. Concordance rates help determine if a trait may have a genetic basis, and, if so, whether it is strong, weak, or moderate. Monozygotic ("identical") twins share 100% of their DNA, whereas dizygotic ("fraternal") twins share only 50% on average. Thus, if a condition is highly heritable, a high concordance rate is expected to be observed among monozygotic twins, nearing 100%, and a much smaller concordance would be observed in dizygotic twins.

According to the CDC, concordance rates of ASD for monozygotic twins and dizygotic twins are 35-95% and 0-31%, respectively (chapter 8A). In addition, among non-twin siblings, concordance rates are 2-18% (1,7). Two recent studies, cited by the CDC, report an apparent difference between concordance rates for male and female twin pairs (8,9). Rosenberg and colleagues reported 100% and 86% concordance rates for male and female monozygotic twins, respectively. For dizygotic twins with at least 1 female, concordance rate for ASD was 20% compared to 40% in male-male twin pairs (8). Hallmayer and colleagues reported concordance rates of 77% and 50% for male and female monozygotic twin pairs, respectively. For dizygotic twins, the reported concordance rates were 31% and 36% for male and female pairs, respectively. Concordance rate for female dizygotic twins of proband males was 5.3%, while concordance for male dizygotic twin of female proband was 50.0% (9). The difference in reported rates between the two studies could be partly accounted for by differences in methodology. Whereas Rosenberg et al. relied on parent-reported questionnaires for their data collection, Hallmayer et al., used both parent interview and direct child observations (8,9) (See Table 2 for the summary of these studies).

Therefore, when interpreting data from twin studies, it is important to note whether separate data for male and female twin pairs are available, since combining these two data sets could lead to inaccurate estimation of concordance rates. Since the concordance rate of ASD in monozygotic twins is typically less than 100%, a role for environmental influence is strongly suggested. In this context, recording and reporting accurate concordance has important implications to our understanding of the etiology of ASD and the environmental vs. genetic contribution to this condition.

Prevalence by country of origin, race, ethnicity, and immigration status

An important area of ASD research is investigation of epidemiological trends in different geographic locations and across different ethnicities. Variability in prevalence between different countries might offer a new perspective on the association of genetic and environmental factors on this condition, which remain largely unclear.

Prevalence of ASD is reported to be lower in countries outside of Europe and North America. However, these data are not controlled for cultural and ethnic influences on ASD assessment and data collection (10). As such, when compared to studies conducted in the US and Europe, statistics reported from other countries might be confounded by the rate of disorder reporting and diagnosis, its classification, and analysis of the data. Current research suggests that the variability in rates of autism across countries is a result of methodological differences rather than a factor of ethnicity and country of origin (5). The extent to which these factors could skew reported numbers is unknown as there is currently a lack of systematic review assessing discrepancies in prevalence rates and methodological styles across countries.

Despite a global rise in ASD research efforts, it appears that the majority of epidemiological data, and the most thorough analyses, arise from studies done in the US and the UK. Wong and Hui (11) cited research from a total of 12 international locations. They included five cities in UK, three cities in US, and one city each from Australia, Canada, Finland, and Sweden. Autism rates in countries outside the US and the UK were either not effectively studied or the results varied greatly from the commonly accepted values that were recorded in the US (11.3 per 1,000) and the UK (15.7 per 1,000). For instance, prevalence of childhood autism was recorded to be 26.4 per 1,000 in South Korea (5), whereas in Oman it was only 0.14 per 1,000 (11). Denmark, Canada, Hong Kong, and Venezuela all reported prevalence of less than two cases per 1,000 children (12). A study from the Faroe Islands reported higher prevalence, with 5.6 – 9.4 cases per 1000 (13). (For complete data from recent studies, refer to Table 1 at the end of this chapter.) These marked lower results were attributed to under diagnosis and use of different methodological approaches in ASD assessment (14). Specific examples include using a general mental screening method which results in lower estimated prevalence compared to values obtained from autism specific assessment measures and multidisciplinary teams (11,15). Much like the variation in ***diagnosed*** ASD cases in relation to parental educational and financial level (chapter 1B), the inter-country range may relate to familial attention of developmental deficiency signs in their children.

The CDC includes data on the race and ethnicity of the children diagnosed, factors often omitted in ASD studies, in addition to their prevalence rates. Within the US population, Caucasian American children are at a higher apparent risk for ASD than other ethnic groups (1). Moreover, a recent study from August, 2013 suggests that children of Latin descent are diagnosed at lower rates and at later ages than their Caucasian counterparts (16) (Table 3).

In the past 30 years, small studies reported that trends in immigration might be a contributing factor to the increased ASD frequency in European and North American countries (17). However, the relationship between immigration status and autism remains poorly understood. European studies indicate that maternal immigration from countries outside of Europe and North America is correlated with a higher risk of having a child with diagnosed ASD (17,20,21). A study conducted in Sweden by Barnevik-Olsson and colleagues demonstrated higher ASD figures among children of Somali background compared to children of other ethnicities. Specifically, Somali children had four-to-fivefold higher rates of ASD diagnosis than children of other descent (20). Other studies conducted in Denmark and Sweden reported that mothers born outside of Europe and North America have increased chances of giving birth to a child with ASD by a relative risk of 1.4 and 3.0 respectively (21). In contrast, investigations in the US have not supported a higher risk associated with parental immigration (18,19).

Keen and colleagues reported similar findings about maternal immigration and risk of ASD in their offspring. In their retrospective study, they found that mothers born in the Caribbean who immigrated to England were at the highest risk for giving birth to a child with ASD, followed by mothers from Africa and Asia. Ethnicity alone was not statistically correlated with increased risk. However, in combination with immigration status, children of black immigrant mothers were at a higher risk for being diagnosed with ASD. No significant effect was observed for mothers migrating from other countries in Europe (17).

Conclusions

Throughout the past seven decades since the first recognition and definition of autism, significant advancements have been made in ASD research, leading to a better understanding of this condition. Despite these developments, challenges remain in the correct diagnosis and epidemiological survey of autism prevalence rates. Currently, the observed apparent upward trend in autism cannot be fully attributed to increases in new cases due to the potential involvement of several confounding variables described in the literature (1,2,4). One of the main variables in surveys of ASD can be attributed to increased awareness and access to assessment services, which have improved the identification of children with autism (1). Another important factor is related to lack of consistent surveying methods, which poses challenges for in-between study comparison and for generalization of findings to the population as a whole (1,2). Nevertheless, the possibility that the reported rise in autism figures could be attributed to a true increase in incidence should not be completely dismissed. Therefore, caution in interpretation of the published data should be used since the nature of the upward trend in autism remains unclear.

Improved reporting and interpretation of prevalence are not only important for better ascertainment of epidemiological trends across time, but also serve as essential tools for elucidating the etiology of the disorder. Since the cause of ASD is thought to be multifactorial, various study designs have been used to examine potential contributing factors. Twin studies have demonstrated that, although autism is highly heritable, there is an important environmental role that cannot be discounted.

In reporting concordance rates in these studies, separate data for male and female twin pairs are not always provided. In this context, recording accurate and sex-specific concordance may have important implications to our understanding of the etiology of this condition and could provide valuable information about autism risk factors to parents, caregivers, educators, and clinicians. The etiological contribution of ethnicity, race, and culture can be studied by performing cross-comparison of different countries and population groups. However, current evidence of lower prevalence rates in countries outside of the US and Europe is confounded by the same variables that lower reliability and validity in US-based studies. Therefore, it appears that attempts to accurately record ASD prevalence are a problem faced by demographers, statisticians, sociologists, health service planners, and researchers globally, and are not limited to studies conducted in the US alone. Consequently, accurate comparison of rates across countries and ethnic backgrounds for the purpose of enhancing our understanding of the etiology of autism remains challenging.

One of the most widely used sets of diagnostic criteria for assessing ASD is the DSM (chapter 1D). Yet, as of now, the effect of the newly revised edition of the manual, DSM-5, on reported autism rates is still unclear. With the readjustment of the definition of ASD, prevalence might actually decrease because some individuals previously classified under the ASD umbrella term may no longer meet criteria for this diagnosis. Care must be taken to reevaluate borderline cases previously diagnosed with earlier criteria. Consequently, these alterations might exert modifying effects on both the individuals no longer meeting the autism criteria, and on the field of autism research as a whole. Reclassification of an individual from ASD to another category might influence special service eligibility and make it challenging for scientists to compare future prevalence rates with data collected to date.

Finally, it is important to note the major social implications that better diagnostic practices may generate. More critical criteria for assessment and classification of ASD will ensure increased accuracy of identification of children with this condition, and thus promote earlier diagnosis and appropriate intervention (chapters 2A-2C). Alternatively, better diagnostic practices should reduce mislabeling of individuals with other developmental deficits as autistic, a label that could have long-term social and educational consequences for the child and his/her family.

Future direction in this field should aim to create a more standardized and accurate system for collecting and reporting ASD statistical trends in order to provide a better understanding of this condition and to help guide research. In the meantime, establishing clear guidelines for assessing children suspected of having developmental disorders in various diagnostic settings - and overseeing their proper implementation - could benefit this field of research.

[A revised report by the CDC (3/2014) now cites the rate of autism in the United States as 1-in-64. This modification may have more to do with the modified criteria in the recently published DSM-5 than an actual increase in the rate of occurrence of the disease.]

Table 1. CDC: Summary of Autism Spectrum Disorder (ASD) Prevalence Studies (12)

Author	Published	Country	Time Period Studied	Ages Studied	Criteria	Methodology	ASD Prevalence per 1000 children (CI)
Lauritsen et al.	2004	Denmark	2001	0 to 9	ICD-10	Case enumeration	1.2 (1.1-1.3)
Oullette - Kuntz et al.	2007	Canada	1996-2004	4 to 9	Special education classification	Case enumeration from special education classification	1.2 (1996); 4.3 (2004)
Wong et al.	2008	Hong Kong	1986-2005	0 to 14	DSM-IV	Case enumeration	1.6
Williams et al.	2008	Australia	2003-2004	6 to 12	DSM-IV	Questionnaires	1.0 (0.8-1.0) to 4.1 (3.8-4.4)
Montiel - Nava et al.	2008	Venezuela	2005-2006	3 to 9	DSM-IV	Case enumeration	1.7 (1.3-2.0)
Baron - Cohen et al.	2009	UK	2003-2004	5 to 9	Special Education Needs register	Case enumeration from survey and direct exam	15.7 (9.9-24.6)
Al-Farsi et al.	2010	Oman	2009	0 to 14	DSM-IV	Case enumeration	0.1 (0.1-0.2)
Kim et al.	2011	South Korea	2005-2009	7 to 12	DSM-IV	Case enumeration from survey and direct exam	26.4 (19.1-33.7)
Kocovska et al.	2012	Faroe Islands	2002, 2009	7 to 16 (2002), 15 to 24 (2009)	DSM-IV, ICD-10	Screening and direct exam	5.6 (2002), 9.4 (2009)
CDC ADDM Network	2012	USA	2008	8	DSM-IV	Case enumeration and record review	11.3 (11.0-11.7)

Table 2. Summary of reported ASD concordance in siblings (7-9)

TYPE	GENDER	CONCORDANCE %
MZ twins	All	35-95
DZ twins	All	0-31
Non-twin	All	2-18
MZ twins	Male	77, 100
MZ twins	Female	50, 86
DZ twins	M+F or F+F	20
DZ twins	M+M	31, 40

M = male
F = female
MZ = monozygotic ("identical")
DZ = dizygotic ("fraternal")
(See text for data sources.)

Table 3. Ethnicity and autism prevalence in US in 2008 (1)

Ethnicity	Prevalence per 1,000
White	12.0
Black	10.2
Hispanic	7.9
Asian/Pacific Islander	9.7

Chapter 1D - DMS-5

Kari Tabag, LCSW-R, Psychotherapist

[A recently published new edition of the Diagnostic and Statistical Manual of Mental Disorders has generated much debate on the classification of manifestations of autism and other neurologic conditions that may or may not be related to it. – Ed.]

Hypothesis

Prior to and following its release in May, 2013, the Diagnostic and Statistical Manual of Mental Disorders, Volume 5 (DSM-5) has ignited a plentitude of debates and controversy among mental and medical health professionals, parents, organizations, advocates, and the like. Presented in an objective manner using current resources, this chapter presents both sides of the debate, provides clarification and explanation about the changes, and discusses if it poses a threat to the delivery of treatment in the mental health, education, and managed care industries relating to the neurodevelopmental disorders.

To be differentiated here are: Asperger's Syndrome (AS), Rett's Syndrome (RS), Pervasive Disorder Not Otherwise Specified (PDD NOS), and Autistic Disorder (AD). Previous diagnosis guides included only children when referring to those diagnosed with AS, RS, PDD NOS, and AD. Therefore, the term "individuals" in this chapter pertains to those previously and currently diagnosed.

A total of 13 new study groups began work on the DSM-5 in 2007. The changes in the new volume were based on comprehensive reviews of scientific advancements, targeted research analyses, and clinical expertise (1). To date, it is the most extensive modification in the DSM series. For example, revisions were made with the hope that the definition of autism spectrum disorder (ASD) is now more specific, reliable, and valid. An individual's history is further taken into account here rather than just behaviors observed during the assessment phase. The age of onset has been extended, thereby including older individuals for purposes of diagnosis.

Observations

Asperger's syndrome (AS)

In 1944, Austrian physician Hans Asperger referred to this syndrome as "autistic psychopathy" (2, 3). According to DSM-IV-TR (Diagnostic and Statistical Manual of Mental Disorders, Volume 4, Text Revision) criteria, AS pertains to the absence of a language delay under the umbrella of Pervasive Developmental Disorders (PDD). Common to all diagnoses in the PDD category are marked delays in the development of socialization and communication skills, with symptoms as early as infancy, although the typical age of onset is before 3 years of age. The average unaffected child should be able to speak words by age two and sentences or phrases by age three, without a delay in cognitive development (one's ability to think and understand) or self-help skills (4).

Rett's syndrome (RS)

Also listed under PDD is Rett's Syndrome, a disorder diagnosed almost exclusively in females, marked by slow head growth from 5 to 48 months (5). Between 5 to 30 months, an affected child is unable to make self-intentional hand movements and develops aberrant hand movements such as hand washing or hand wringing, loses interest in her/his environment, presents with poorly coordinated movements of the upper body, exhibits a delay in thought patterns, and displays a reduction of physical movements as well as a visible slowing of physical and emotional reactions. (Refer to chapter 8A for further information about RS, especially its differentiation from autism.) Some research suggests a possible connection between Down's syndrome, Rett's syndrome, and autistic disorder in some cases (4). This may be due to a common factor, yet to be defined, underlying the etiologic mechanism in such neuropathologic events.

Autistic disorder (AD) and autism spectrum disorder (ASD)

Three of the four disorders, Autistic Disorder, Asperger's Syndrome, and Rett's Syndrome, are eliminated as separate diagnoses with distinctive criteria in the DSM-5, and are now included under ASD. Derived from DSM-IV-TR's Autistic Disorder criteria, autism spectrum disorder is the title of a new section which incorporates four separate disorders: (Autistic Disorder (AD), Asperger's Syndrome (AS), Pervasive Developmental Disorder - Not Otherwise Specified (PDD-NOS), and Childhood Disintegrative Disorder) with differing levels of symptom severity (4,6).

As explained by the American Psychiatric Association (APA) Board of Trustees (December, 2012), ASD severity levels (defined in later sections of this chapter) are based on the amount of support services required as determined by diagnosable criteria (7). As stated in the DSM-5, the severity of symptoms of ASD will be more closely monitored, rather than referring to symptoms from a list of criteria, such as repetitive speech and/or language delay. In effect, this will reduce misinterpretation and possible confusion with other disorders such as Attention Deficit Hyperactive Disorder (ADHD) (8).

As listed in the DSM-5, to meet diagnostic criteria ASD is characterized by and requires three persistent deficits in the areas of

1) social and emotional reciprocity,

2) non-verbal communication behaviors,

3) developing and maintaining appropriate relationships,

4) repetitive speech, movements, or employing of objects,

5) excessive maintenance of routines, formalized patterns of verbal/nonverbal behavior, or excessive refusal to change,

6) highly restricted, unusual, fixated interests, (e.g. strong preoccupation with atypical objects), and

7) hyper- or hypo-reactivity to sensory input or extraordinary interest in appreciated aspects of the environment.

Symptoms must be present in childhood and cause significant impairment in customary social, occupational, or additional areas of functioning (1, 4). Diagnostic criteria are divided into two groups (A and B). All criteria in group A (listed above as one through three) need to be met, and at least two criteria need to be met in group B (listed above as four through seven).

Affected social and language interactions, as well as communication impairments as observed in autistic patients, are often manifested with a rigidity of interests, "restricted repetitive behaviors (RRB's), and interests and activities" (8). RRB's are co-morbid with Obsessive Compulsive Disorder (OCD), symptoms involving hyperactivity, Attention Deficit Disorder (ADD), Mood Disorder, severe isolation and sometimes suicide, adolescent cannabis and alcohol abuse, gastrointestinal problems and sensory integration disorders (1, 9). Due to social and language impairments, it is important to note that ASD individuals are also often the object of bullying because of being viewed as different.

The APA cites the reason for establishing ASD this way due to previous versions involving different clinicians diagnosing the same individual with different disorders. Some clinicians have been changing their patient's diagnosis (of the same symptoms) from year to year. Additionally, the APA contends that the new criteria based on data, or lacks thereof, are clearer and "inclusionary" (8). For example, the new criteria include:
1) gestures and verbal communication,
2) change the definition of social behavior from "failure to develop peer relationships, and
3) abnormal social play" (DSM-IV TR) to "difficulties adjusting behavior to suit different social contexts" (DSM-5). It should be noted the first three criteria echo that of the standards listed in the DSM-IV-TR for Asperger's syndrome.

Currently, school districts and managed care companies do not fund therapeutic services delivered to children diagnosed with AS. Therefore, a specific diagnosis of ASD would help in gaining aid for such services. The APA emphasizes that those who were diagnosed prior to DSM-5's release will not need to be re-diagnosed unless there exists an obvious, sensible, and clinical reason to reevaluate such an individual (10).

Historically, autism is defined by a common set of behaviors and, as previously mentioned, is now *ranked according to severity of defective social communications and repetitive behaviors* (7). Ranging from 3 to 1, the severity levels are illustrated as:

"3" requires very substantial support and includes severe deficits in verbal and nonverbal communications (the individual rarely initiates speech or minimal response to communicative initiative of others);

"2" requires substantial support (the individual displays a marked deficit in social communication skills and social impairments even with supports in place). There are limited interactions or responses to communicative initiative of others. The individual may speak simple sentences and odd non-verbal communication; and

"1" requires support services without the services in place. The individual exhibits difficulty initiating social interactions with others, are unsuccessful in responding to social interactions from others, and are able to converse with disconnection to others (1, 5).

Among restricted repetitive behaviors (RRB's), level "3" pertains to an inflexibility of behaviors with extreme difficulty coping with change and repetitive behaviors that interfere with functioning in all spheres. "2" relates to a difficulty coping with change, inflexibility of behavior, distress, and/or difficulty changing focus or action. Such individuals exhibit observable repetitive behaviors. "1" pertains to inflexible behavior; the individual has difficulty switching between activities and problems of organization that hinder independence (1, 5).

Given all these points, information now becomes confusing. According to the DSM-5, if an individual does not meet the criteria for ASD (as previously described), they should be assessed for Social Communication Disorder (SCD) or Pragmatic Language Disorder, neither of which are considered a form of autism. Therefore, based on the criteria for SCD, those who currently (*not* historically) present with Asperger's syndrome could very well receive a diagnosis of SCD instead (6,8). This conflicts with APA's statements.

What if an individual does not meet ASD criteria or present with social communication problems? If they do not meet the defined criteria, what should their diagnosis be? Additionally, SCD does not warrant funding for services as it is not listed under the umbrella of ASD and is a separate diagnosis, thereby reinforcing the proposal that Asperger's disorder will eventually decline and the diagnosis of SCD will increase dramatically (11).

Many experts question how these changes will affect those previously diagnosed or affect diagnoses in the future, and if an individual will lose her/his diagnosis and services which they currently receive from public sources (e.g., behavioral therapy) (11). On the one hand, ASD marks the merging of autism with Asperger's syndrome. For years, researchers and medical professionals have referred to AS as "high functioning autism". Until recently, Asperger's syndrome has not been included under the category of autism. It is proposed that some of these changes will allow diagnosing practitioners to spend more time focusing on ASD criteria and specific traits an individual is exhibiting (9). As previously stated, under DSM-IV-TR criterion, autism (ASD) presents as three or four different disorders. Parents will now be able to refer to the DSM-5 criteria and see if a description describes their child's behavior.

On the contrary, changes in the DSM-5 do not prevent anyone from receiving treatment and services. In many cases, it may actually improve these opportunities as some states provide services to those diagnosed with ASD (11). According to the DSM-5, a diagnosis of ASD can occur prior to the age of seven, whereas, the previous (DSM-IV-TR) requirement was prior to the age of three. This change eliminates the requirement of symptoms presenting in early childhood even though warning signs may not become fully manifest until social demands exceed limited capacities (12). Additionally, according to the first three criteria for ASD (social and emotional reciprocity, non-verbal communication behaviors, developing and maintaining relationships to the appropriate developmental level), some isolated Asperger's syndrome criteria continue to exist without the name.

On the other hand, the severity levels ignore any mention of intellectual disabilities in the definition. This broadens the spectrum at the high functioning end, as the first two levels of severity (as described earlier) describe typical variations in human behavior and personality, such as "no significant interference or impairment". Some experts believe this limits the assessment of severity, as it gives an impression that not many individuals would be diagnosed with a high level of severity (11). Others feel the changes ignore the public perception of AS and ASD (10).

A fear exists among those diagnosed and their families that change from a diagnosis of AS to a diagnosis of ASD may affect the manner in which they receive services and are perceived by others. This situation reinforces families' concern about whether or not their loved one will be stigmatized by clinicians who have no information about them upon first meeting. There is a large number of those already diagnosed with autism who have co-morbid intellectual disabilities and worry that the grouping of diagnoses may change the perception of those formerly diagnosed with AS. Many view AS as part of their identity (11).

By grouping all spectrum individuals together, it is projected they will lose their uniqueness and be unable to relate with a majority of those newly diagnosed with ASD. There may be more service options for those defined as autistic, particularly educational. However, are most of the services provided appropriate for those previously diagnosed with AS? The severity levels illustrate that along the autism spectrum, there are differences in abilities and working treatment options for helping these individuals (11).

An EEG study published in July, 2013 (two months after DSM-5's release) reported that AS and autism are biologically distinct. Neurologists at Boston Children's Hospital studied EEG data of children with ASD, with whom they compared children with normative cognitive development (12). They found that AS "manifests" with specific patterns of brain connectivity in children, suggesting biological differences between the two conditions (12). According to the lead investigator Duffy, "It is essential to separate these two groups because they need different education and training opportunity" (13). It is important to note that this study was only in reference to children. Additionally, it failed to suggest that Asperger's syndrome is fundamentally different from classical autism. Rather, it identified little differences between Asperger's and autism (1).

Conclusions

Since 1952, the DSM, with volumes and text revisions published by the APA, has been viewed as *the* manual for evaluation and diagnosis. Based on research by the APA, revisions of the DSM have been published approximately every 10-19 years. DSM III-R was published in 1980 and DSM-IV-TR was published in 1994 (8). It seems likely that the DSM-5 will be revised as well, thereby stoking concerns, controversy and debate. In fact, at the time of writing this chapter (October, 2013), the recently published edition of DSM-5 is already under revision. Some equate the DSM-5 with the DSM-II, published in 1968 (1).

A majority of sources debating the changes and their effects were projections, published prior to DSM-5's release. The changes have created many protests and have led to the filing of law suits (13). Arguments on one side claim that funding was placed mainly into research on AS and not enough into autism, while the other side posits that the DSM-5 promotes further research. Further time and research will tell just how much those with historically diagnosed AS and RS will be affected by the changes.

It is the uncertainty about the diagnostic criteria for autism that may, in part, account for the apparent rise in occurrence of the disorder (chapter 1C). Such indecision makes a comparison of statistics from one population to another or from one era to another ineffectual, without well-established criteria. As more is learned from research on the etiology and course of autism, the more likely stronger, reproducible diagnostic measures will be established and generally accepted. Serial modifications of the analytical standards without fundamental increases in the comprehension of the basic bio dynamics of the disease decreases, rather increases, understanding and progress in dealing with it.

ADDENDUM

When it comes to diagnostic and screening instruments for autism, there are many acronyms. Most clinicians consider the Autism Diagnostic Observation Schedule (ADOS) and the Autism Diagnostic Interview-Revised (ADI-R) as the gold standard tests for diagnosing the disorder. However, only a fraction of the hundreds of autism studies published each year use them to confirm the disorder in study participants. Hopefully, the DSM-5's definition of Autism (ASD) will make it easier for clinicians to use and diagnosis. Autistic behavior and symptom scales tests attempt to screen for or diagnose autistic-spectrum disorders. They may also be used to determine the level and severity of autistic behaviors (14).

Autism Behavior Checklist of the Autism Screening Instrument for Educational Planning (ABC-ASIEP): The score is presented as a scale indicating the existence and severity of autistic behavior, as contrasted to other disorders.

Autism Diagnostic Interview-Revised (ADI-R): It is used to conduct a standardized parent interview. It's based on the World Health Organization's definition of autism. Score is expressed as a scale.

Autism Diagnostic Observation Schedule (ADOS): This is a format for conducting a diagnosis via direct observation of the patient.

Autism Research Institute (ARI) Form E-2: Diagnostic Checklist: Parents who send the completed checklist to ARI will receive scaled test results, interpretive information, and information on autistic spectrum disorders at no charge. Form E-2 rates behaviors frequently seen in autism on a scale, and also asks parents to rate the results of any treatments they have tried. It is available in several languages. An optional ARI questionnaire, Form E-3, asks questions about treatments tried and their results. This is not a diagnostic tool, but part of ARI's efforts to build a large database on autism for research purposes.

Behavior Observation Scale for Autism (BOS): The BOS checklist is a direct-observation format intended to help evaluators distinguish autistic-spectrum children from normal or mentally retarded patients. Score is expressed as a scale.

Behavior Rating Instrument for Autistic and Other Atypical Children (BRIAC): This observation-based diagnostic tool looks at the areas of relationship to an adult, communication, drive for mastery, vocalization and expressive speech, sound and speech reception, social responsiveness, and psychobiological development. Additional scales are available for nonverbal and/or hearing impaired children. Scores are expressed as scales.

Childhood Autism Rating Scale (CARS): The CARS is a direct-observation format for evaluating the behavior of children and adolescents. Results can be scored on two scales, one with a range from "age appropriate" to "severely abnormal," the other with a range from "not autistic" to "mild-moderate autistic" to "severely autistic." An excerpt from the CARS is included in Appendix F.

Gilliam Autism Rating Scale (GARS): Three GARS subtests cover behaviors and their frequency in the areas of stereotyped behaviors, communication, and social interaction. A third subtest asks parents about developmental disturbances in the child's first three years. Scores are expressed as scales and percentages.

Parent Interviews for Autism (PIA): This set of questions for parents is frequently used when diagnosing younger or nonverbal children.

SOCIAL ISSUES

Chapter 2A - Family Dynamics

Jeffrey Gardere, Clinical Psychologist

[The effect of autism on intrafamilial interactions is profound because of the complexities of the disorder and the extra efforts needed by family members to deal with added pressures and responsibilities. – Ed.]

Hypothesis

With regard to disorders diagnosed in childhood, autism continues to capture the public attention and is ranked among the most stressful of disorders diagnosed in childhood for many reasons. With this disability we see problems with communication, emotional expressions and antisocial behaviors which in totality place an extreme amount of stress on every member of the family (1). Often this disorder can be considered a double disability because 80% of the cases also involve mental retardation, ranging from mild to severe. Therefore, autism is a disorder where a child can receive a DSM-5 diagnosis within the autism spectrum disorder and an additional diagnosis of mental retardation. A diagnosis of autism alone is a major challenge for both the autistic child and the family. But with the additional component of mental retardation, it becomes even more challenging.

Observations

There have been some recent developments in the news and on the scientific front which in their own way that illustrate, contribute or may even increase the stress that families face when they have a child with autism:

The new and controversial DSM-5, is causing ripples among parents in the autism community. Much to the chagrin of parents who have an autistic child(ren), the DSM- 5 eliminates Autistic Disorder, Asperger's Disorder, Childhood Integrative Disorder and Pervasive Developmental Disorder now has now been combined into Autism Spectrum Disorder (ASD) (2). Many of these parents believe that there may now be an over-diagnosis of ASD, resulting in more competition for therapeutic and educational services that are already in short supply. They are also fearful that children who have Aspergers or a very mild case of autism, may be diagnosed and placed into the new DSM category of Differential Diagnosis of Social (Pragmatic) Communication Disorder, which is not part of ASD (3).

There has been a questionable rise in the incidence rates of autism (chapter 1C). In March, 2013, the CDC reported that 1 in 50 school age children were diagnosed within the Autism Spectrum Disorder (4). That is a dramatic rise from the 1 in 88 statistic in 2008. The

New Jersey area still continues to baffle the experts with statistics that are closer to 1 in 33 (5). Of course, the issue here is the etiology; what may be causing the increased numbers in New Jersey and some other areas of the country. Many experts believe the increased numbers may be due to increased awareness and detection (6).

The increase in reported rates also has the unintended consequence of giving more momentum to those who believe environmental factors, including pollution and toxins, are involved with the etiology of autism (chapter 4E). There are also a number of parents who still believe that vaccines, especially the measles, mumps and rubella vaccine (MMR), may be a cause of autism (chapter 7A). This controversial belief was stoked by the work of gastroenterologist Andrew Wakefield and his colleagues. Their 1998 study (7), claimed that the MMR vaccine causes a series of events that include intestinal inflammation, followed by loss of intestinal barrier function, and the entrance into the bloodstream of encephalopathic proteins, and consequently, the development of autism. In support of his hypothesis, Wakefield described 12 children in his study with neurodevelopment delay, 8 with autism. All of these children had gastrointestinal complaints and developed autism within 1 month of receiving the MMR vaccine. To be clear, he emphasized a correlation (link) instead of causation.

At a press conference sometime after that, he suggested that the MMR vaccine was inadequately tested for safety as compared with the single vaccines(the measles vaccine, the mumps vaccine, the rubella vaccine), and therefore recommended that parents should have the option of one vaccine at a time, instead of all three combined in one vaccine at a time (8). However his research was discredited by a majority of the scientific community. Subsequently The British General Medical Council (GMC) conducted an inquiry into allegations of misconduct against Wakefield and two former colleagues (9). On Feb. 2, 2010, *The Lancet*, which published his first paper, officially retracted it and called it a flawed study. But the genie was out of the bottle.

There were many parents who went into fear and panic mode, and prevented their children from getting some if not all, of their inoculations. This resulted in diseases such as measles, which was almost eradicated, now making a resurgence, with serious outbreaks in different parts of the world (10). Quite recently there have been several news stories where scientists and epidemiologists attribute this resurgence directly to Wakefield (11). Though the mainstream scientific community has categorically stated there is no link between the MMR vaccine and autism, the controversy lives on. The recent rulings and monetary awards from the U.S.Vaccine Court for plaintiffs in two recent cases which contended that vaccines had caused brain injury leading to an ASD diagnosis (12), has kept this controversy going. Allegedly, the MMR vaccine was the common denominator in these cases (13). There are also parents who are diehard in their beliefs that vaccines, such as the MMR, have played a role in their child's autism. In addition, Wakefield continues to defend his research, while others are attempting to replicate his original study (14). Though the MMR vaccine is much less of a worry for most parents, it is still is a source of anxiety for newer parents who are wrestling with the decision whether to vaccinate or not. For those who believe their children were affected by the MMR vaccine a cause for guilt for allowing their children to get the vaccine, and anger at the pharmaceutical companies who they believe are much more concerned about profits than the health of children.

In another major development, in a study published online in the journal *Nature* in August, 2012 (15), researchers in Iceland found that as many as 20-30% of cases of autism and schizophrenia may be linked to the father's advanced age. This may be based on the supposition that as men age, their sperm may have acquired more mutations than when they were younger. The researchers studied 78 families and found that children born to 20 year old fathers had 25 mutations which were directly linked to the father's genes, while those born to 40-year-old fathers had 65 mutations (16).

The reality is that the overall risk to a man in his 40s or older fathering a child with autism is in the range of 2 percent, at most (17). There are still many unknown contributing biological factors. Certainly, older men should not be discouraged from having children, though they should be cognizant of the risk factors of advancing age in siring a child with developmental delays. For older fathers who have children with autism, this finding may fuel the guilt that a father may now feel in conceiving a child who develops autism. This is both a stunning and sobering finding, given that in the past, only the mother's and not the father's advanced age was the sole determinant as to whether a pregnancy will be high risk, especially for a developmental delay (18).

With regard to mothers, a new study from Harvard School of Public Health (19) shows women who experienced physical, emotional, or sexual abuse as children are more likely to have a child with autism, as compared to women who were not abused. Those who experienced the most serious abuse had the highest likelihood of having a child with autism — three-and-a-half times more than women who were not abused. The study authors believe that to a lesser extent, factors such as gestational diabetes, preeclampsia, and smoking, and to a larger extent, the effects of abuse on women's biological systems, such as the immune system and stress-response system, are responsible for increasing the likelihood of having a child with autism. Here the issue is not just about the guilt a woman who was abused may experience regarding her child having autism, but the dynamic of perhaps having depression, or even Post-Traumatic Stress Disorder related to that past abuse, on top of the overwhelming stress of raising her autistic child.

Often making the news are sensational yet tragic cases of filicide, sometimes along with attempted or successful suicides by the parents. The twist here is the murders of children with autism by their overwhelmed parents, primarily the mothers, who are often the day-to-day, stay-at-home caregivers. The general public has decried these parents and mourned the children. Still, blogs by parents who have children with autism put a human face and more complexity as to why these tragedies happen. These bloggers discuss the many severe challenges they, themselves have faced in raising a child with autism, including the incredible amount of emotional pain and stress they have experienced from financial hardships, marital issues, and the various other hardships that now become part of their daily lives.

The small number of parents who have killed their children and or themselves, had these very same issues. It could very well be that these parents most likely were not getting help or psychological treatment. Just as importantly, the blogger parents also share the dedication and love they have for their child with autism, including the incremental triumphs they are able to achieve. Their stories become a primer and lifeline and needed emotional support to other parents and their families who experience the very unique struggles and dynamics of raising a child with autism. These unique family dynamics, how they impact the family as a whole, as couples, parents and siblings, will be the focus of this remaining discussion in this chapter.

Stages of dealing with the diagnosis of autism

For many parents, accepting the initial diagnosis that their beautiful and beloved child is autistic, given what little they may know initially about autism, can be both terrifying and devastating. Though every parent and family handles this diagnosis in his or her own way, generally there are various stages that many parents experience in order to finally and fully accept a diagnosis which will forever change their lives, the lives of the present or future siblings, and, of course, the life of the affected child.

Denial and rationalization

Without knowing much about autism, most people generally understand it is a lifelong disability that requires a complete realignment of parental and family priorities. There are many parents who suspect their child may have a developmental disability such as autism and want a diagnosis so they can begin to address it right away. It is understandable that there are also other parents who want to avoid or delay this traumatic diagnosis for as long as they can. Even though they may observe some language, interactional or motor delays or even odd or reptitive behaviors, they either ignore or explain them away as being something more innocuous or insignificant. Some parents will hope that these behaviors will improve or even disappear. In essence, they put off getting a formal diagnosis for as long as they can, until one parent, family member, friend or most likely the pediatrician insists on their taking some action.

Fear and shock

Once the diagnosis of autism is made, it is again understandable that some parents may initially feel that their beautiful child is damaged or broken; for life. For parents accepting this diagnosis, it's implications and the fact that their child will have life long challenges can initially lead to feelings of shock, dread, apprehension and fear of the unknown. It is not just the initial diagnosis of autism, which is the problem, but the concern as to the level of autism, as well as the possibility of an accompanying mental retardation. Adding to this trauma is the reality that in many cases, unless the child is in the extremely high functioning range of ASD, he will require intensive therapeutic, educational and child care services for years to come. Depending on the severity it may extend through his adulthood. This child will now and for the foreseeable future, become the complete focus of the parents and family. That is certainly much for any parents , no matter how resilient, to accept without experiencing some emotional trauma.

Confusion

As part of this trauma, many parents also experience confusion as to the manifest and latent symptoms of autism in their child, as well as the progression of these symptoms emotionally and behaviorally through the coming years. The true confusion comes from the subject of our initial discussion at the beginning of this chapter, the definitive cause of autism. This question will be discussed in detail in other chapters of this book. It is this lack of information, the incomplete picture, not having definitive answers, which makes the autism diagnosis even more difficult to accept. Initially, with this incomplete clinical picture, parents are not confident as to where to start or what to do. To better accept a diagnosis one should have a cause and just as importantly a prognosis; often missing from a diagnosis of autism.

Blame and guilt

This incomplete clinical picture, the unanswered questions also has other emotional consequences. It is a natural tendency to want to know who or what may be the cause for an event or situation, especially one that is significant and life changing, such as autism. For the parents of an autistic child, one of the first targets of blame for the disorder is themselves. Then this blame causes guilt. Kanner (20) has posited that parents believe their own behavior is the cause of their child's autism. Furnham and Buck (21) and Gray (22) state that some parents believe they are being punished for the wrongs they committed prior to the birth of their child. Some parents ponder whether they may have a defective gene that causes autism. As part of this self investigation, some parents attempt to retrospectively determine what may have gone wrong or was missed with regard to a risk factor during the pregnancy. Even further, they consider whether there were pregnancy or delivery complications which may have been missed or masked. Some parents look outward to the environment either immediately or after, not being able to make any headway or get answers from the aforementioned avenues of query. These parents may question or believe that the environment or known or unknown toxins may have played a role in causing their child's illness. As mentioned earlier, even though the mainstream scientific community states that there is no link between the MMR vaccine and autism, there are still many parents and advocates who still trust Wakefield's conclusions. Thus the parents may blame the medical establishment and governmental agencies for giving a vaccine which they believed may have caused their child's problem

Gray (22) posits mothers are more likely than fathers to believe they are at blame for their child's autism To compound this self-guilt, finger pointing goes on between the parents especially when it comes to a condition such as autism. Fathers may be proclaiming many "I told you so's" to the mother for not breastfeeding their babies.

There are additional studies with risk factors (24,25) or links to autism (female sexual abuse, advanced age of the father) which may also cause both mothers and fathers, to blame themselves for their child developing autism (chapter 8A). In time, that guilt does pass when they realize that not only are they not at fault for their child's condition, but even if they are, to whatever extent, this accusation or self blame becomes wasted energy which should be better focused towards the care of their child.

Anger

Anger can follow or accompany the blame and guilt, especially as is evident in most cases of autism there is no clear cause or etiology. Parents ask,"why our child, why our family, why us?" This anger becomes even more magnified during times of stress and frustration, especially related to getting good educational and therapeutic services for their child. Parents complain that the services are too few and far from each other, and are embedded in a complex maze. Many parents have expressed frustration with the system and the lack of cooperation they receive from the institutions that provide or even fund these programs. This, of course, leaves parents feeling abandoned and isolated. Too often, that anger and frustration can be aimed at the other spouse, close family members, and, sadly the sick child.

Depression

The classic psychodynamic definition of depression as being anger turned inwards is very true, especially in dealing with autism. There is only so much anger one can carry before he/she becomes exhausted and the depressed, especially if that anger accomplishes nothing constructive. In addition many parents dealing with the initial diagnosis of autism have expressed that their depression has been fueled by the "dream deferred." Specifically, this can be described as the disappointment that the diagnosis of autism has turned all of the hopes and dreams they had for their child upside down. They will not be attending award ceremonies for academic achievement and excellence, the play dates may be far and few in between, and their child may not get married or have children. The "normal" happy family they envisioned will now be different with its very unique challenges.

The other part of this depression is that for their child with autism, the world may be a hostile and cold place. Even if they have very little experience with autism, these parents realize that their child will have to face a world that emphasizes "sameness," and, therefore, there will be times that he/she will be isolated, marginalized, discriminated, made fun of by other children, and faced with discrimination. It is quite understandable that this heartbreak can easily lead to depression. In time, parents of autistic children learn that it is not a dream deferred but rather a re-imagining of the dream. The child may not win scholarships to colleges, but will learn and achieve in a way that is self-fulfilling. At times he may be treated or viewed differently, but will gain confidence, believing in and loving himself. Maybe he will not grow up to become a doctor, but if he can find a good job, live independently, and have a loving mate, that would be a dream realized. Again, it takes time to get to that place emotionally and parents soon realize that it is their love, perseverance, managing, and controlling their frustrations, and accessing proper services and supports that will lead to the best possible outcome for their child with autism, as well as their own stability and happiness. Once they are able to get to this stage, they will have reached the stage of acceptance.

Acceptance

Once the parents get to the phase of acceptance, they are in a much better position to face the reality that their lives will be forever changed. This is where the hard work truly begins, because they now must reorganize and rearrange their lives to attend to the needs of their child who has autism. This phase of acceptance may not totally obliterate the previous phases, in that the anger, frustrations, guilt, and blame, especially during periods of stress, may very well present themselves repeatedly through the process of caring for their child. However, the acceptance of the autism diagnosis, the acceptance that the child with autism is special and therefore has a lifetime of special needs, the acceptance that life will never be the same again, the acceptance that this child will be the main focus of the family, the acceptance that they have been blessed with a loving child who will be different from most children, is the healthiest place for them to be emotionally.

Before going any further, it is important to point out that the phases previously described do not always apply to all parents. Though many parents do go through these phases, perhaps not even in the order presented, there are also many parents who are able to accept the autism diagnosis head-on and immediately empower themselves through information, education, support groups, and mobilization of family, to dig in and take on the Herculean task of caring for their child with autism.

Personally and clinically, I have encountered couples who during the pregnancy, discovered through the amniocentesis that their unborn child may have chromosomal abnormalities. No matter the consequence or manifestation, these parents have made the choice and conviction, to not abort, but to have the child and move forward as a family. In preparation, they have done their research and know what it takes to the best parents possible, and helping their child succeed in life.

At this point, let us address how having a child(ren) with autism specifically affects the family unit, mother, father and siblings.

The Family - toxic family, friends, and isolation

Having a child with autism has a major impact not just on the parents but if there are other children, on the entire family unit. Quite often the family can become a self contained unit, often isolated from extended family members and friends. Part of the reason is because the parents are going through the aforementioned phases of dealing with the autism diagnosis and may want to do this privately. Often times extended family members and friends may not have the understanding or patience to interact with the child who has autism. This is not to say that they are insensitive, most likely they may feel inadequate or incompetent in reacting to the child in an effective manner. Sad to say, they may be embarrassed to have the child with autism at their social gatherings, because he may act out and perhaps disrupt the occasion. Families often report how they may be invited to family or friend's parties or get-togethers, but it is suggested that the autistic child stay at home. All it takes is one snub for the parents of the autistic child to become skittish and overly sensitive to the point of withdrawing from any socially events regardless of whether they are invited or not.

Yet another part of this isolation may come from the fear that the child with autism may act out or even be out of control behaviorally in a restaurant, on public transportation, or some other public space. In these situations, especially in the early years, the parents may be extremely embarrassed by people staring or complaining about their child's behavior. Thus in order to avoid these situations they may no longer eat out or take family vacations, instead becoming more homebound and isolated. They begin to build a world that is more comfortable and circumscribed for the family. One that is safe and manageable, but also isolated. That may also mean eliminating unsupportive or even toxic friends and family. No family is an island and thus by sheltering themselves and their autistic child, which is psychologically unhealthy for the child and goes against the benefits of mainstreaming, their solitary life is often an unhappy and constricted. That is why it is recommended that they should make every effort to surround themselves with sympathetic individuals and supports networks, which makes the life mission of raising their child much more manageable and fulfilling.

Stress and depression

While it is known that parenting of a child with autism is stressful, this situation may become even more stressful for those who are poor, dealing with other emotional issues or are single-parent homes. Regardless of the aforementioned situations, whether a single or two parent home, families who are raising a child with autism have been found to have a higher risk for depression. In addition, the two-parent home appears to have marital discord, which is most likely related to the extreme amount of stress they experience raising the child with autism. (26). Contrary to the 80% divorce rate for married parents of an autistic child that has often been a topic of discussion in the autism community, we now know that the marital discord does not result in an inordinate divorce rate as compared to married couples without an autistic child. In fact, researchers at the Kennedy Krieger Center released the results of their study in May, 2010 (27) that showed 64 percent of children with an autism spectrum disorder (ASD) belong to a family with two married biological or adoptive parents, compared with 65 percent of children who do not have an ASD. However, the study does point out what is common knowledge and what has been shown in past studies: couples with a child with autism experience more stress in their marriage than couples with typically developing children or couples with children with other types of developmental disabilities, such as Down syndrome. One reason being that there are more resources made available for children with Down syndrome versus children with autism.

In addition to the depression and social isolation we tend to see in these family units, the parents are constantly emotionally aroused and vigilant, in caring for the physical and emotional needs of their child(ren) with autism, resulting in their being generally exhausted. Quite often they are not paying attention to their own needs as individuals or a couple tend not to take time off, relax, engage in hobbies, or nurture the romantic relationship. In other words they must be "on" all the time. So even though partners in the marriage or committed relationship can take shifts sharing the work, or have different work functions with regard to caring for the child with autism, it is still an overwhelming, all-consuming task. That is why even when the marriages stay intact, they tend to be very troubled and dysfunctional. . For the single-parent who has to raise an autistic child(ren) by him or herself: as one can imagine, it is more than overwhelming.

Financial issues

It is a well-known fact that the family who is raising a child with autism quite often may face financial ruin. According to *CNN Money* (28), the cost of providing care for a person with autism in the U.S. is estimated at $1.4 million over a lifetime. When you factor in a child with autism who is also mentally retarded, the cost jumps to $ 2.3 million, and that's in addition to the already existing cost of $241,080 associated with raising any child and which includes food, education and housing (29). The families who are fortunate enough to have insurance, have to pay at least $1000 out-of-pocket, monthly, for the therapies. President Obama's Affordable Care Act contains important provisions for individuals with autism and related conditions and their families (30). Under this new health care law, the financial burden should ease up to some extent. Nevertheless being under this kind of financial stress further adds stress to the family, and to the child with autism, especially if it is cost prohibitive for him or her to get all the services he needs.

Fighting for services

Therapeutic, educational and social services are essential for the autistic child and his family, especially early interventions services. The lack of a full compliment of such services may negatively impact the autistic child, as well as exacerbating the depression and burn out that accumulates over time within the family. The reality is that even though these services and supports are available through the educational and social system, navigating through the maze of delivery, insuring that the child is getting appropriate, adequate, and effective services, is extremely stressful for parents. There are then day to day struggles of making sure that the child is being treated fairly by students, teachers and administrators at school.

Historically, parents have had to keep up the pressure on provider entities to make sure that the child is also receiving adequate mainstream educational services since it is important that the child learn interactional skills outside of special education instruction. This effort places the parents in the role of caseworker, which can be a fulltime job, on top of the fulltime job of working out side the home, and in the home, caring for the autistic child and the family. As one can imagine, this constant and diligent work also contributes to personal frustration and burn out.

Fighting for therapeutic and educational services are a significant dynamic, given that in the first several years of the autism diagnosis, parents rely on these services as a major lifeline, for their child with autism. As the autistic child grows to young adulthood and is less in need of these services , the parents rely much more on their own emotional and familial supports.

Religion and spirituality

Because the task of raising a child with autism is so enormous and overwhelming, it is not surprising that these families find solace, inspiration and support through religion and or spirituality. This point is supported by Bristol (31) who found that families with a child with autism, were more likely to utilize strong moral or religious beliefs for coping, versus the families who did not have a child with autism. There are families who may already have a predilection towards religion, while other families may turn anew to religion, or rediscover their old one, in order to renew their faith as a source of strength and or relief to raise their child with autism.

Many families dealing with autism have found comfort, energy, hope and joy from their religion and/or spirituality. It helps them cope with the situation that at times can seem impossible; but most importantly gives them a perspective that goes beyond psychology, but into a spiritual realm, where everything is possible, including the peace and happiness of their child with autism.

Mothers

Women, whether married or single, are traditionally the stay at home parent versus men, in the raising of children with or without autism. Of course, this landscape is changing as more men than ever before are also accepting the stay- at- home role. Given that women are more prone than men to depression and anxiety in general, it should still be noted that mothers of autistic children, experience higher levels of anxiety and depression than fathers with autistic children (32-34). To be clear, this is not about which parent is more affected, but more importantly how they are affected differently and specifically to their gender.

Because mothers are more likely to believe that they are more at fault for their child's autism then the fathers (23), they may consciously or unconsciously believe that their one mission in life is to care for that child, even if it means ignoring their own emotional or physical health. It should be stated that there are many mothers who do not feel that guilt, but because they are the stay at home day to day providers, they engage in the same behavior of completely dedicating their every waking hour to the care of their autistic child and not fully tending enough to their own needs. Because of this lack of attention to their own health, a good number of these moms put themselves at significant risk for physical and emotional illness (35). This is why it is important that mothers and, of course, fathers of children with disabilities or significant illness are constantly advised to take time out and care for themselves.

Women, in this case mothers of children with autism, tend to express their feelings more than fathers. Therefore, it is easier for them to verbally express their frustrations and grief, and can cry, which is a great catharsis. In addition, these mothers engage much more in healthier coping behaviors than fathers, by actively seeking out social supports (36). For the single mother dealing with autism, it can be much harder raising a child with autism alone, without a spouse or partner. They have the additional worry of staying healthy so that their child with autism is taken care of for as long as possible, even into adulthood.

Mothers who have careers outside the home report that they have serious limitations to the time dedicated to their workplace, given the hours they must give to their child with autism. Therefore they are unable to fully excel in their chosen occupation or profession. This frustration can perhaps put them more at risk for depression, substance abuse, and or other mental health issues (37).

Fathers

While mothers have higher levels of anxiety and depression, fathers of children with disabilities have higher levels of stress associated with the child's lack of ability to communicate (38), which may then negatively impact their feelings of attachment for the child. To be clear, it is not, that these fathers do not love their children with autism fully, it is just that fathers tend to bond with their infants differently than mothers. Because the fetus develops within the mother, they develop a visceral bond. In fact a one week old baby can recognize the smell of the mother over that of the father (39). On the other hand, men tend to bond with their infants through verbal and social exchanges. Children with autism in many cases interact much less with the parent, versus a child without autism. Autism, therefore, interferes with the verbal/interactional bonding between father and child. When stressed by the day to day rigors of raising a child with autism, this lack of verbal and social bonding, may put these dads at emotional risk to questioning their love for their child. This often results in the dads having overwhelming guilt about these feelings. But surely as the years pass these fathers are better able to overcome these issues and bond with their autistic child just as well as the moms.

DeMeyer (40) believes that fathers have the same stressors and issues as the mothers but are unable to express them and internalize them, as fathers do in general, regardless of the presence of autism in their children. Houser and Seligman (41) found that father's of children who are mentally retarded use more withdrawal and avoidance behaviors than fathers raising unaffected children. Therefore, fathers are not affected less than mothers, by the reality of having a child with autism, it is that they process and react to the experience along gender lines.. Historically males are socialized from youth to avoid crying, or showing too much emotion. Instead they are taught to be stoic and be that emotional rock that their families can lean on. That is why men often suffer "silently" when dealing with many types of stressful situations, including raising a child with autism; they just do not want to express their feelings about it. Thus many fathers say that their child's autism does not affect them greatly, when, in fact it does, though they may not recognize it, or choose to not address it. That it is also why in the two parent home it is not surprising that many fathers say that they are not concerned about themselves but are much more concerned about the stress on their wives or partners.

Fathers tend to also withdraw more than mothers and may engage in coping behaviors such as all consuming work outside of the home, which may be why some mothers tend to complain of the "lack" of participation in the caring of their child with autism. Again looking at gender roles, many males are socialized into believing that their job and worth, is to earn money, and provide safety and security for their family. However with or without a child with autism, men are redefining their roles and doing more of the hands on parenting, finding that balance between work outside and within the home (42). The most important point to be made here is that fathers may appear to be less affected by the stress of raising a child with autism, but they ARE affected, they do care, and they do love their children with autism as much as the mothers do.

Siblings

The siblings of a child with autism are also affected in both negative and positive ways. Often times they isolate themselves from friends because of being too embarrassed to be associated with their autistic sibling. They may be too afraid to have friends over, or take that sibling out among their friends because they are unsure as to how their sibling with autism may behave. The reality is that their friends may be very uncomfortable with the autistic sibling and may in turn withdraw from the unaffected sibling. For these reasons the sibling of the autistic child may have higher levels of loneliness and problems with peers. This loneliness is often times directly related to the lack of social support from peers (43). Such loneliness may also contribute to depression and academic failure.

This is a very difficult situation, given the strength of peer pressure and being like other youngsters during this timer in their lives. At times they may feel the need to dissociate from their affected sibling so as to have periods of a "normal" childhood. The sibling without autism also develops feelings of anger, jealousy, and hate towards their autistic brother or sister, who have become the center of the family (44). These feelings are especially strong when going through the emotional, and hormonal, fueled angst of the adolescent and teen years. At the same time these thoughts and feelings eventually give way to guilt, because of the true love the sibling without autism does have for their autistic brother or sister.

The unaffected sibling is often required to pitch in and be part of the working family in taking care of the needs of the sibling with autism. That means missing some of the activities and significant events that kids should enjoy as part of growing up: such as family vacations, meals at restaurants, etc.

On the positive side, because of their exposure to the realities and stress of assisting in the care of their sibling(s) with autism, these siblings develop maturity , empathy, responsibility, and the acceptance of those who are different, quicker than their contemporaries who do not have a sibling with autism or another developmental disability.

Factors which contribute to healthier outcomes for the family and the autistic child

The old adage of "what doesn't kill you only makes you stronger" is quite true when it comes to dealing with autism. The diagnosis of autism in one's beloved child can be a shock initially, one that can change the previous life plans of the family. Yet despite the incredible amount of stress and hardship these families experience, they not only survive, but eventually thrive. Still there are families who struggle mightily in this situation because of a lack of financial, educational and therapeutic resources. While those who are more successful in taking care of the needs of their child with autism along with the needs of the entire family have learned to access a full range of resources and supports.

In addition, these families have been able to establish coping and empowerment strategies in order to get the best outcome for the child(ren) with autism at the same time as maintaining the emotional, physical and financial stability of the family. The following are the traits, habits, practices and strategies that these successful and healthier families utilize.

Seek a quicker diagnosis

Though it is a natural tendency to be in denial when first witnessing the initial signs of autism in one's child, never the less, the "clock is ticking." and time moves on. Research studies have shown that early identification and intervention can make the critical difference in a more positive and therapeutic outcome for the child with autism (44). The families who are able to get a quicker and more definitive diagnosis of autism, also are at a healthier place emotionally to not only care for their child with autism, but also are more empowered to begin seeking and accessing services, treatments, and both formal and informal support groups.

As parents, they do not engage in the blame game against one another. Again, though it is natural to try to place blame on one another as parents, as to the cause of autism, this does become a very futile and frustrating approach. Though there may be cases where a genetic factor or an identified environmental toxin may yield an inordinate number of autism cases, the reality is that ~~many~~ most parents may never know the definitive cause of their child's autism. Even if the parents do find a definitive cause, at the present time, in most cases, there is no viable cure. Therefore, parents are better served by directing their full energies and focus towards the best services and practices for getting positive outcomes for their child with autism.

Get early intervention services as quickly as possible

As discussed previously, an early diagnosis and acceptance of that result will yield a quicker intervention and better long term outcome for the child with autism. That is why once a parent suspects autism, or a general disability, or a physician or mental health clinician, has made an autism diagnosis, Early Intervention Services should be established immediately. The Early Intervention Program (EIP) is mandated by the Individuals with Disabilities Education Act (45). This act states that all children in the U.S. have a right to a "free appropriate public education." Early Intervention Programs are specifically designed for children at risk for or diagnosed with a disability; in this case, autism. Studies have shown that children, regardless of their disability, who receive such services on the whole, show better emotional, physical and social functioning during their academic and future years (46,47).

Fully explore and participate in various therapeutic and social services

In addition to Early Intervention Services, which are essential for the child with autism, parents should also explore many other social services and treatments, including: nutrition, music, dance, art, yoga, sports, play therapy, behavioral therapy, speech therapy and family therapy. All of these approaches, individually, or in combination, have provided some degree of assistance and therapeutic gain in the treatment of autism (47). Also, as stated earlier, parents, perhaps with the guidance of a trusted health professional, should research and explore the standard and new, traditional, alternative, and holistic treatments.

It is also important that parents become an equal and deciding partner with all treatment professionals in making decisions and participating in the delivery of services both outside and inside the home (chapter 2C). In essence, parents should become the co-physician, the co-speech therapist, the co-behavioral modification specialist, etc. This assures a continuity of care as well as full and enthusiastic participation from the providers. This is especially important because children with disabilities often fall through the cracks, in the treatment and educational services maze, resulting in haphazard treatment and attention.

Finally, being involved as a co-partner to the professionals, in helping treat the child with autism, brings a sense of mastery and self-empowerment to the parents. As well, the child with autism, also gains a sense of security, comfort, and mastery, knowing his or her parent is involved in the treatment and educational programs. Dr. Robert Nadeef, a clinical psychologist who wrote the book, *Special Children*, and who has a grandchild with autism, states that once you begin in the direction of helping your child through these services and there is progress, the mood brightens and hope is there again.

Financial planning

Given the high cost of treating autism, over the lifetime of the child, in addition to the cost of raising an entire family, it is wise to consult with a financial planner who specializes in the costs of the treatment of autism. It is just as important to use a certified accountant/ tax preparer who can help with every possible tax advantage and or deduction regarding the related costs of autism. For those who cannot afford these services, joining autism support groups for parents, is a viable way to learn helpful financial strategies.

Emotional supports

Support groups either formal or informal provide families dealing with autism, the opportunity and catharsis to address their stresses, frustrations, and other feelings. With the support group they can vent, cry, and even learn and share empowerment strategies.

Online interactive and support groups are also a great resource when one is in crisis and cannot wait for their group to meet in person, or for various reasons it is not convenient to join an in-person group, or the in-person group is too far away geographically. The online groups also have the advantage of have access, 24 hours a day of a global community of a fully diverse group of parents and families who are dealing with autism.

Taking care of oneself

A major problem and even downfall for couples/parents of the child with autism is focusing only on the child and not taking care of themselves. These parents then place themselves at risk for psychological and medical illness. Their marriages, relationships and family lives also begin to suffer. That is why it is vitally important that parents, siblings and other family members who are taking care of a child with autism, also take the time to address and care for their own needs. We hear it every time we fly on an airplane: "in case of an emergency landing, pull down the oxygen mask, place it around your nose and mouth, then do the same for your child." My point is that if you as the parent do not take care of yourself, eventually you will not be able to provide care in a healthy, loving and efficient manner for your child and your family.

Every expert recommends that parents of a child with autism should take some personal time, to pursue a hobby, exercise, eat well, and make time for simple pleasures. For parents who are married or in a committed relationship, take the time for simple niceties such as: a daily kiss, flowers in the bedroom, or if possible, an overnight or long afternoon at a nearby hotel.

Taking care of the needs of the siblings without autism

Families who have both survived and thrived in raising a child with autism, are mindful that their children without autism, wherever possible, also need to be equally and individually loved. A good strategy in the two-parent home is to have one parent spend time with the child with autism and, the other parent can spend one-on-one time with the unaffected child. Of course with a single parent, achieving this task can be a bit more daunting. Here, perhaps another family member or friend can baby sit the child with autism, while the parent spends time with the unaffected child.

Given that everyone in the family should do their part in caring for the autistic child, it is also important to not overburden the unaffected child with the caretaking duties of the autistic sibling. The fact is every child should have the luxury of experiencing and enjoying a childhood. Therefore it is also recommended that the child without autism also be afforded the opportunity of getting their own psychotherapy, in order to address and process their feelings concerning how their lives are being impacted by having a brother or sister with autism.

An attitude of gratitude

Parents who are successfully coping with raising their child with autism have an "attitude of gratitude." In other words, no matter the hardships brought on by the autism, they are able to appreciate every little bit of progress that is made by their child. They appreciate his nuances, strengths and his unique beauty. Most importantly they appreciate his or her existence.

Conclusions

The families that have made it through the maelstrom of receiving the diagnosis of autism as well as living the daily struggle and triumphs of having a child with autism seem to agree on one thing: it has been the most challenging but yet satisfying experience of their lives. In essence, they have been able to bring love and care to their affected child, the child they love, the child they adore, and the child they would give their lives for. It is the same thing that any parent should do as they would for any child.

Chapter 2B: Societal Implications
Katherine Triplett, Dana Libov, Jean-Paul Leva

[The difficulty faced by medical professionals in trying the ameliorate the status of children with autism can test the confidence of families in their educated, trained partners to achieve some improvement in the performance of affected siblings and offspring. – Ed.]

Hypothesis

The unsubstantiated proposed etiologies of autism spectrum disorders (ASD) have been propagated through society by many unreliable sources, especially the media. Rhoades, Scarpa and Salley suggest that parents of children with ASD admit to relying on the media for information regarding their child's diagnosis rather than turning to healthcare professionals (1). Additionally, many parents openly admit to lacking confidence in physicians with their ability to correctly diagnose their ASD child. This is evidenced by one parent's concern stating, "it was a lack of knowledge on the physician's part that delayed a diagnosis for [their] child" (2).

Observations

The role the media has served poses two problems: the misinterpretation of available information and the abandonment of physicians as a reliable resource. Given the recent changes to the Diagnostic and Statistical Manual of Mental Disorders' (DSM) criteria of ASD, physicians have been presented with the unique opportunity to recover the role as the primary source of information for those with ASD (chapters 1C,1D).

The media has long been responsible for perpetuating the myth of an 80% divorce rate amongst parents of children with ASD, despite the absence of an epidemiological study to corroborate this claim (3). Upon hearing a statistic of this sort, the parents of a child with ASD may believe they are faced with a double prognosis – the difficulty of raising a child with ASD and the possible disintegration of a marriage. Hartley et al., studied 391 parents of a child with ASD and compared divorce to those parents of "same-age typically developing children" (4).

Although parents of an ASD child are indeed at an increased risk of divorce (23.5%), as compared to those parents in the control group (13.81%), it is important for them to be reassured that that this is not the daunting 80% that is constantly cited (3). This statistic, however, should not be interpreted to mean that raising a child with ASD does not come with unique challenges.

Parents raising a child with ASD are often faced with an increased financial burden on top of dealing with a unique set of stressors that may not be present in the family dynamic of those without a child with ASD (chapter 2A). In fact, it has been recognized that "few disabilities appear to be more taxing on parents than ASD" (5). Though there have been attempts to improve insurance coverage for individuals diagnosed with ASD, caregivers are still faced with increased expenses to ensure their child's needs are being met.

Furthermore, over half of the parents with ASD children have had to reduce or even completely eliminate their working hours in order to adequately provide for their affected child's needs (6). In a study examining the stressors mothers of children with ASD faced compared to those of children without disabilities, it was found that mothers of ASD children experienced more "fatigue, arguments, avoided arguments, and stressful events" (7). These mothers also reported spending more time on childcare, as well as up to one additional hour attending to household chores, compared with mothers without an ASD child (7). These stressors are sure to not only impact the mothers themselves, but also the rest of the household. These results highlight the need for support services from both the community and physician for families caring for an ASD child.

Effective May, 2013, the DSM-V criteria comprised a broader definition of ASD, which now includes the "previous DSM-IV autistic disorder (autism), Asperger's disorder, childhood disintegrative disorder, and pervasive developmental disorder " (8). This changing definition of ASD will have societal implications, as it will also redefine society's current understanding of ASD. Thus, it is an opportune time for clinicians to change the ASD community's dependence on media as a primary information and advisory resource.

This opportunity is supported by the fact that the DSM criteria are aimed at medical professionals. As per the American Psychiatric Association, the Diagnostic and Statistical Manual of Mental Disorders, Fourth Edition, Text Revisions (DSM-IV-ITR) has been used by professionals in a wide array of clinical and research contexts; they include "psychiatrists and other physicians, psychologists, social workers, nurses, occupational and rehabilitation therapists, and counselors" (9). As the intended readership is similar for DSM-V, this problem is two-fold. First, the patients and their families have neither a reliable clinical resource to recognize early indicators of ASD nor a reference to understand the implications of this diagnosis. Second, the DSM criteria assume the professional's role in educating patients about the guidelines. As aforementioned reports indicate, the ASD community's weakened trust in physicians' ability to recognize ASD. This suggests an inherent conflict in the clinician-patient relationship. In order to redirect the ASD community's dependency from media outlets and local resources to clinicians and professionals, we need to improve the medical community's understanding of ASD diagnoses and provide meaningful, scientifically based care for those affected by ASD.

Many parents distrust their physician's ability to properly diagnose ASD (chapter 1A). The misdiagnosing of ASD may be due to "lack of familiarity with the disorder or underutilization of standardized clinical measures" on the part of physicians (10). Delayed diagnoses may result in families seeking outside resources for care (2). Furthermore, physicians are "concerned about the effects of labeling children as autistic" because there are neither concrete, standardized criteria for diagnosis nor a known etiology (10). According to Rhoades, Scarpa and Salley, this may also be attributed to a lack of experience and training in those working with such patients. As a result, children with ASD often go undiagnosed until early childhood. These authors recommend that physicians should receive specialized training regarding autism spectrum disorder in order to improve early diagnoses (1).

The need for directed training and diagnostic criteria is echoed in the American Academy of Pediatrics' (AAP) desire for early screening, diagnosis and intervention. The AAP "recommends that surveillance begin with the first visit to the pediatrician", along with subsequent "universal screening at 18 and 24 months" (6). Improving physician's specialized training in ASD and systematic, earlier screening should decrease delays in diagnosis and, in turn, reestablish the faith in the physician's role as the primary diagnostician and educator.

The establishment of this role is further recognized in the medical home model. A medical home is defined by the Agency for Healthcare Research and Quality (AHRQ) "as a model of the organization of primary care that delivers the core functions of primary health care." According to this definition, the medical home should have the following attributes: "Comprehensive care, patient-centered, coordinated care, accessible services, [and] quality and safety" (11).

The obstacles faced by individuals with ASD and their families are difficult (chapters 2A-2C). According to Kogen et al., "Children with special health care needs" (CHSCN) with ASD, compared to those without ASD, have a significantly greater amount of challenges. CHSCN, along with their families, "have greater financial, employment, and time burdens compared with other children with special health care needs." The finding that families of ASD children who did not have access to a medical home "had a higher burden on almost every indicator" as compared to the families with access to a medical home led these authors to suggest that the procurement of a medical home could help to benefit the ASD community (6). This approach to medical care caters to a medical community who is currently dependent on sourcing their own resources. The Primary Care Physician (PCP) as a comprehensive care provider, serving as a liaison for coordinated patient care, would help to lessen the burdens expressed by individuals with ASD and their families.

Included in the "patient-centered" attribute of the medical home model is addressing the patient from a whole person vantage and "understanding and respecting each patient's unique needs, culture, values, and preferences" (11). This approach is particularly relevant given the aforementioned desire for resources and support by individuals with ASD and their families. In concordance with Thomas, et al., this model should be tailored to the individual in order to account for the child with ASD's individual strengths and deficits (12). "In order to define meaningful treatment goals and strategies," the whole person vantage of the child and the child's family should be considered (12).

In order to create an open conversation between parents of children with ASD and their PCP, physicians need to tailor their care to the racial, ethnic and cultural value system of the individual and their family. By improving the physician's central, coordinating role in the advocacy and provision of care of the patient with ASD and their family, physicians will be able to regain the trust of the affected individuals. Additionally, physicians can serve the important role of dispelling myths and false information regarding ASD, misconstrued and or misinterpreted through pop sources of information.

Conclusions

The ASD community has drifted towards a reliance on resources other than the clinician or primary care physician. Facilitating more clinician involvement would provide more accurate, comprehensive and valuable information to individuals with ASD and their families. In turn, the individuals with ASD and their families would rely more upon and better trust the physician. Lastly, this change in behavior would also help to improve early diagnosis and intervention in accordance with the goals of the DSM-5.

The popular media has an important role to play in bringing to the attention of the lay public advances in science and medicine. Now is the time for physicians to regain the affected community's trust by becoming better educated on the diagnosis and early intervention options available to deal with affected individuals, while educating caregivers about the realities of raising a child with ASD.

Chapter 2C – Therapy Difficulties

Venus Steinman, Speech Pathologist

[The complexities involved with trying to assist autistic children in overcoming their social and functional limitations emphasize even further the urgent need to solve the question of the origin of this neurologic disorder – Ed.]

Hypothesis

From the "red flags" that are detected, to the official diagnosis, to the countless hours and money spent on specialists, a diagnosis of Autism Spectrum Disorder (ASD) is life-changing. This is because the child affected will have specialists working with him/her for many, many hours to facilitate his ability to communicate (in this social world in which we live). For as many research and written articles there are written on autism, many people still do not have a good understanding of what autism is and how it affects the person labeled with it. Sadly, in most cases, this disorder is disrupting. The affected child will be judged by the label "autistic" that he/she carries first and not by what is offered to the world as an *individual* with autism.

Dealing with families of children with ASD, I have witnessed the difficulties that the families have endured and the problems of the children, who either cannot verbally communicate or struggle socially. As a speech-language pathologist, I have worked with several children diagnosed with ASD. According to the American Speech-Language-Hearing Association (ASHA), a "Speech-Language pathologist is responsible for the diagnosis, prognosis, prescription, and remediation of speech, language, and swallowing disorders; a speech-language pathologist evaluates and treats children and adults who have difficulty speaking, listening, reading, writing, or swallowing. The overall objective of speech-language pathology services is to optimize individuals' ability to communicate and swallow, thereby improving quality of life" (1). Because difficulties with communication and social skills are symptoms that are (initially) noted, a speech-language pathologist (SLP) takes an active role in aiding the all-encompassing life of an individual with ASD (2).

Observations

In managing affected children, the professional can assist in the assessment and diagnostic process as well as in the therapeutic aspects which involve improving communication and social-language development. Diagnostically, SLPs define and determine what are an individual's communication and social deficits. Therapeutically, they plan and set goals to work towards that are suitable for each individual treated, focusing on communication and social language.

Although ASD is a disorder characterized by deficits in social skills, communication, and the way that the individual relates to the world around him, (2), the severity and the behaviors of each individual vary. For essentially all of the children with ASD evaluated and/or treated by SLPs, the core difficulties are similar; however, their symptom expression and severity of deficit are different. The challenges to the therapist are:

1) assessing and providing the goals, techniques, and strategies that work for each individual child,
2) collaborating with other specialists and educators on the best learning style/environment for the child,
3) educating parents and educators, and
4) advocating for individuals with ASD to provide them with a better quality of life.

In this section of the book, I will describe the difficulties that children with ASD and their families encounter from the perspective of a Speech Language Pathologist. I have provided therapy in both home and school-based settings for children with ASD. With regard to evaluations, members of an interdisciplinary team in schools help reaffirm the diagnosis of ASD that had been made, as well as reading paperwork that families are asked to fill out and speaking with the guardians of children that have exhibited "red flags" are always difficult. Typically, the children that have been seen by the professional team (i.e., neurologist, psychiatrist, developmental specialists, speech-language pathologist, occupational therapist, physical therapist, social worker, and special education teacher), accompanied by their guardians. Typically, they have had the same nervous looks on their faces, a look that expressed imparted that they did not want their biggest fear confirmed. There have been times in which guardians have broken-down and cried as I was doing my evaluation because they were witnessing my attempt to elicit language skills that their children did not successfully achieve. I highlighted and pinpointed aspects of prelinguistic and linguistic skills, as well as social skills, that their child was unable to (or in many cases, they would exhibit scattered skills) demonstrate. Fear, nervousness, and anxiety were often emotions that were expressed.

When an initial diagnosis is made (typically, by a pediatric neurologist or developmental pediatrician), the guardians/parents usually need time to understand what ASD means and what the diagnosis entails. Many are bewildered, wondering what the next step is. Some are overly verbal and ask many follow-up questions, desperate to take an initiative. On the other hand, many appear to be very overwhelmed and remain quiet. All are extremely concerned about their child's daily life and about what the future may hold for them and the family. No matter when a child is diagnosed with ASD and how the professionals who are part of the interdisciplinary team try to educate the parents/guardian about what steps come next, no one could truly prepare a person about the challenges that lie ahead for their child and their family.

In working with parents of children diagnosed with ASD in the public school system, I have stressed to them that my role is not only to provide therapy for their child, but also to collaborate with them and with the rest of the child's team to educate and advocate for their child. A child's team varies as symptoms vary. Therefore, a team could consist of, but is not limited to, a general education teacher, a special education teacher, speech-language therapist, administrators, paraprofessionals, psychologist, occupational therapists, physical therapists, a social worker, and, at times, a nurse. It is important that the team works together, *not* separately, as it pertains to the child. Each professional can impart knowledge about what is thought to be best for the child with ASD based on the practitioner's area of expertise. In turn, the team needs to periodically reassess, discuss, and update what works best for each child. The professionals strive to provide an optimal experience for the affected subject in his/her academic setting.

Although the specialists within the school make up the primary team, the parents and/or guardians are very much a part of the team as well. The parents/guardians of a child with ASD are their lifeline. No one knows a child better than his/her own parent or guardian. They are able to update the therapist with information that may not otherwise be known. New behaviors that they have noticed in their child when in certain situations, changes in family dynamic, new medications that the child may be taking, or simply what the child's sleeping pattern has been like over a matter of time is important. Conversely, parents/guardians require feedback from those who work with their child professionally in order to reinforce skills and therapeutic strategies that are being incorporated in the academic setting. With everyone working together, the child with ASD will, hopefully, be more successful in achieving functional goals.

The team in the school must be in constant contact with the family. Being a school-based therapist, knowing that caseloads are often full, I am aware that there is not much time to communicate via phone calls with parents. Therefore, I make occasional phone calls. However, I typically use a notebook designated for communication between myself and my children's parents/guardians as a primary source of communication. In my experience, parents/guardians have many questions about the progress of their child. "Will my child ever be able to-------?" "What is your opinion about ------?" "Do you think that my child is in the appropriate learning environment?" are often questions that are asked. The continuous concern and worry in conjunction with the hope that their child will be able to relate to his/her environment and/or communicate and improve his social language skills is always on the minds of the parents. Therefore, setting appropriate goals, achievable goals and goals that are functional, should always be a priority of the team.

In setting goals for a child with ASD, it is vital that the objectives are appropriate for *him/her*; ASD is not a "one-size-fits-all" diagnosis. With that in place, a child with ASD is able to make gains in his communication and social skills. According to ASHA's (American Speech-Language-Hearing Association) National Outcomes Measurement System, a study was conducted that concluded that 2/3 of the preschoolers (the study did not indicate where on the spectrum these students fell) who participated in this study made progress towards specific goals provided with 2-5 times more therapy intervention than children who received no intervention. Functional communication gains were made on one or more levels on a series of a seven-point rating scale. Moreover, progress was made in the area of spoken language (73%) and in the area of pragmatics, (64%) after receiving intervention by an SLP (3). However, collaboration between the professional team and the child's parents, as well as continued reassessment of appropriate therapeutic approaches, is imperative toward the child's communication and social progress.

As stated earlier, children's improvements towards particular objectives are based on appropriate targets being set for each individual child, as well as the teamwork that is implemented thereafter. It is not uncommon during the course of the school year that I am speaking on behalf of a child with ASD to educators about the core difficulties that are dictated by the disorder. A child's Individualized Education Plan (IEP) is a particularized proposal that is prepared by a team of educators, professionals, and parents that includes the present educational status of the child, outcomes of evaluations that have been conducted by the school, and goals for the child. The team meets annually to discuss the progress that the child made and whatever additional concerns there may be of the parent and/or educator. The SLP not only modifies speech-language goals, but also discusses changes in the way that information is being presented in the classroom as well. The therapist analyzes what he/she knows about the child, talks it over with the team at the meeting, and, together, sets appropriate modifications and accommodations on the IEP.

Modifications are "changes in what is being taught to or expected from the student and accommodations are changes that help a student overcome or work around his disability." (4)

Both are extremely important as they are the key to helping the child with ASD progress in the classroom. An example of an accommodation for a child with ASD who may have difficulty with loud noises (i.e., noisy auditorium, noisy cafeteria) would be earplugs (or headphones); Ear plugs that would dull down the noise and make the child more comfortable. However, for another child this may not be appropriate. He may need to have lunch with a small group (to encourage socialization and only if possible) in the classroom, as the ear plugs may not be suitable to him. Choices of this nature need to be discussed and considered, as the child with ASD, in certain respects, often cannot advocate for himself in that his world around him is too overbearing. Furthermore, he may not be able to state in a socially appropriate manner that he is overstimulated and, perhaps, needs a break.

Typically, when a child with ASD is overstimulated, tantrums, outbursts and refusals to cooperate are evident. As an SLP, as with other professionals that work with the child, it is one's job to help enlighten the educators on what is the best way to approach a situation that will, hopefully, prevent a breakdown from occurring in the academic setting. Although this may be challenging for educators to deal with, we must do our best in trying to facilitate an environment and situations that will prevent such behaviors. The team must also realize that while professionals and educators are dealing with these challenges in school, parents of children with ASD face and cope with these behaviors at home, afterschool, on weekends, holidays, and summers. Additionally, they are aware of what is being done within the schools as well, and are at times asked to be involved in making choices that will assist in their child's ability to get by in school. To attempt to comprehend what a parent and family of a child that has ASD go through, one has to realize and respect what they are faced with on a daily basis and the difficulties that impact their lives.

For the parents, their children's rigidity, breakdowns, and refusals to cooperate are often extremely difficult for them to handle. Parents often appear to be frustrated, saddened, and stressed from what might not typically faze a child without an ASD diagnosis. Parents of children with ASD who are enrolled in general education schools have the added stress of dealing with other children who do not have a diagnosis of ASD. They may be notified of behaviors that range from uncooperativeness because their child is agitated by topics that do not interest them in the classroom, to their child screaming because a peer got too close during a lineup, to a child having difficulty with transitioning between activities.

It is a challenge to educate people who do not work closely with affected children. This may be due to the nature of the disorder; ASD is a communication and social language-based disorder. Therefore, socially it appears as though children with ASD are being "difficult," or "rigid," as all children can be at one time or another. However (and this is where it may be difficult for society at large to understand with regard to higher functioning, verbal children with ASD), their social struggles and their challenging behaviors are not personal. They are not attempting to manipulate a situation to achieve getting what they want. They are not purposely inattentive (or minimally attentive) because they want to be. It is part of their disorder.

It is not easy to enlighten others about this because social (verbal and non-verbal) language is very much a part of how one perceives others and how he/she may interact with them. For example, non-verbal language such as eye contact, joint attention and physical body space between a speaker and listener are all examples of non-verbal language that a child with ASD may not have.

While reflecting on conversations that one has had with others, how many people came near to you while they spoke? If they have, you might have felt uncomfortable. Verbally, language skills consist of, but are not limited to, having both communication partners contributing to the topic being discussed, and being able to detect when a breakdown in communication has occurred. This may be due to the listener being confused as inadequate background information is given. These are scenarios in which one could find himself/herself in a conversation with an autistic child.

The feelings that one may have while going through these experiences are the reasons why informing others about the core language difficulties that a child with ASD has is a challenge. Communication, social nuances, and social language rules are all deeply embedded into our culture. Therefore, trying to dissect, analyze, and explain a social language skill that may be a challenge for a child with ASD is not easily accomplished.

It is helpful to take a closer look at case scenarios involving two different (hypothetical) individuals on various parts of the autism spectrum. The reader should consider the challenges that families of children with ASD experience on a daily basis. (Each case does not describe or reflect any *one* client/student directly; both are fictional characters with made-up names that have an ASD diagnosis and portray children with characteristics consistent with the diagnosis.)

In the first case, Peter is a 10-year-old male who demonstrates scattered pre-lingustic (0-12 months) and linguistic (12-17 months) skills with regard to comprehension and expression. For example, he demonstrates fleeting eye contact, turns his head to locate a sound, responds to "no", shakes and bangs objects in play, vocalizes sounds (but usually to protest), and communicates non-verbally, using gestures such as pushing or pulling. Additionally, he is able to point to a familiar toy, has a vocabulary of one word, and identifies familiar objects from a group of objects. Alternatively, he is unable to babble syllable strings (i.e., ba-ba, ma-ma), actively look for a person who is talking to him, look at people or objects to which the caregiver calls attention, look intently at a speaker, or play simple games. Moreover, he is unable to demonstrate appropriate use of an object, use more than one object in play, initiate turn-taking games, or produce a variety of consonant sounds (5).

As a result of Peter utilizing almost no words, and due to his ability to willingly use gestures like pointing and identifying familiar objects from a group of objects, he was assessed and supplied with an Alternative Augmentative Communication (AAC) device (used with individuals who have limited-no verbal expressive language to facilitate their communication needs [6]). Provided with therapy and consistent carryover with the device both at home and at school, Peter is able to identify the foods that he prefers to eat and toys that he likes to play with, and to make simple requests. However, he is unable to smile at his family members upon seeing them walk into a room, hold eye contact long enough to look at his parents face when they are talking to him, or verbally call his caregivers by their name - *mom* or *dad.* (With advanced technology, children who have AAC devices may have an electronic one that can be programmed to express what the individual would like to say, producing mechanical verbal output. However, the child needs to be taught to request, initiate, and/or comment as a social language foundation in order for him to call for his caregivers or family members).

Whereas parents of non-autistic children worry about balancing birthday parties or scheduling play dates, Peter's parents worry if he will ever care to notice others in the room, if they will ever be able to roll a ball back and forth with him, or if he will ever say," *I love you*" to them.

In the second case, the child, named Kaitlin, is a 13-year-old girl who presents with high functioning ASD. She is in an ICT (Integrated Co-Teaching) classroom that consists of approximately 40% of children with various disabilities and 60% who are considered general education students. A couple of her classroom peers also have an ASD diagnosis. Kaitlin works best when she can anticipate what the activities are for the school day, when she is provided with a written check-off schedule to facilitate her ability to fluidly go through her day, and when provided with concrete directives that reflect what behavior is expected of her (not too wordy, no sarcasm, and no rhetorical questions). Conversely, she does not greet her classmates or her teacher upon arrival, initiate or engage in an ongoing reciprocal conversation with her peers or teachers, and presents with fleeting eye-contact. Furthermore, she will insist on speaking about her favorite topic – *rainforests.* She exhibits agitated behaviors if follow-up questions are asked by the listener, will sit without needed materials to complete an activity unless it is specifically noted to do so on her written schedule, becomes upset, tantruming if there is a sudden change in her schedule (i.e., fire drill), and rocks back and forth with her hands cupping her ears while school announcements are being made.

Because Kaitlin is verbal, her speech-language pathologist has mandated her to twice a week receiving speech and language in a small group that focuses on social language, and one time a week where speech-language skills are being taught one-on-one. Goals to work on with Kaitlin consist of greetings and salutations in her small group, initiating a request for a desired object from her peer or teacher, and incorporating therapeutic tools that would help with decreasing behaviors due to sudden changes in schedule.

Kaitlin has difficulty with the traditional methods of teaching social-language skills, such as learning by observing her same-aged peers who do not have a diagnosis of ASD, or simply through direct instruction. She requires other therapeutic techniques used by SLP's that focus on concrete visuals, concrete language, and concrete social situations where she may require a role-playing script to assist her to be successful socially. While parents of children Kaitlin's age are consumed with worrying about their daughter dating or the group of friends that their daughter is surrounding herself with, Kaitlin's parents are worried about whether or not Kaitlin will have a conversation that reflects interest of another person's feelings and/or experiences, if she'll ever have a group of friends, or if she'll learn to comment with such enthusiasm about anything other than her favorite topic, *rainforests*. Moreover, in thinking about the future, they wonder if she will be able to interview for a job because she presents with fleeting eye contact and does not verbally or non-verbally greet others. She speaks only of her interests and does not like when someone asks follow-up questions about what she is speaking.

In the event that she does get a job, the parents would worry if she will isolate herself from everyone else because she has no desire for camaraderie. Perhaps she will be reprimanded because she refused to cooperate in a group project, insisting that everyone else's ideas were not as good as hers. Worse yet, would be being fired because of continually "insulting" clients or co-workers about choices that they were making, comments that they had made, or because of their appearances. To Kaitlin's parents, she does not demonstrate the behaviors that she does because of what some might say are "rude." She does not look to hurt people's feelings or appear aloof. She is a child, soon-to-be adult, who has ASD, a disorder with core difficulties in social-language skills. However, how will the parents be able to reach everyone who may come in contact with Kaitlin to let them know that they should not blame her, judge her, or mistreat her?

Conclusions

Working on dealing with and coping with these concerns of all the *Peter's* and *Kaitlin's* in the world and those on the spectrum that fall in between are exhausting for a family. The integration of siblings in this therapeutic effort is especially important. Society at large, in our daily interactions, may have difficulty understanding and interacting appropriately with individuals with ASD. This is an ongoing fear as well.

Presently, professionals can build awareness and improve society's understanding of what ASD entails and how to act towards individuals who are diagnosed with ASD: with respect and patience. It should always be remembered that individuals with ASD are *individuals* first, with an ASD diagnosis. They are a part of someone's family and they are loved as is anybody else's child. In the future, it is hoped that the cause and a treatment for ASD are found to enhance the quality of life of families that struggle with children with ASD, and to help prevent or curtail the occurrence of ASD in future generations. Possible approaches to this question are discussed in the chapters that follow in this book.

Chapter 2D: Refrigerator Mothers
Shelley Co, Milena Kaufman

[Early proposals that autism was the result of inadequate mothering and emotional support of young children have since been refuted, as bearing no relevance to the probable etiology of this neurobehavioral disorder. – Ed.]

Hypothesis

The term "refrigerator mothers" was first used around the 1950s to refer to mothers with an autistic child [1]. It was believed by many, including doctors and lay people, that childhood autism was caused by mothers who were supposedly unaffectionate and "cold" towards their children [2]. Some of the people who contributed to the popularity of the refrigerator mother theory of autism include Leo Kanner, a psychiatrist who led the Behavior Clinic for Children at Johns Hopkins University [3], John Bowlby, a psychiatrist who worked for the World Health Organization in the 1950s [4], and Bruno Bettelheim, a psychologist who worked as a professor at the University of Chicago from 1944 to 1973 [5]. That these individuals worked at prominent institutions and were considered experts in their fields gave credence to their writings and postulations about childhood mental development. This led to the persistence of the refrigerator mother theory, in spite of works and studies suggesting the theory's falseness [6]. By the time the refrigerator mother hypothesis fell out of favor with the public and the medical establishment, the damage was already done. Mothers had already been stigmatized and the feelings of guilt, shame, and disgrace could not be easily erased.

The term, "autism," was initially coined in 1911 by the Swiss psychiatrist Eugene Bleuler, who thought of autism as a subset of schizophrenia, which was another term that Bleuler established [6]. But it was Leo Kanner who is credited with first identifying autism in his 1943 paper, "Autistic Disturbances of Affective Contact," where he described eleven cases of children eleven years old and younger [5]. He noticed that these children from the moment they are born exhibited an extreme aloneness and didn't respond to external stimuli [7]. Additionally, they are "anxiously and tensely impervious to people." In describing the similar behavior displayed by the children, Kanner also noticed that they are from "highly intelligent families." He stated that the fathers of this group of children were psychiatrists, lawyers, chemists, plant pathologists, and professors, while the mothers were mostly college graduates who worked as physicians, psychologists, nurses, and teachers. He noted that from this group of parents, few could be characterized as "warmhearted." The parents seemed to be more interested in their work whether in science, literature, or art and were "limited in genuine interest in people." Kanner also observed that in the group of parents, the marriages seemed to be "rather cold and formal affairs" and so he questioned to what degree this could impact a child's well-being [8]. In doing so, Kanner not only became the first individual to describe autism, but also became the first individual to suggest that perhaps parents themselves had a role in triggering their child's disease.

Kanner reiterated this idea in a 1949 paper in which he observed the similarities among the fifty-five autistic children whom he studied. Again Kanner noted that these children were exposed to "parental coldness, obsessiveness, and a mechanical type of attention to material needs only." The children "were left neatly in refrigerators which did not defrost." Kanner continued by saying that their autism or their withdrawal seemed to be a mechanism in which the children could escape from the coldness of their parents [9]. Throughout the next decade, the metaphor would stick and the persona of the "refrigerator mother" would unfold.

Observations

Rise of the "Refrigerator Mother" theory

However, the focus on the "refrigerator mother" and not on the "refrigerator father" during the 1950s seems to have been due to underlying factors beyond Kanner who described both mother and father as cold. One such issue was psychoanalysis, which gained widespread popularity around the mid-twentieth century and after World War II in the United States. In psychoanalysis as established by the Austrian physician Sigmund Freud, mental disorders are not thought of as diseases, but rather "disturbances in the development of the ego" and so psychoanalysis concentrates on how psychological disorders are a result of "the infant's failure to develop a differentiated sense of his- or herself." In psychoanalysis, the primary factor that shaped the development of the infant's ego was the infant's mother. Additionally, psychoanalysis, after World War II, was strongly aligned with the medical community, thus reinforcing "its claim of expertise over childhood mental health and mental disorders," especially autism and schizophrenia [10]. Thus, psychoanalysis played a prominent role in perpetuating the authenticity of the refrigerator mother theory with its emphasis on the role of the mother.

Another factor which primed the public and medical professionals to accept the refrigerator mother hypothesis was the work of John Bowlby, a British psychiatrist. He was commissioned to prepare a monograph on the mental health of children, particularly homeless children, by the World Health Organization (WHO). The result was *Maternal Care and Mental Health*, which was published in 1952. Peppered with psychoanalytic concepts in its emphasis on the mother, the monograph also laid out Bowlby's maternal deprivation hypothesis, which states that what is necessary for good mental health is that the child and mother have a "warm, intimate, and continuous relationship" in which both find "satisfaction and enjoyment." A lack of such a relationship is what Bowlby terms "maternal deprivation," which has varying consequences, some being "symptoms of neurosis and instability of character." Complete deprivation yields even more serious consequences and "may entirely cripple the capacity to make relationships" [11].

In regards to the child's father, Bowlby states that "in the young child's eyes father plays second fiddle." Reinforcing the exceptional role of the mother, Bowlby asserts that "almost all the evidence concerns the child's relation to his mother," which he considers to be the most important relationship during the child's early years. To support his claims, Bowlby's monograph contains a discussion of the several types of studies that were conducted and their results. One involved direct observation, another was a retrospective study, and the third type of study was a follow-up study involving groups of children who suffered deprivation in their early years. They would later be examined on their mental health status. From these studies, Bowlby asserts that "the prolonged deprivation of the young child of maternal care may have grave and far-reaching effects on his character and so on the whole of his future life" [11].

Bowlby's monograph also has elements of psychoanalysis. Bowlby even directly mentions Anna Freud, the daughter of psychoanalysis' founder, Sigmund Freud when speaking about the age at what which maternal deprivation is most damaging. After reviewing the cases,

Bowlby concluded that "separations and deprivations in the first six months of life were less important for the child's welfare than later ones," a view that Anna Freud also shared. The blending of Bowlby's maternal deprivation hypothesis and psychoanalysis is also evident when Bowlby discusses the "ego" and how its proper development is influenced by the "the mother who in the child's earliest years fulfils the function of his ego and super-ego" [11].

In 1958, Bowlby would build upon and refine his maternal deprivation theory and formulate what is known as the attachment theory, stating that a baby becomes attached to the mother because she fulfills the baby's physiological needs for food and warmth. The psychologist Mary Ainsworth in the 1960s and 1970s would then test this theory in the Baltimore Project, an observational study involving twenty-six families in Baltimore [12]. One aspect of the study included what was called the "Strange Situation" protocol, which involved observing the responses of children to their mothers and to strangers. Ainsworth's work would give credence to Bowlby's ideas as her studies showed that the degree of attachment that a child has to his/her caregiver was positively correlated to how well the caregiver responded to the child's needs [13].

While Bowlby and Ainsworth made important contributions to the attachment theory, it was Bowlby's statements on maternal deprivation in the 1950s that helped the refrigerator mother hypothesis grow in popularity. At every turn, it seemed that mothers were to blame for any irregularities in their child's behavior; it was evident in Kanner's writings in the 1940s and it was reinforced in Bowlby's 1952 monograph with psychoanalysis gaining recognition in the meantime. This was the setting that mothers with autistic children had to face. In addition, by the 1950s, the "job" of American middle class women was to nurture healthy, normal children. This was underlined by the fact that women were pushed out of the workforce and placed back in the home after World War II. Because of this, it was easy for the refrigerator mother idea to take hold and persist in people's minds, especially since it was the mothers who were responsible for taking care of the children. That many women looked to advice columns and books for guidance on domestic affairs, many of which had psychoanalytic undertones, additionally guaranteed the presence of notions concerning refrigerator mothers during the 1950s [10].

What further propelled the popularity of the refrigerator mother theory in the 1960s was Leo Kanner once again and Bruno Bettelheim. In 1960, Kanner, in the magazine, *Time*, portrayed the autistic child as "the offspring of highly organized, professional parents, cold and rational" [13]. Kanner further describes these parents as "just happening to defrost enough to produce a child" [14]. By the time Bruno Bettelheim published *The Empty Fortress: Infantile Autism and the Birth of the Self* in 1967, the public would be receptive to what Bettelheim had to say about autism as they had already been exposed to Kanner's ideas, psychoanalysis, and Bowlby's work. The legitimacy of Bettelheim's ideas was further solidified as Bettelheim was already considered an expert on child psychology as he was the head of the Sonia Shankman Orthogenic School for disturbed children at the University of Chicago beginning in 1944 and received a grant from the Ford Foundation to study autism and possible treatments from 1956 to

1962 [14]. Bettelheim was also an advice column writer in *The Ladies Home Journal*, securing his place in the realm of familial issues [10].

Bettelheim's perspective

Bettelheim emphasized the role of the environment early on in *The Empty Fortress*. First, he discussed his own experience in German concentration camps and his dehumanization as a result of what he described as an "environment that seemed focused on destroying my independent existence, if not my life." It seems that Bettelheim thought that just as environments can be manipulated to dehumanize maybe they can also be constructed to humanize. As head of the Orthogenic School, Bettelheim tried to create an atmosphere that "might undo emotional isolation in a child and build up personality" [15]. It is from the cases that he observed at the Orthogenic School that Bettelheim developed his ideas on autism as set out in *The Empty Fortress*.

Just like Bowlby's *Maternal Care and Mental Health,* the impact of psychoanalysis in shaping the thinking concerning childhood development and mental health is evident throughout the pages of Bettelheim's *The Empty Fortress,* especially in the analysis he provides of the behavior of three autistic children at the Orthogenic School. However, before delving into the three cases, Bettelheim discusses the importance of nursing and feeding, stating that how the infant is held and "whether he is carefully 'heard' or emotionally ignored" will impact the child's development." Additionally, "nursing and what happens around it seem to be the nuclear experience out of which develop all later feelings about oneself and other persons" [15]. This stresses the significance of the interaction between mother and child, an important psychoanalytic concept.

Bettelheim also talks about the mother's role in teaching her child to eat independently. He describes how mothers may push their children to be independent too early to which Bettelheim responds, "I do not say such a child will become autistic. But his pattern of relating to others may become constricted." On the other hand, if the mother too much inhibits her child's attempts at independence, the consequences are also serious and "infantile autism is a possible outcome" [15]. It is here where Bettelheim touches upon the fundamentals of the refrigerator mother theory - that a mother's behavior towards her child will likely determine whether her child will become autistic.

In his discussion of breast-feeding and nursing, Bettelheim not only evokes psychoanalytic principles, but he also inserts his own thinking about the affect the mother's behavior will have on the infant's behavior and whether the infant will become autistic. Bettelheim does the same when he analyzes the behavior of the Laurie, Marcia, and Joey, three autistic children, at the Orthogenic School as described in *The Empty Fortress*. First, he describes how the first child, Laurie, tears paper in such a way that the torn edges interlock with each other. Bettelheim speculates that this interlocking paper represents teeth and the child's obsession with feeding as an infant. Laurie also in some of her drawings will create two dark circular figures and in other drawings will color in the background of a piece of paper and leave two circular white spaces. Bettelheim interprets the two dark circles as the "bad breast" or the "bad mother" and the two white circles as the "good breast" or "good mother" [15], ideas that had been established by the psychoanalyst Melanie Klein as part of her object relations theory. Bettelheim admits that these interpretations are speculative, yet he continues to say that Laurie had been torn "between her overwhelming desire for the good breast (the good mother) and her despair because, in spite of all her efforts, there seemed nothing there for her, not even a "bad breast." The result was that Laurie "knew only one defense - to do nothing at all by not acting" and so reverted to the autistic state [15].

Similar analyses are offered for the behavior of Marcia and Joey. Marcia was observed to play with water using a bucket, glass, and bottle. Bettelheim said that the three objects represented Marcia's family. The bottle was symbolic for Marcia's mother and Bettelheim acknowledges that the bottle's shape seemed to conform to a womanly figure. Marcia was represented by the bucket and Marcia engaged in play in which the pouring of water from the bottle to the bucket "suggests that she was again recreating events out of infancy, such as being fed." Joey, on the other hand, was obsessed with machine parts. He attached a battery, speaker, and cardboard wheel around the headboard of his bed to form what seems like a car. When he would enter the dining room, he would lay down imaginary wire connecting himself to an imaginary outlet. Bettelheim says that these imaginary electrical connections had to be constructed before Joey could eat because "only the current ran his ingestive apparatus." In the spirit of psychoanalysis, Bettelheim continues by stating that just as an infant has to be physically connected with his mother in order to be nursed, "so Joey had to connect with electricity, had to plug himself in, before he could function" [15].

Another instance of psychoanalysis' influence on Bettelheim occurs when he criticizes Kanner for supporting the idea that one was born with autism over the theory of an environmental cause of autism. Bettelheim states that Kanner failed to ask, "why does a person behave in this way instead of some other?" which to Bettelheim was an important notion to consider when examining psychological behavior ever since the rise of Freud and his ideas. Thus, Bettelheim emphasizes that autism is a condition that is developed. To him, it is not genetically acquired as he states that he finds it difficult to believe that "autistic children are different 'from the beginning of their extra-uterine existence'." To support this, Bettelheim asserts that from the cases at the Orthogenic School, there was "no tangible evidence that autism was recognized at birth or right afterward" [15].

Bettelheim in *The Empty Fortress* also affirms towards the end of his book that "the precipitating factor in infantile autism is the parent's wish that his child should not exist" [15]. Such an inflammatory statement reverberated throughout people's minds and maybe even some parents painfully shared in this feeling already. Additionally, since it originated from Bettelheim, people believed it [1]. It reinforced the notions of the refrigerator mother theory, ideas which had been in existence for nearly two and a half decades. Because of this, *The Empty Fortress* would overshadow the work of Bernard Rimland who sought to disprove the refrigerator mother theory three years prior in *Infantile Autism: The Syndrome and Its Implications for a Neural Theory of Behavior.*

Fall of the "Refrigerator Mother" theory

Rimland was one of the first people to challenge the refrigerator mother theory as the cause of autism. He provided a counter-explanation to the established misconceptions surrounding the theory by presenting evidence-based data that the disorder was rooted in biology and not cold mothers. Rimland's book explores the lack of authenticity behind the idea that an emotionally closed-off parent is to blame for the root of autism [17]. Rimland argued that the cause in fact was biochemical in nature, and that with the aid of behavioral and biomedical therapy, these children's symptoms could be improved. The book emphasized that the defect behind autism was rooted in genomics and compounded by environmental factors [18].

Rimland was a psychologist with a personal interest in the study of autism, because he himself had a son diagnosed with autism. After his son turned two years of age, Rimland and his wife knew their son was exhibiting a variety of concerning, developmentally delayed behaviors. In the 1950s, autism was far from a well-known diagnosis. Rimland even had a doctorate, but had yet to come across the term. Symptomatology such as "staring into space and "not recognizing people," offered vague clues as to what the disorder entailed [18]. Rimland was only able to diagnose his son using ambiguous criteria from an old college textbook . At the time of his son's diagnosis, physicians and lay people believed that it was due to the lack of a loving, warm mother in the autistic child's life. Rimland buried himself in research to uproot this conventional view and find what really was behind the cause of his son's illness [19].

In the public eye, Rimland's work was the first to question the widely held beliefs of Bruno Bettelhiem's refrigerator mother hypothesis. As time passed, Rimland's theory grew acceptance and gained popularity within the autism community. This was the first time that these mothers were not identified as the cause for the child's autism. These mothers who had previously suffered countless guilt were now opening themselves up to learn about Rimland's research.

In 1969, a few short years after his publication, a group of parents of autistic children founded the National Society for Autistic Children, now better known as the Autism Society of America (ASA). The group publically rejected the "refrigerator mother" and sought to begin the movement of educating families on Rimland's research and the scientific causes behind autism. Rimland shifted the very core of the original medical views of autism, taking it from an illness based on lack of emotion, into that of a scientific cause based on biological and environmental roots. Rimland states, "For years we have heard the experts say that autism is a lifelong disability, … This is simply not true anymore" [19].

Kanner's shifting views

What is interesting is that the forward for Rimland's book *Infantile Autism: The Syndrome and Its implications for a Neural Theory of Behavior* was written by Dr. Leo Kanner, one of the first physicians to be known as a child psychiatrist as well as one of the first to speak of autism. However, Kanner also struggled with what the root of autism was over the decades.

Kanner began his autism research in the 1930s. At that time he described the cause to be hereditary in nature. His early descriptions of autism, coined "Kanner syndrome," described children born with an inability to relate to others. Kanner writes, "with these extremely detached children, you must give them the chance to relate to a limited number of people and to come into the world - to thaw out," demonstrating that his early views on autism stemmed from internal causes [19].

His work, *In Defense of Mothers,* was written in 1941, to disprove the psychoanalytic theories of Freud that stated these children were emotionally disturbed individuals due to their experiences early in life with their caregivers. In his book, he also emphasized to mothers, "regain that common sense which is yours, which has been yours before you allowed yourselves to be intimidated by would-be omniscient totalitarians," encouraging mothers to believe in themselves and not take blame [18]. Kanner's views took a turn in the 1940s, however, when he published, "Autistic Disturbances of Affective Contact," which first suggests that refrigerator mothers were the cause of autism. The idea that the mothers who were lacking in warmth, compassion, and love produced autistic children who isolated themselves in their own world grew in popularity over the years. The 1940s were a notable era heavily influenced by theories that proposed that behaviors were the result of certain experiences. In addition, since the 1940s was a time period when gender roles were re-evaluated, the view of the working woman during World War II taking on a "man's job," instead of home raising children, made the idea of the "refrigerator mother" rather popular at that time [10]. Dr. Kanner continued looking into the mannerisms of these parents, which reinforced his belief that many of the developmental difficulties the children were experiencing were directly caused by stiff and cold parental environments [8].

Later in the 1960s, Kanner's views began to change again and move away from the refrigerator mother theory. The influence of the families he was working with began to sway his opinions, as he came upon numerous loving warm families whose children had autism. Also during this time Kanner began a friendship with Jacques May, a French physician, who himself had two children with autism. In the end, Kanner rescinded his previous statements supporting the notions of the refrigerator mother hypothesis and agreed with Rimland's research. Through his own continued research, Kanner came to believe that autism was brought upon by a neurological cause as opposed to refrigerator mothers. He continued to spend much of his life dedicated to further studying and proving this research [7].

Personal connections to the theory

Dr. Jacques May was a physician known best as the father of "medical geography." Originally from France, he spent the 1930s and 1940s studying cause and effect between environments across the globe and the diseases they caused. His studies emphasized the causal role of environment on disease [21-23]. In the 1950s, Jacques and his wife, Marie-Ann, immigrated to the United States with their two twin boys who were diagnosed with autism. Upon moving to Massachusetts, they sought to create an environment where children with autism could grow, learn, and receive appropriate care. In 1959, working with other parents in the area, they opened the Parents School for Atypical Children. The goal was to create a live-in school for these children where they could be provided with a loving environment with continuous art and play therapy to help their development [24].

From the beginning, May took a distinct stance against psychoanalytic views of autism, rejecting the refrigerator mother theory. In 1958, he wrote "A Physician Looks at Psychiatry," where he criticized the very concepts of psychoanalysis, stating its views were non-scientific. May also believed that the refrigerator mother theory did nothing to better the lives of these children. Having personally experienced their approach on his two twin boys, he wrote about his own family's battle, and the slew of child psychiatrists who did nothing to enrich his boy's lives. He also went on to be the founder for the League for Emotionally Disturbed Children, which gained significant popularity. Through the league, he was able to fund further autism studies and publish his research, which publicly rejected the ideas of the refrigerator mother being at fault for their child's autism. This was one of the key events that began to shift the blaming finger away from mothers [7,24].

Another person who took a personal stance against the refrigerator mother theory was Clara Clark. In the book, *The Siege*, Clara Clark writes, "if today I were given the choice, to accept the experience, with everything that it entails, or to refuse the bitter largesse, I would have to stretch out my hands—because out of it has come, for all of us, an imagined life. And I will not change the last word of the story. It is still love." Clara Claiborne Park mothered an autistic child and like many, felt feelings of guilt due to wildly held accusations of the refrigerator mother. She, however, denounced these "shortcomings," with her book, which was published in 1967, the same year that Bettelheim's *The Empty Fortress*, was published. Ms. Clark wrote about her personal struggle to raise her eight year old daughter in a loving, warm home, shattering the perceptions of Bettelheim's "refrigerator mother" stance [25].

Love is what Clara Park was able to bring to countless mothers with her book *The Siege*. Park refused to believe that mothers like herself, who would do anything for their children were in fact the cause of autism. Her writings went on to inspire mothers to no longer take fault, and feel guilt for this illness. *The Siege* became much more than just a personal story of her daughter; it became an important resource for educators, physician, and families. Fred Volkmar, a child psychiatrist and the director of the Yale University Child Study Center, spoke of Clara Park, stating that "since she first published her book, wider recognition of autism and early diagnosis have led to new treatments and improved outcomes" [25]. Her book encouraged families to believe in themselves, and fight for their children [26]. It also gave professionals in the field a documented firsthand look into the experiences these mothers were having, truly exemplifying a much deeper-rooted cause to autism.

Conclusions

After the refrigerator mother theory began to withdraw from popularity, autism research began to center itself on the biologic and genetic causes. In 1977, Michael Rutter, and Susan Folstein published a groundbreaking twin study, "Infantile Autism: A Genetic Study of 21 Twin Pairs" showing that in fact there may well be a genetic component to autism. Their research proposed that there was a higher concordance of autism in identical twins, as compared to those that were fraternal [27] (chapter 1C). This monumental research provided the framework for modern autism research.

Although Bernard Rimland was one of the first researchers to believe in the genetic role of autism, in later years he ironically began implying that these children had an innate genetic susceptibility compounded by environmental triggers (chapter 8A). In more recent publications, Rimland began to point the blame at environmental factors such as pollution, car emission, processed foods, and ultimately vaccines. These triggers were "polluting" the children's bodies. He held a firm belief that the answer lay in the mercury preservative, thimerasol, a compound used in vaccinating children early on (chapter 7B). Rimland went on to become a supporter to the MMR vaccine theory created by gastroenterologist Andrew Wakefield, whose proposal in time also proved to be false [26] (chapter 7A).

Research involving the neurological aspects of autism was also underway. In the 1950s theories suggesting that autism may be linked to injury or infection to the CNS had emerged (chapters 6B,6C). The theory behind the cause of autism had evolved to a more medical etiology, focusing on perinatal implications. Studies were done to evaluate the amount of oxygen fetuses were exposed to *in utero* as a potential cause (chapters 3G,3H). In 1973, in the *Journal of Autism and Childhood Schizophrenia*, DeMyer and colleagues concluded that "viral disease during or after gestation, birth trauma, malnutrition, oxygen lack or generally any of the events known to damage the brain may be the cause of the autistic syndrome" [27]. These early studies redirected the view of autism away from the psychoanalytic shadow and onto the science behind the disease [24,28].

Modern interpretations of the theory

It has been decades since the etiology of autism was proposed as an ill-treated child; however, there are still aspects of the theory that linger despite research favoring the genetic-related etiologies of autism. Korea is known to have one of the highest rates of autism spectrum disorder in the world with a prevalence of one out of every thirty-eight children [29] and although many scientific research articles have been published recognizing autism as a cognitive disease, there is a cultural belief that autism stems from a "cold" mother. Some psychiatrists in Korea have claimed that children who carry a diagnosis of autism are experiencing these symptoms due to attachment issues between mother and child [30,31]. They believe the children are suffering from maternal neglect, that these mothers are not providing the emotional warmth and compassion children require, and that these mothers were not engaging with their children. They also contended that these women became too involved in their roles at work, causing them to lack in their role as a mother, causing their child to become autistic. Anthropologist Roy Richard Grinker, a father of a child with autism, had watched video recordings collected by these researchers in Korea. The videos displayed the interactions between the children with autism and their supposed "cold" mothers. However, Grinker felt different. From his book *Unstrange Minds,* Grinker states "what I saw was the mother's reaction to her child's autism. I saw a mother demoralized by months of futile and unrewarding attempts to communicate with her child" [32]. In the eyes of the researchers, however, what they saw was an example of the classic refrigerator mother theory.

While there are some people who still subscribe to the fundamentals of the refrigerator mother hypothesis, contemporary manifestations of the theory also exist. One example is from a 2008 study entitled, "Insulin and Insulin-Like Growth Factor 1 (IGF-1) Increased in Preterm Neonates," which evaluates infantile growth patterns after receiving massage therapy. Such infants who received said therapy developed dramatically quicker compared to those whom did not. These babies put on more weight and increased their insulin, as well as IGF-1, levels, as compared to the premature infants that did not receive the massage therapy [32]. The study might be compared to what a "warm," affectionate mother would do with her own child, like caress, touch, and massage her child. Has the refrigerator mother theory evolved and returned? Could it be speculated that mothers whom had spent less time having this sort of physical bonding with their children affect the growth and development of the child?

The etiology of autism has been largely debated for decades, and we are still in search for what is really at the root of the illness. Many avenues have been explored and a clear-cut cause has yet to be identified. Current research suggests that autism is strongly related to the genetic coding of the affected individual, as well as environmental factors, perhaps affecting individuals with a more vulnerable genetic infrastructure. Could the twentieth century "refrigerator mother" theory actually be signs of autism in the parents themselves? Or did the physicians and psychiatrists of the 1900s have it all backwards? Were they witnessing a mother's reaction to her child's autism? Were these mothers' "distant" behaviors only secondary to countless attempts to coddle their children who had not reciprocated their emotion? Were these mothers just learning to keep an arm's length in an effort to create as comfortable of an environment for the child as possible? Although it is clear there is no direct cause and effect of a "cold mother" bringing about autism in her child- the question remains, could emotionally, absent mothers in the twenty-first century interpretation of the refrigerator mother theory have an impact on the further development and progress of children?

BRAIN/NERVE DISORDERS AND INSULTS

Chapter 3A – Brain imaging

Victor Hoang, Mario Flores, Alexis Sandoval

[The development of a number of sophisticated electron devices to aid in the imaging central nervous system structures has greated aided the establishment of more objective methods for diagnosing autism and exposing neurologic changes that may hold the key to understanding the cause of this disorder.]

<u>Introduction</u>

Autism is described as a disorder of social interaction. The understanding of the social brain is key in studying autism. It is no coincidence that many key neuroanatomical structures involved in social interaction have been found to be abnormal in individuals with autism Spectrum disorders (ASD). Autism spectrum disorders have demonstrated a wide variety of identifying characteristics, which provides a basis for diagnosis. However, these guidelines are nonspecific making ASD a very large umbrella term encompassing: Autism Disorder, Asperger's Disorder, and Pervasive Developmental disorder. The diagnosis based solely on these characteristics seems outdated especially now that it is possible to use advanced neural imaging technologies to demonstrate variations in brain activity, structure, and connectivity between these distinct disorders.

History of brain imaging

Neuroimaging had its origins in the early 1900s; the first technique was called the pneumoencephalography. This procedure drained cerebral spinal fluid (CSF) and filled it with air, oxygen and helium, which would help visualize the brain in an x-ray. Unfortunately, this procedure was poorly tolerated, causing headaches and severe vomiting among other side effects. For this reasoning, pneumocephalography is no longer in use and has been replaced by more modern imaging techniques. Today, the field has dramatically improved with the use of functional magnetic resonance imaging (fMRI), positron emission tomography (PET), electroencephalography (EEG), magnetoencephalography (MEG), and voxel-based morphometry (VBM).

Overview of imaging modalities

There are several main neuroimaging procedures that are used to study autism. Some common methods include PET, fMRI, EEG, and MEG. Imaging modalitiesare divided into structural and functional techniques. Structural techniques are used to find gross anatomical abnormalities, such as, tumors or hemorrhages. In contrast, functional neuroimaging is used to measure neural activity during mental stimulation, such as looking for regional neural activation when listening to music. Functional imaging can be further broken down into measurements of changes of blood flow (PET and fMRI) and changes in electrical currents (EEG) and magnetic fields (MEG).

There are several key points that have to be considered when evaluating neuroimaging studies including the age of the subjects, the imaging modality and the neuroanatomical structures being evaluated. First, the age of the subjects has major limitations on what can be elucidated from the data. For example, the primary pathophysiology is only seen in younger children during critical neurodevelopmental stages. Second, it is important to be aware of the limitations of each imaging modality. For example, blood flow based imaging (PET and fMRI) has the advantage of great spatial resolution, but has poor temporal resolution due to slow changes in blood flow versus the rapid changesin electrical current imaging seen in EEG and MEG.

Purpose of the chapter

In this section our objective is to evaluate studies and the imaging modalities that are used to distinguish normal developing brains from those with ASD. In this section we seek to answer the following questions: What are the latest developments in neuroimaging with ASD? How is imaging currently used to diagnose and treat ASD? When can ASD be firstidentified through brain imaging? Could the use of neuroimaging indicate if a child is at risk for having ASD? What are the changes seen in the brain of an autistic individual?

Observations
MRI

Magnetic resonance imaging (MRI) is a safe, noninvasive neuroimaging method used to study brain morphology with greater resolution than other imaging modalities. This imaging technique is useful in providing gross neuroanatomical changes. In studies involving autism, MR imaging is being used to identify structural differences in patients with autism spectrum disorder (ASD) versus the normal population. It is also being looked into as a possible tool to diagnose ASD earlier in children. A MRI scan is particularly useful in studies involving children and adolescents because of its high sensitivity and spatial resolution in the absence of radiation exposure (1). However, obtaining high quality MRI images in young patients can be challenging because the patient must remain absolutely still during scanning and eventhe slightest head movement can distort brain images and change the structural analyses (2). Due to this sensitivity, children with ASD are normally placed under general anesthesia during MRI scanning to obtain high quality images (3,4). Sedation is done to ensure that the patients remain motionless during scanning and to avoid any unnecessary agitation or nervousness (claustrophobia) while inside the MRI machine. In addition, the MRI magnet generates loud acoustic noises during the scanning process and children with autism often have auditory sensitivities, which can increases levels of agitation (5). In contrast, the imaging process in the control group can occur either while the patient is asleep, awake or under sedation (6,7).

MRI studies have consistently found abnormal regulation of brain growth in ASD patients during development. At birth, brain size in children with autism is relatively normal (1). This normalcy in volume begins to rapidly change in early childhood. In young children with autism, imaging studies have demonstrated that there is an increase in overall brain volume (megalencephaly) compared to normal aged-matched children (1,6). In addition, there is evidence that demonstrates the greatest period of brain enlargement in autism occurs during the toddler years and early childhood (8). It is during this critical age range that a child really begins to increase in their development of language, cognitive, social, and attention skills. Recent studies also show overgrowth occurring mainly in the cerebrum, hippocampus, cerebellum and amygdala in the brains of children with autism while other structures remain unaffected (4,7).

Macrocephaly, which is an enlarged head, has been found in multiple studies, but no clear evidence has been shown whether it causes developmental delays. A study demonstrated that increased head circumference found between 5-12 months increases the risk of developing autism (5). One of the possible explanations for macrocephaly is due to rapidly growing brain during the first year of life, although no study has evaluated this hypothesis (9).

In the cerebellum, the overgrowth remains proportional to the overall total brain volume. There is also evidence to suggest that the disproportionate enlargement of the amygdala is present by 3 years of age in ASD patients (4,7,10). In addition, the overgrowth of the amygdala has been linked in a few studies to severe anxiety and the worsening in social and communication skills. In older patients with ASD, the enlargement is replaced with a total brain volume that appears more normalized which has been attributed to a period of slower growth and even degeneration (1,8).

fMRI

Functional Magnetic Resonance Imaging (fMRI) is a neuroimaging procedure that measures brain activity. Neurons, like all cells, require a blood supply to deliver oxygen and nutrients. When brain activity increases more active neurons have a higher demand for oxygen, which will increase the blood supply. fMRI takes advantage of this principle by measuring the blood supply which correlates withneural activity. Therefore, more active regions of the brain can be detected. For example, with auditory stimulus such as listening to someone speaking, fMRI can detect increases in blood flow to brain regions such as the temporal lobe. There are many advantages of fMRI over other imaging modalities such as safety since there is no radiation involved. However, disadvantages of fMRI include the high cost, low availability and low temporal resolution.

The fusiform gyrus (FFG) is known as the face area, essential for facial recognition. Repeated studies have shown that individuals with ASD have hypoactivation in the FFG when looking at faces. It was found that ASD patients have a dysregulation rather than a deficit in the fusiform gyrus. When ASD subjects were instructed to make face contact, they consistently avoided looking at the eyes of facial images, which the study suggested was the reason why the FFG was hypoactive during this task (11,12).

Furthermore, patients with ASD have anxiety when looking at eyes and do not develop expertise for faces. When ASD patients were instructed to look at faces and told to look specifically at the eyes FFG activation increased to normal levels, leading to the notion that the FFG is not damaged.A study by Kliemann found that when ASD patients looked at faces there was a dysfunction in the activation of the amygdala. The amygdala is critical in emotional processing and therefore contributes to the anxiety experienced during this task (11,12).

Sleep fMRI

Sleep fMRI is a promising new procedure that is beginning to be used to study ASD. This new procedure uses fMRI to measure neural activity ofchildren with ASD during sleep. An advantage to this method is that it avoids the controversial use of sedation, as well as the bias that sedation can create. The procedure takes toddlers that are in a normal sleep state and measures regional changes paired with auditory stimulus.

Studies using sleep fMRI have shown defects in the superior temporal gyrus (STG) in children as young as 14 months (13). Normally, the superior temporal gyrus is an important structure involved in perception of emotions in facial stimuli, auditory processing, and language. In addition, STG has connections to the amygdala and prefrontal cortex and other brain regions affected in autism.

MEG

Magnetoencephalography (MEG) uses the magnetic field produced within brainas current flows through neural dendrites. Approximately 50,000 neurons, specifically pyramidal neurons in the cortical surface are needed to give a measurable signal on MEG. The benefits of magnetoencephalography, is the rapid ability to resolve events compared to functional MRI techniques, although the use of functional MRI and MEG are often used simultaneously. More interestingly, MEG can localize and map neural activity with high spatial resolution after an auditory and visual stimulus has been introduced (14). This allows precise measurements of the auditory and visual responses through neural signaling.

In MEG, the magnetic fields produced by electric currents flowing in neurons are measured with multichannel SQUID (superconducting quantum interference device) gradiometers, an extremely sensitive detector that measures magnetic fields.The sites in the cerebral cortex that are activated by a stimulus can be detected from the magnetic-field distribution (15).

There have already been studies done to demonstrate variability in magnetic responses from auditory stimulus due to aging. For instance, one study looked at three responses after using a tone-burst to stimulate the auditory field. They recorded neural magnetic responses 30milliseconds (M30), 50 ms (M50), and one at 100 ms (M100) after the stimulus. They found that the amplitude of the contralateral M50, often used to study the association of aging and hearing loss, was shown to enlarge with age (16). Researchers are now interested in investigating auditory variations using magnetic neural imaging in ASD.

Evidence has already shown that MEG could be used to demonstrate the effects of psychiatric disorders and neural connectivity or processing changes. For example, MEG has been used to identify relationships between brain function and behavior in patients diagnosed with schizophrenia showing that they have auditory deficits to human voices (17). In addition, MEG was used to model auditory activity in the left and right superior temporal gyri by examining the effect of changes in source strength, orientation or latency of the superior temporal gyri (18). Specifically, it was shown that there was a large variability of the superior temporal gyrus between the left and right hemispheres.

Well-characterized ASD subjects were examinedby MEG to examine auditory impairments. Their MEG method consisted of three head-position indicator coils that were attached to the scalp. These coils provided continuous specification of the position and orientation of the MEG sensors relative to the head. They were able to stabilize the subject as well as account for eye blinking and heartbeats that would alter the magnetic fields and data. Researchers were interested in using MEG to identify differences in the auditory delay in children/ adolescents that were diagnosed as typical ASD. They found that the main effect indicated right hemisphere latency prolongation at all frequencies in ASD (19).

Roberts used MEG and investigated the 50 ms (M50) and 100 ms (M100) components of the auditory evoked field to explore changes during development in ASD. Roberts found the M50 amplitude was increased more in children than in adults, which suggested a developmental trajectory with M50 amplitude decreasing and M100 increasing with age. Child M50 and M100 latencies were prolonged relative to adults. Children with autism did not differ from the control children with respect to these observations.

PET

Brain PET is a nuclear imaging technique that uses a camera and tracer injected in the bloodstream to produce multi-dimension images of the distribution of chemical throughout the brain. It was the preferred method of functional neuroimaging before fMRI, but it is still used in neuroscience research and diagnosing certain types of dementias and other neurological diseases. An advantage of this technique is good spatial resolution, which measures regional neuronal activity based on blood flow changes. A limitation is that it is only useful for monitoring short tasks due to the quick radioactive decay of the injected tracer.

PET scan studies have found abnormal brain serotonin synthesis of ASD children within the ages of 2 to 15 years. The frontal lobe was affected the most, but decreased synthesis was also observed in the temporal, parietal and occipital lobes. Another patter observed was lateralization of serotonin synthesis. There were marked decreases on the left hemisphere, which is the dominant side of language (20).

Voxel-based morphometry

Another neural imaging technique used to better define differences in the neuroanatomical structure of patients with ASD is Voxel-based morphometry (VBM). Voxel-based morphometry is a technique that is able to measure the volume of the whole brain or specific regions allowing researchers to compare structural differences between ASD and non-ASD controls as well as asymmetries within ASD patients. Morphometry has previously been used to study brain structure and changes that occur due to aging or during learning (21,22).

Previous autism studies used voxel-based morphometry (VBM) in adults with ASD to study brain volumes however, individually data collected from these studies had been inconclusive.

Furthermore, VBM has been applied by a number of studies to help quantify ASD in hopes of improving future diagnostic tools for these diseases. In 2011, Radua focused on white matter (WM) differences in ASD versus healthy controls. Previous Voxel based morphometry was limited by relatively small sample sizes, resulting in insufficient statistical power. Radua was able to overcome these limitations by performing a meta-analysis that consist of 13 previously conducted VBM studies and used a new method of interpreting VBM data called signed differential mapping (SDM) (23). Signed differential mapping used greatest points of VBM measurements in order to recreate maps of brain volume differences between patients and controls. This technique prevented biased results across studies and helped to better compare patients with controls.

Radua's collection of data and interpretation of the results showed that patients with ASD had an increased in white-matter volume in the right arcutate fasciculus and left inferior fronto-occipital and uncinate fasciculi (24).

The arcuate fasciculus is bundles of nerves that connect the frontal, parietal, and temporal lobe. Specifically this region on the left side of the brain connects what is called Broca's and Wernicke's area, which are involved in speech and language interpretation. On the right side the arcuate fasciculus are known to be involved in visuospatial processing, where damages have been shown to involve impaired understanding, pitch production, tempo and loudness (25).

The uncinate fasciculus is a bundle of nerve fibers that connects the frontal lobe with temporal lobe whose function is involved in the limbic system, involved in human emotion as well as language, which Schmahmann mentions are all functions impaired in ASD patients. In addition, Damasio and Maurer, believed that the abnormal limbic system was responsible for the social and communication problems faced by ASD patients (26,27).

Individually, VBM studies were inconclusive however, by using a meta-analysis and use of signed differential mapping (SDM) Radua has been able to identify significant differences in areas of the brain whose functions seem to correlate with specific symptoms seen in ASD.

Conclusions

ASD is disease that affects brain development. Some of these abnormalities demonstrated include brain connectivity, increased brain size, structural differences, hemisphere lateralization, cognitive processing, decreased serotonin synthesis, and white and gray matter volume.

Limitations of Neuroimaging

Since ASD is such a heterogeneous disease, there is variability across patients and finding global brain abnormalities can be a challenge. Many studies show abnormalities in a large percentage of subjects but it is quite difficult to see the exact changes within each and every patient. Therefore finding a suitable biomarker for diagnostic value has been troublesome.

Current use of modalities for screening and diagnosis

Currently imaging modalities are not used for diagnostic evaluation for Autism. Refer to chapter 9 for the current guidelines for diagnosis. Some studies have shown promise in finding brain abnormalities in children as young as 6 months before the sign of symptoms. Understanding the pathophysiology is critical, nevertheless imaging has great promise for developing biomarkers to classify young children into high and low risk groups. If therapies such as stem cells or IGF therapy prove successful, children in high-risk group can potentially be of benefit.

Future Research

Neuroimaging has lots of promise for aiding in diagnosis in the future. A search for a clear biomarker in all children will be important for clinicians working with ASD. With early neuroimaging biomarkers, therapy can be started during critical developmental stages. It is clear that starting therapy too late after symptoms have started to show will have little effect, therefore it is crucial to detect abnormalities as early as possible. Once a biomarker is found, neuroimaging has the potential to be a major component in diagnosis and possibly also in evaluating the success of treatments (3).

Glossary

MRI- magnetic resonance imaging

fMRI- functional magnetic resonance imaging

MEG- magnetoencephalography

PET- positron emission tomography

ASD- Autism Spectrum Disorder

FFG- fusiform gyrus

STS- superior temporal sulcus

STG- superior temporal gyrus

VBM- voxel-based morphometry

SDM- signed differential mapping

Chapter 3B – Brain Macropathology

John Farag, Andrew Rudin

[Efforts have been made to identify the affected areas of the brain which distinguish autistic patients from neurologically unaffected ones. One of the characteristic observations is the head enlargement found in youngsters with this disease. - Ed.]

Introduction

Autism was defined by the American Psychiatric Association in 2000 as a "neurodevelopmental disorder characterized by poor social communication abilities in combination with repetitive behaviors and restricted interests". This broad definition allows for a wide array of clinical presentations and patients can be diagnosed with mild, moderate, and severe forms of autism. As such, autism is now categorized as Autism Spectrum Disorder (ASD) to incorporate the various clinical manifestations. Furthermore, the Diagnostic and Statistical Manual on Mental Disorders, part five (DSM-5) has been revised to include autistic disorder, Asperger's disorder, childhood disintegrative disorder, and pervasive development disorder under the umbrella of ASD. The reason for this change from the DSM-IV is that researchers found that clinicians were not consistent in their diagnoses of the separate disorders (1) (chapter 1D).

The variations in clinical symptoms of ASD are due in part to the range of macro-brain pathology findings present in ASD. First, we will explore the "growth dysregulation hypothesis" presented by Akshoomoff et al. in 2002 (2). We will then examine other studies which support or contradict this hypothesis. Finally, we will compare and contrast the activation and deactivation of specific brain function areas in children, adolescents and adults with ASD (3,4).

Observations

The growth regulation hypothesis follows the idea that in the early years of ASD, there is excess brain growth which gradually reverses, resulting in decreased growth. One such paper set out to determine when exactly brain enlargement occurs. The study looked at a group of boys and girls ages 2-4 years and further divided them into early onset or regressive ASD (5). Some children exhibit autism in the first few months of life (early onset), whereas others appear grossly normal but experience a later (15-30 months of age) loss of previously acquired social functions (regressive). The authors of this study performed a retrospective review of head circumference from birth until 18 months. What they discovered was the head circumference of the sixty-one children with regressive autism began to increase at approximately 4-6 months. This was an increase of 2-3% relative to the control (unaffected) group (n = 66). However, this change was not noted in children with early onset autism (n = 53) or those normally developing children.

Comparable findings were also evident when total brain volume was examined with MRI in the same cohort (5) (chapter 3A).

Another study examining brain volume among ASD and controls found no difference. However, when the group was divided by age, older than 18 versus younger than 18, they found something interesting. Children and adolescents with ASD have increased brain volumes. As they age, the brain volume decreases relative to the controls (6).

The volume of grey matter (GM) in ASD followed a similar trend as brain volume. GM was increased in children and adolescents but decreased in adulthood. Significant decreases of GM were evident in the frontal, parietal, and occipital lobes. Brain thickness and surface area were also examined. These manifestations also declined in a similar fashion to that of brain and GM volume. The increases were greatest at about 7.5 years of age and the decreased growth appeared around 14.5 years (6).

The change in cortical thickness noted in this study was discovered to be the opposite of another study in 2010 by Raznahan et al., in which cortical thickness decreased overall in children and increased in adults. On the other hand, Hardan et al. had results consistent with Mak-Fan et al. (7). In a study on 41 males with ASD at the National Institute of Mental Health, increased gyrification in the left lateral occipital region, left precuneus, and the right temporal occipital region were found (8). Of these three areas, the left precuneus and the right temporal occipital regions had the most gyrification whereas the left lateral occipital cortex had the greatest gyral depth. In the controls, increased gyrification of the left inferior parietal cortex was associated with increased vocabulary performance, but no such relationship was seen in ASD individuals. Doyle-Thomas et al. claimed that in those studies that stated there is a decrease, the age range was very narrow, whereas no difference was seen in groups with a wide range (9).

The orbital frontal cortices (OFC) and the rostral anterior cingulate cortex (rACC), which are just superior to the CC, cause social impairment with different cortical thickness profiles (10). In the OFC, thinner cortices were found in cases with more affected social function, whereas the rACC was associated with diminished social function and thicker cortices. The researchers proposed that the thinning in the OFC occurs in childhood and continues into adulthood.

The external portion of the human brain is grey matter (GM), brain tissue composed of cell bodies. To accommodate the excess GM and the large surface area of brain tissue, the brain folds upon itself, forming a gyrus (pl: gyri). Studies examine the gyrifications of the brain in ASD patients found that there was no difference compared to unaffected cases. When cases were divided by groups based on age, those under the age of 18 had increased gyrification in the prefrontal area of the brain relative to the controls (11). Such a difference between ASD and controls was absent in adulthood.

Underlying the GM is the white matter, an area composed of myelinated nerve fibers whose job it is to carry signals from neuron to neuron at an extremely high rate (see chapter 6B). Hua et al. compared the growth of two 11-year-old boys, one with ASD and the other unaffected. What they found was that the boy without ASD had many regions of the brain composed of white matter in a state of active growth. The boy with ASD lacked this growth pattern (12). Even across a large study, the same presentation was seen. The CC, corticopontine tract, and the thalamic radiation of the frontal lobe all showed a reduced growth rate. The inferior longitudinal fasciculus, and the optic radiation of the occipital lobe, posterior thalamic radiation of the parietal lobe, as well as their continuation into the temporal lobe, also showed decreased growth rates. This loss of numerous areas of white matter and the associated tracts only provides more evidence that autism is a disorder not just of abnormal growth but also lost connections between various regions of the brain.

Minor physical anomalies (MPA) are commonly seen in children with neurodevelopmental disorders because of the shared origin by the face and nervous system; the neuroectoderm. MPAs are markers of neurodevelopment which result in particular phenotypes. One such MPA seen in autism is an increase in the distance between the eyes known as hypertelorism. There is a subjective nature in the description and classification of an MPA and to reduce this bias, the researchers used T1-weighted MRI (see chapter 3A). When the head expands, it results in contraction of the optic chiasm. During development, the angle of the optic chiasm progresses from 180° to 71°, and finally 68° by adulthood (9). The distance between the orbits gradually increases. By the age of 3, this distance is 50% of that of an adult. Therefore, by measuring the distance between the eyes, one may extrapolate neurodevelopmental abnormalities.

Individuals with ASD (n = 36) had a much larger distance between the eyes relative to the controls (n = 55). Furthermore, the increased distance had a positive correlation with the bilateral volume of the amygdala, which results in expansion of the amygdala in a ventro-medial fashion toward the uncus and posteriorly to the inferior pole of the superior temporal lobes (7). These areas are involved in the memory, social, and emotional aspects of human nature. When the uncus is lesioned in Rhesus monkeys, they lack nearly all emotion and become indifferent to their surroundings. Thus, the involvement of the amygdala on the uncus may partially explain the reason for the clinical presentation of patients with ASD.

Research from the University of Missouri has further examined brain shape by focusing on the corpus callosum (CC). The CC is the "highway" that connects the left and right hemispheres controlling thoughts and actions between the two regions in a smooth, coordinated fashion. In ASD, this crucial area of the brain is misshapen. The CC typically forms a "C" shape, and in ASD, the ends are curved inward, decreasing the anterior to posterior length. Previous studies have shown that the anterior region is involved in cognitive information (13) and the posterior is involved in language and hearing (14). The posterior region may also be involved in sensory information, which may help explain the extremes in sensation that ASD patients experience (15).

Functional magnetic resonance imaging (fMRI) studies have started to utilize cognitive and emotional tasks to map the brain regions associated with the symptoms of ASD (3). These studies compare the brain's regional development in children, adolescents and adults with ASD and typical developing control (TDC) participants. Comparisons were made to their functional abilities in social interaction, qualitative impaired communication, and restricted, repetitive, and stereotypical patterns of behavior.

While studying social interaction, it was found that abnormally developing children (ADC) demonstrated greater left pre-central gyrus (controls voluntary movements of the right side of the body) activation than in TDC children, at the same time it was observed that these children have decreased activation of the right superior temporal gyrus (associated with hearing and speech), parahippocampal gyrus (memory storage and recall), bilateral amygdala (memory and emotional reactions), and right fusiform gyrus (facial, body and word recognition). Adult only studies demonstrated significantly greater activation of the left superior temporal gyrus in ASD adult vs TDC adults, as well as less activation in the left anterior cingulate gyrus and culmen. When comparing this group of studies together, it was noted that the activation of these areas in ASD children was significantly greater then ASD adults in the left posterior central gyrus (especially clusters of Brodmann areas 3 and 2 in the primary somatosensory cortex). Hypo-activation of the right para-hippocampal gyrus/hippocampus and the right superior temporal gyrus was noted in ASD children compared to ASD adults. (3).

The testing of nonsocial tasks had a slightly different results pattern. ASD children, versus TDC children, demonstrated hyperactivity in the insula (Brodmann area 13 – a bridging area between the lateral and medial layers of the brain) and right middle frontal gyrus (Brodmann area 46 - motor planning, organization, and regulation), while demonstrating hypoactivity in right caudate (learning and memory) and superior frontal gyrus (self awareness and laughter). Adult testing found ADC adult to have hyperactive right medial front gyrus (Brodmann area 8 - planning complex movements), and inferior occipital gyrus (visual areas). Possible link to certain forms of epilepsy), in the left middle frontal gyrus (Brodmann 11 - planning, reasoning, and decision making) and anterior cingulate gyrus (Brodmann area 32 - rational thought processes). There were no areas where TDC adults had significantly greater activation over ADC adults. The convergence of hyper-activation of autistic children over affected adults in regions including the insula (Brodmann area 13) right middle frontal gyrus (Brodmann areas 9 and 46) and left cingulate gyrus (Brodmann area 24). Hypo-activation was greater in ASD children over ASD adults in right middle frontal gyrus (Brodmann area 10 and 11). (3)

Finally, we considered structural neuroimaging studies utilizing voxel-based morphometry (VBM). This method compares the local concentration of gray matter between two groups and then separates gray matter from the normalized images while smoothing the gray-matter segments. The final step, smoothing the gray-matter segments, is vital because the voxel-wise parametric statistical tests compared this particular component among the two groups. The theory of Gaussian Random Fields was used to make corrections for the multiple comparisons being made (16). This technology allowed comparatives to be performed for grey and white matter in children to adults with ASD and their age matched TDC counterparts (17).

These studies demonstrated that children/adolescents with ASD were more likely to have decreased grey matter density in the left putamen and the right cerebellum in comparison to their age matched TDC counterparts. In addition, this group had significantly reduced grey matter in several frontal lobe regions including the medial prefrontal cortex, inferior frontal gyrus, insula and regions within the parietal and temporal lobes. The same children demonstrated increased grey matter in right anterior cingulate cortex (Brodmann area 32) and fusiform gyrus. Adults with ASD showed decreased grey matter bilaterally in the putamen, superior frontal gyri, and the right superior and middle temporal gyri, with significant reduction in grey matter in the medial prefrontal cortex and anterior cingulate cortex. These adults had increased grey matter in the left anterior cingulate cortex (Brodmann area 24), middle frontal gyri, middle temporal gyri, and hippocampi. (17)

The white matter finding for ACD children and adolescents demonstrated a decrease in cingulum bundle, superior and inferior longitudinal fasciculi, and several portions of the corona radiata. The same group had increased white matter in the internal and external capsules, cingulum, and corpus callosum. The white matter finding for ASD adults included decreases in the cortical spinal tract and cerebellum, with increases in the external capsule and corona radiata (17).

The medial prefrontal cortex, the superior parietal lobe and the putamen all have less grey matter in individuals with ASD, regardless of age, when compared with their TDC counterparts. A similar comparison of the superior frontal gyrus, middle temporal gyrus, and cerebellum showed increased gray matter. There were few similarities in the ASD group when examining the white matter with the exception of the external capsule which showed an increase in concentration.

Conclusions

This chapter has discussed the hypothesis that ASD is associated with atypical neural connectivity. This seems to be a valid hypothesis because, as reported studies have indicated so far, there are communication problems between different areas of the brain in autism. Difficulty is associated with the amygdala, where its increased size creates a problem with the uncus and inferior pole of the superior temporal lobe. The misshaped CC further causes poor communication between adjacent regions of the brain that cooperate to control language, hearing, emotions, and sensation. This observation further supports the hypothesis that brains of individuals with autism handle situations much differently than typically developing brains. When the attention of ASD individuals is directed toward an internal stimulus, there is increased brain network connectivity. When the stimulus is external, there is decreased connectivity. In the resting state there appears to be decreased intrinsic connectivity. What this has shown is that the brains of individuals diagnosed with ASD function much differently than those with typically developing brains, due to changes in connections across different regions of the brain.

To further evaluate what exactly causes these changes, two major areas should be of particular focus in future studies. The first is that there must be a large longitudinal study that follows patients for several decades. A study of this sort will surely involve multiple institutions. One factor that must be consistent in such a study is the tool by which the study population is examined. As seen earlier in this chapter, there is contradictory information on the same subject, likely due to differences in age and subjects, but also partly because of different imaging modalities. Even within the same imagining procedure, there are numerous protocols by which examination can be performed. There must be standardization of the protocol to ensure any meaningful information for comparison between research groups.

Previous studies in this subject have had very small cohorts, making the establishment of cause and effect very difficult. However, with the changes made to the criteria for autism in the DSM-5, the study population can now be much larger. Those with Asperger's disorder, childhood disintegrative disorder, and pervasive development disorder can now be examined under the umbrella of ASD. There is one potential fallback to including patients diagnosed with this group of diseases: Like autism, little is known about these other disorders; their inclusion in ASD studies could hinder any meaningful conclusion about cause and effect.

The second area of importance is the study of females. ASD affects males and females at a rate of 4:1. This has resulted in many studies focusing only on males. There must be a reason for higher rates of ASD in males as opposed to females, examining the disease in women should shed some light on the pathogenesis of this poorly understood disorder.

fMRI studies demonstrate age-related changes in both social and nonsocial tasks, with neurological differences associated with ASD constantly in flux from childhood to adult life (3)(see chapter 3A). This may support the theories of early cerebral overgrowth that have been corroborated by Schumann, et al.'s longitudinal structural MRI study of ASD, which demonstrated enlargement of grey and white matter, but no growth in occipital grey matter in 41 ASD and 44 TDC children serially scanned between ages of 18 months to 5 years (4). This was corroborated by post mortem studies done by Courchesne et al. which showed higher total PFC neuron count and brain weight in ASD children when compared to TDC children (18).

When looking at the results related to social tasks, we see less activation in children in the parahippocampal gyrus and hippocampus. This was also corroborated in another study that utilized structural MRI to show that ASD children, with and without mental retardation, had larger right hippocampal volume than TDC children (19). Another study showed that hippocampal abnormalities could play a role in visual abnormalities associated with ASD (20, 21). ASD adults have aberrant hippocampal-fusiform pathway white matter neural connectivity, as demonstrated by diffusion-tensor tracking (22). All cases have significant left versus right hippocampal asymmetry connected to laterality of visual perception (23).

As for nonsocial tasks, children with ASD have increased activation of right insula, middle frontal gyrus, and left cingulate gyrus when compared to ASD adults. This correlates with prior studies by Di Martino et al. who demonstrated the insula's involvement in ASD. The middle frontal gyrus in combination with both the temporal and parietal cortex has been implicated in the pathophysiology of ASD (24,25). This seems to be substantiated by the other studies noted above.

Longitudinal neuroimaging studies will be necessary to confirm he developmental trajectories of the neural alterations associated with ASD as children become adolescents and, ultimately, adults (3).

The voxel-based morphometry (VBM) studies are generalized to higher functioning individuals with ASD. Children and adolescents are more likely to demonstrate altered brain morphology in the hippocampi, cingulate gyrus, insula, and the fusiform gyri, brain regions that have been implicated in memory, social communication, attention, affect and social cognition. Adults demonstrate morphological variation in motor fiber pathways. Both groups demonstrated changes in regions related to fronto-striatal communications and repetitive behavior, being the prefrontal cortex and putamen respectively as can be seen in the executive function impairments that are stereotypical for this group. The morphological changes to the prefrontal cortex and striatum can explain the inability to maintain a plan in working memory while inhibiting an inappropriate response. Since these alterations were seen in both children and adults once can deduce that they occurred developmentally, contributing to a life-long deficit of executive functions (17).

Children with ASD show decreased grey matter in the hippocampal region, an area often associated with memory impairment and possibly linked to impaired episodic memory (26). Social communication impairment has also been related to deficits in this area (27). The areas of social communication and episodic memory may be related when one considers that episodic memory is utilized to evaluate and predict social behavior in others.

Chapter 3C - Brain Pathology and Behavior
Daniel Herzog, Katie Williams

[Attempts to relate areas of the brain affected in autistic patients and their behavioral disturbances are described, especially the interconnection of these centers, in order to gain an overall understanding of neural aberrations in this disorder. – Ed.]

Hypothesis

There are many areas of the brain that are abnormal in structure/function in autistic individuals. Given the diverse symptoms associated with autism and the many brain aberrations, it is possible that there is perhaps one underlying abnormality that ultimately leads to the widespread neuropathological changes causing the many signs/symptoms of autism. Despite all the research that has been conducted, however, as of now the exact cause of or a single pathologic location in the brain with autism is unknown. It still remains difficult to definitively associate brain pathologies with specific autistic behavior. The present chapter will not cover all the brain abnormalities that have been identified in patients with autism. We will primarily discuss areas that integrate information from various regions of the brain and have responsibilities that correlate with the behavioral abnormalities seen in autism (chapter 3B).

Observations

Anterior cinglulate cortex

One of the main areas of the brain that is thought to be abnormal in autistic individuals is the anterior cingulate cortex (ACC). It is located towards the anterior and midline of the brain. The ACC is responsible for a number of emotional and cognitive functions (1). It is involved with emotional learning through experiences, vocal expression of internal states, and emotional value assignment to internal and external stimuli. Additionally, it is accountable for evaluating the efficacy of an individual's response to external stimuli and, if needed, adjusting that response to ensure a more favorable outcome for future encounters with those stimuli (2). Also, the ACC is involved in motivating a person to perform actions for the purpose of later receiving a reward (3).

With these functions, it is plausible that abnormalities in the anterior cingulate cortex can contribute to some of the aberrant behaviors seen in patients with autism. These abnormalities may lead to a lack of personal motivation since the individual may not grasp the value of behaving in a favorable way for a later reward (4). Similarly, a person will exhibit repetitive behaviors if he lacks the ability to properly monitor the efficacy of his actions the first time they are performed (5).

A number of studies have been done to compare the anterior cingulate cortex of autistic people with those of unaffected individuals. There are significant differences which are thought to contribute to some of the anomalous social behaviors seen in autism. The surface area of the cingulate cortex is generally greater in individuals with autism than in normal individuals (6), although it is not clear exactly how this has an effect on the functionality of the ACC. However, there have been a number of studies that were able to directly relate abnormalities in the structure and function of the anterior cingulate cortex to specific behaviors (chapters 3B,3D).

An investigation using functional MRI (chapter 3A) to measure brain activity found that the anterior cingulate cortex is activated in unaffected individuals primarily when they respond incorrectly to a question. In autistic individuals, however, the ACC is activated equally regardless of the accuracy of their response. Furthermore, it was also found that the autistic subjects with stronger activation of the anterior cingulate cortex to correct responses had more severe symptoms of repetitive behavior. This abnormal activation in some cases contributes to the type of repetitive and rigid behavior seen in autism. Firstly, autistic individuals may think that there was something wrong with their response to a stimulus even if it were, in fact, an acceptable response. They may continue to react to the same stimuli despite having already responded to it appropriately. In addition, they lack the flexibility to adjust their responses to slight differences in repeated exposure to similar stimuli, as they will have difficulty analyzing which aspects of their behavior were appropriate for the stimuli (5).

The ACC is also connected to the prefrontal cortex. This area is the most anterior part of the brain and is connected to the anterior cingulate cortex through a bundle of nerve fibers called the forceps minor. The forceps minor is part of the corpus callosum, the main bundle of nerve fibers connecting the left and right hemispheres of the brain. When a person is in a situation that he can respond to in more than one way, it is thought that the anterior cingulate cortex evaluates the conflict between the possible responses, but the prefrontal cortex biases the choice of one of the possibilities (7). The volume of the forceps minor in autistic individuals is significantly less than in normal individuals. Furthermore, a greater reduction in the volume of the forceps minor correlates with stronger symptoms of rigid behavior (8). Difficulties in resolving the conflict between possible responses may also lead to rigid behavior, as the individuals will have difficulty analyzing new and different approaches to stimuli.

One of the behavioral features of people with autism is a lack of social motivation, which presents as a diminished interest in seeking and enjoying social interactions (9). Autistic individuals show less activation of the anterior cingulate cortex than unaffected individuals in response to the offer of social reward (4). Since they do not attribute value to social reward, they will not look to socialize or seek interactions with others. This is yet another example of an anterior cingulate cortex abnormality appearing to contribute to the behaviors seen in autism.

Amygdala

The amygdala is a collection of nuclei located in the medial temporal lobe near the anterior end of the parahippocampal formation. Since the amygdala is not one single entity, it is sometimes referred to as the amygdoloid complex. The amygdala is connected to many other areas of the brain. It receives visual, auditory, and olfactory sensory information. Interestingly, the anterior cingulate cortex, which has been mentioned earlier in this chapter, also projects into the amygdala. The amygdala, in turn, connects with other regions of the brain through two main pathways, the stria terminalis and the ventral amygdalofugal pathway (10).

The amygdala is involved in emotional stimulation and affects social behavior. Stimulating the amygdala in conscious humans evokes feelings of fear, irritability, and anger. Imaging studies have shown that there are variations in the amygdala activation when a person is shown facial expressions that induce different emotional feelings. Furthermore, the amygdala shows greater activation when the person is shown faces expressing stronger emotions (11). It is also involved in reading social signals from the face and the comprehension of expressive body movements (12). Clearly, our understanding of the body language and the facial expressions of the people around us affects how we respond and interact with them.

Abnormalities in amygdala growth in autism seem to indicate its involvement in this disorder. Until about age 7 years, the amygdalae in autistic people grow abnormally quickly and are larger than the typical amygdale (13). At about age 7, the growth rate in autistic individuals slows, at which point the amygdalae of neurologically normal individuals grows faster than those of autistic individuals. In later adolescence and early adulthood, the autistic amygdala decreases in size compared to the typical structure (14). The relationship between its size and the symptoms of autism is unclear, as autistic children with larger amygdalae generally have more severe behavioral presentations, while in adults the situation is reversed. However, the greater the departure from normal, the more severe is the neurologic problems in either case.

Difficulties in the recognition of facial and body expressions in autism also point to amygdala involvement. When determining the trustworthiness of people from their facial expressions, autistic people and people with amygdala lesions regard people in general as more trustworthy than do normal individuals (15). Emotional body movements and expressions lead to increased amygdala activation in normal individuals. However, in autistic individuals, these do not lead to greater activation than a neutral body stance does (16).

Another abnormality in the amygdalae in autism is the lack of habituation. Normally, when a person is exposed to a given stimulus for an extended period of time, he/she becomes acclimated to that stimulus, and the effect that such stimulation has on the recipient is decreased. In autistic individuals, however, such response decreases at a much slower rate than in normal individuals. Since old stimuli continue to activate the person's brain, new stimuli will not be perceived as the amygdala is still activated from the previous stimulus. Therefore, changes in body expressions will not be appreciated as much (17).

This phenomenon of habituation has been used to explain conflicting studies as to the level of activation in the autistic amygdala in general. Although most such studies indicate that the amygdala is activated less in autistic individuals than in unaffected individuals (18-20), some observations have found there to be increased activation in the amygdalae of autistic individuals (21,22). A possible explanation to this apparent contradiction is the amount of time over which the amygdala activation was measured. Overall, the studies that measured amygdala activation for a shorter period of time found there to be decreased activation, whereas in studies that measured for a longer period of time there was increased activation. This can be explained by the apparent lack of habituation in autistic people. Since the amygdala stimulation continued longer in the autistic individuals, it gave the impression of having greater activation (17).

Cerebellum

The human nervous system is divided into two major parts (10):
1) The central nervous system (CNS) includes the brain, brain stem and spinal cord.
2) The peripheral nervous system (PNS) encompasses all the nerves traveling to and from the central nervous system carrying sensory and movement (motor) information.

The cerebellum is located posterior to the brain stem and below the parietal and occipital lobes of the brain. The cerebellum is attached to the brain stem via three pairs of cerebellar peduncles. These peduncles are made up of many nerve cell axons allowing communication between the cerebellum and other areas of the brain. It is through these connections the cerebellum is able to influence CNS and, ultimately, PNS function.

A role of the CNS is to interpret the incoming data and generate an appropriate, coordinated response. The cerebellum is believed to play a part in coordination through synchronization of muscle contractions and relaxation to form useful movements (10). Further, imaging of the cerebellum has revealed increased cerebellar activity in non-motor tasks, suggesting the cerebellum plays a role in cognitive functions as well. Anatomical and functional magnetic resonance imaging (chapter 3A) confirms the role of the cerebellum in cognitive and visuospatial functions as well as its influence on affect (the experience of emotion) (23).

Damage or developmental changes to the cerebellum can result in deficits in language, decision-making and affect, as well as uncoordinated or erratic motor function (24). Because of these generally accepted functions, current research continues to identify links between pathological changes in the cerebellum and symptoms of autism. Over the last few decades, many researchers have identified neuropathologies of the cerebellum of autistic individuals. These findings include augmented cerebellar size (25), decreased numbers of Purkinje cells, abnormalities in deep cerebellar nuclei, increased oxidative stress, as well as multiple abnormalities involving neurotransmitters (26). Additionally, functional imaging techniques have especially enhanced the ability to assess specific brain area activation while certain tasks are performed. However, relating cerebellar pathologies to specific autism spectrum disorder symptomatology remains difficult.

Although there are several changes consistently noted in the autistic individual's cerebellum, one of the most commonly agreed upon findings is an abnormality with Purkinje cells. Reduced Purkinje cells in the cerebellum are the most reproducible pathology found in autistic brain autopsies (27). Therefore, this discussion will address how changes in the Purkinje cells in the cerebellum potentially play a role in causing the symptoms of autism.

Purkinje cells are the principal cells of the cerebellar cortex (10). Based on incoming inputs, they can produce a cortical output via the deep nuclei of the cerebellum (24). Essentially, they are the cells that ultimately determine the influence of the cerebellum on a task after it receives input from other parts of the body. In some autistic individuals, the most pronounced areas of Purkinje cell loss are in the archi-cerebellar cortex (which corresponds to the functional division known as the vestibule-cerebellum) and the neocerebellar cortex (also known as the lateral cerebellar hemispheres) (28).

The vestibule-cerebellum is associated with muscle tone adjustment and coordinates muscles that maintain balance (10). The vestibule-cerebellum also coordinates eye control and neck muscle function and thus is important in controlling gaze (24). On the other hand, the neocerebellar cortex receives input primarily from the cerebral cortex. Then the Purkinje cells project into the dentate nucleus (one of the deep nuclei) before the axons leave the cerebellum to their final intended site of action. Although these connections are typically related to coordinated motor function, recently functional imaging has indicated that the dentate nucleus is also involved in non-motor functions, such as cognition.

Autistic individuals typically have cognitive deficits, which include impaired social interaction and communication, as well as restricted and stereotyped behavior (29), and altered motor behavior (30). The more recent acceptance of the non-motor role of the cerebellum has made it an area of the brain of particular interest in attempts to identify autism's etiology. Additionally, the Purkinje cells are the only cerebellar cortex output and are consistently abnormal in autism (31). The cerebellum communicates with many cortical regions of the brain to modulate cognitive, motor, language, sensory, and emotional functions (26). This function, coupled with frequently noted cerebellar pathologies, such as decreased Purkinje cells, suggests the cerebellum ultimately is involved in the autistic individual's symptomatology. However, it is clear that the cerebellum is not the only change noted in autistic brains, and thus, is only one piece of the etiologic puzzle.

Corpus callosum

The human brain is divided into left and right hemispheres, and the interconnectivity is extensive. The cerebral cortex is connected via numerous intra-hemispheric and inter hemispheric fibers. These connections include association fibers which connect one cortical area to another within one hemisphere, projection fibers between the cortex and subcortical structures, and commissural fibers that connect cortical areas of the two different hemispheres (10). Generally, the fibers are made up of myelinated neuronal axons and are referred to collectively as white matter (chapter 6B). The corpus callosum, located in the midline of the two hemispheres, is one of the most extensive bundles of commissural fibers.

Interregional interactions of the brain are vital for appropriate function. Neurons interact in such a way to coordinate cognitive and sensorimotor tasks (32), including language processing (33). More recently, proposed autism neural models have evolved from a lesion-based approach to that of abnormal connectivity between the CNS structures (34). More specifically, this model has been dubbed the Under-connectivity Theory. This theory proposes that autism is associated with decreased functioning of the circuitry of the brain, which results in deficits of both neural and cognitive integration of information (35) (chapter 6E). For example, several neuroimaging studies suggest decreased brain area coordination in autism and that abnormal connectivity between social brain areas could play a role in the socio-emotional troubles of autistic individuals (36).

In studies of the pathophysiology of autism, identifying locations of underconnectivity via a variety of radiological imaging techniques has revealed several candidate regions of pathology (chapter 3A). Some studies have focused on the white matter microstructural properties, others on tract (bundle of axons) development, while still others address the size and length of axonal fibers. A frequently addressed area is the corpus callosum.

Although there remains some controversy, the possibility of abnormalities of the corpus callosum in autism seems to be relatively well accepted, and generally research has shown that it may be smaller in volume in autistic individuals (35). As neuroimaging studies continue to determine the best mode of analyzing white matter scans, many other researchers are working to determine the ultimate symptomatology of a smaller corpus callosum. However, with increasing evidence that deficits in connectivity play a role in autism and the number of researchers finding decreased corpus callosum volumes in ASD, it appears this may be one of the contributing issues of the behavioral manifestations of this disease.

Key features of autism are social and emotional deficits; integrated brain activity is necessary to engage in appropriate social interactions (37). Because the corpus callosum is the primary structure connecting the two cerebral hemispheres, decreased volume (and thus decreased connectivity) may contribute to some of the behavioral dysfunctions of autism (38). One of the more compelling comparisons has been in the behavioral manifestations of autistic individuals to those with agenesis of the corpus callosum. With some exceptions, people with such pathology have frequently shown deficits in some of the same areas as ASD patients (39). This strengthens the argument that decreased connectivity between the left and right cortex may play a role in autism symptoms.

What is important to note is, currently, no studies have been able to definitively relate changes in the corpus callosum or in other intra-hemispheric white matter fibers to be the sole cause of specific autism symptoms. However, evidence is growing to suggest that pathological changes in interconnectivity between hemispheres and within hemispheres may be a contributing factor to the autistic phenotype.

It is interesting to note that in normal individuals and those with early onset autism, there occurs an increase in head circumference after infancy, but yet the change is less in regressive ASD. In addition, probably because autism occurs much more often (4 to 1) in males than females, the latter deserve targeted study as well to determine if neurologic changes in both genders with ASD are similar or if this is a distinct difference.

Conclusions

As has been thoroughly noted in this and other chapters of this book, changes on both the microscopic and macroscopic levels of the brain characteristically occur in autism. Research is ongoing in the verification of some of the pathological differences already identified and in locating new areas of interest. Neuroimaging techniques have evolved in such a way as to allow greater analysis of function and structure of the autistic brain, in addition to the pathologies noted via techniques done post-mortem. What remains one of the more difficult areas of ASD research is relating the anatomical and cellular changes of the nervous system to idiosyncratic behaviors found in autistic individuals.

It is apparent that there is no one difference in the brain that can be specifically and individually linked to autistic behavior pathogenesis. Rather, it seems that a variety of microscopic and macroscopic changes contribute to the persistent behavioral characteristics that define autism. The anterior cingulate cortex, amygdala, cerebellum, and corpus callosum are only a few of the brain regions that potentially allow linking of structural deficits and developmental modifications to autistic behavior. Whether the degree of pathologic change is proportional to the extent of involvement on the autism spectrum remains to be determined. As research techniques and autism knowledge grow, it will be fascinating to see how the relationships between autistic brain pathology and autistic brain function determine characteristic behaviors.

Chapter 3D – Brain Micropathology
Y. Irene Li, Sebastian Jofre

[To better understand the underlying changes in the autistic brain, microscopic evaluation has identified specific modifications. Of special interest are hyperplasia, hypoplasia, and dysgenesis which may hold the key to explaining overt characteristics of this disease. – Ed.]

Hypothesis

Autism spectrum disorder (ASD) is a neural developmental condition classically characterized by stereotypical repetitive behavior and pronounced deficit in social interaction and communication. It is generally diagnosed within the first 1-3 years of life. Patients often present with a wide range of classical symptoms of varying severity, as well as co-morbidities such as mental retardation, Fragile X Syndrome, Down's Syndrome, and epilepsy (1-3). These additional disorders commonly associated with ASD are not seen in all patients and have limited prevalence among certain age groups. Due to the variegated presentation of symptoms identified upon diagnosis, several areas of the brain have been implicated as potential sources of pathology mediating the development of the disorder. These include functions involved in regulation of higher thinking, communication and social interaction, as well as emotions and memory formation (1).

The human brain, a complex circuitry and integration center, includes the cerebrum, brainstem and cerebellum. Injury or morphological changes due to aberrant neuronal development in any one area can cause the formation of inappropriate or immature circuitry and, ultimately, deregulation of function. In recent years, research findings have led scientists to believe that the underlying genesis of autism corresponds to disruptions in the mechanisms of early brain development. This perspective highlights the importance of genetics, immunology, and biochemistry in influencing neuron development, as well as the fundamental anatomy and physiology of the brain. In such a way, it is likely that any event causing disequilibrium in the crucial, balanced mechanisms leading to proper neuronal maturation would have widely disseminated and compounded effects on the concurrent development of the brain.

By examining the micro-pathology of the autistic brain, researchers endeavored to answer the fundamental question of "What is changed?" At the same time, they strove to be mindful of the heterogeneous changes seen throughout several areas of the brain in formulating their observations and conclusions. The identified variability, coupled with the inherent complexity of the brain's circuitry, pose the ultimate challenge that scientists today face in their attempts to pinpoint the etiological mechanism for the development of autism.

In 1985, Kemper and Bauman reported changes in cellular density within areas of the limbic system, which functions in the generation of emotions, behavior, and memory, to name a few (4). This study highlighted the involvement of the limbic system as a potential contributor to autistic development and behavior. The limbic system is a closed circuit composed of the hippocampus, amygdala, anterior thalamic nuclei, septum, habenula, limbic cortex and fornix.

By relating the pathology observed in the neuronal cells, as well as the lesions seen in various regions of the brain to the expressed patterns of behavior, these scientists sought to correlate lesion and outcome. Since then, investigators have continued to study microscopic changes and lesions affecting neurons and their supportive glial cells, while observing the contributions these deformations make to the development of ASD. Such findings have led several research groups to place especial emphasis on the cellular changes occurring in the limbic system, the cerebellum, and the frontal and temporal lobes.

Several hypotheses have emerged with the advancements of technology and the availability of post-mortem brain samples. Although no one particular hypothesis has produced sufficient conclusive supportive data, current findings have focused on three cumulative trends of evidence attributable to abnormal neurogenesis: cellular hypoplasia, hyperplasia, and dysplasia/dysgenesis. These three areas of study will form the primary focus for this chapter.

Observations

Born from past observations of variable neuronal dimensions in the brains of autistic patients, several prevailing bodies of thought have sought to explain the underlying pathology. Of these, three hypotheses have emerged as the most prominent. One proposes cellular hypoplasia, or decreased cell number, as the process responsible for autistic behavior. Another focuses on hyperplastic changes, or increased cellular numbers, as they contribute to aberrant neuronal pathways. A third hypothesis proposes that dysplastic, irregular, and disorganized cellular changes are at fault.

Several explanations for these over-arching themes of tissue morphology changes have become popular. Note, however, that because extensive cross-over and inherent inter-connectivity exist between sections of the brain, a change in any one area would inevitably impact the proper function of other areas of the brain as well.

Hypoplasia and neuronal loss

The hypoplastic changes associated with autism can be observed in the neocortex. This area is of special importance because it houses neurons that serve as two-way connections from the outer surface of the brain to the thalamus. The neocortex is composed of six layers (I – VI), each distinctive in cellular composition and distribution. Current research suggests that the spectrum of symptoms currently associated with this disorder may be linked to the under-development of the neurons housed in this region.

The primary cell functioning in transmission of output signals from the cortex is the pyramidal cell. These neurons reside principally in layers III and V of the neocortex and are especially populous in the regions associated with motion. In layers II and III, these cells give rise to commissural fibers that communicate between the right and left hemispheres. Interestingly, the brains of autistic patients present with pyramidal neurons of smaller size. A recent study by Tang et al. has, furthermore, found evidence to implicate mitochondrial abnormalities in the immature function of autistic pyramidal cells (5). Notable morphological changes have been seen in cells of most types when there was insufficient energy production by the mitochondria, the powerhouse of the cell. The neuron is no exception to this principle.

Normally, the mitochondria are central to many physiological processes within cells. For one, they are able to produce energy necessary for cellular function, development, and survival via oxidative phosphorylation. This generates more than 95% of neuronal adenosine triphosphate (ATP) under normal physiological conditions. Improper ATP generation interrupts normal ATPase-regulated maintenance of the electrochemical gradient between internal and external environments of the neuron, making neurons more excitable (5). Without energy, neurons are unable to properly traffic neurotransmitters and hormones across their axons, rendering neuronal communication inefficient. Secondly, defective mitochondrial membrane further promotes the formation and accumulation of toxic radicals and reactive oxygen species (ROS) that contribute to DNA damage, as well as disrupted neuronal development, structure and communication.

Alternatively, abnormalities in the cerebellum, which is involved in unconscious regulation of motor abilities, have an association with the physical symptoms of autism. Loss of Purkinje cells in the cerebellum and vermis in the post-mortem brains of autistic patients of varying ages, some with presenting comorbidities such as mental retardation or seizures (4,6). The cerebellum, which regulates unconscious motor control, balance and posture, among its other functions, is also thought to contribute to stereotypical patterns of behavior associated with autism, particularly in response to environmental stimuli, cognition, and orientation.

Purkinje cells are large neurons responsible for transmitting signals from the cerebellar cortex to the cerebellar nuclei located at its core. Under normal circumstances, Purkinje cells manage input and output of information through inhibitory neuronal signals. In autism, however, these neurons are often smaller and less numerous. Certain conjectures to the cause of this loss of cell number have been focused on the activation of microglia. Microglial cells form an essential part of the brain's immune system. Descending from myeloid progenitor cells, they share common attributes with macrophages and take part in mediation of pro-inflammatory and anti-inflammatory responses upon the introduction of hypoxic stress or other sources of injuries (chapter 6D).

Morphological changes seen in these cells include, but are not limited to, increased cell body size, process thickening and retraction. Extensions of filopodia necessary for proper microglial sensing and detections of injury as well as of chemokines and cytokines have been suggested to be impaired by these changes. As these microglial cells are associated with the maintenance of synaptic integrity in the brain, their modifications have been implicated in the development of neuronal connections and plasticity (7). Descriptions of this pathology is very similar to those observed in Bergmann's gliosis in which hyperplasia of astrocytic cells contribute to and are associated with loss of Purkinje cells.

Indeed, past observations of the activation of microglia have included the cerebellum, as well as the cortical and subcortical regions of the brain. Current studies have focused on certain regions of the brain that have shown increased levels of microglial activation through the use of magnetic resonance imaging (MRI) and positron emission tomography (PET) imaging (chapter 3A) with a detectable tracer administered in regions of the cerebellum, midbrain, and thalamus (8). Increased presence of tracer and microglial activity were found in the cerebellum, midbrain, pons, the subcortical region of the corpus callosum (region of white matter that forms the medial borders of the lateral ventricles of the two cerebral hemispheres), the anterior cingulate cortex of the limbic system, and the frontal, temporal and parietal regions. The greatest elevation is seen in the left cerebral hemisphere, specifically in the regions associated with Brodmann Areas (BA) 44, 45 and 22 that are involved with speech, language and hearing. Microglial cells in the dorsolateral prefrontal cortex were also described as being markedly activated in young patients less than six years of age (9).

(Of special interest is the reduced axonal diameter and myelination found in neurons of the central nervous system in brain biopsies of autistic individuals as it relates to IGF-stimulated activity of oligodendrocytes. This is discussed in detail in chapters 6B & 6E.)

Hyperplasia

One prevalent pathologic finding observed in the brains of autistic patients is their increased dimensions, suggesting a potential link between large brain size and the incidence of ASD. Consequently, many studies have focused on the hyperplastic changes of the cerebral cortex (4,6,10,11). Macroscopic and MRI imaging studies have indicated cortical thickening in several key areas. It has been suggested that abnormalities in any one of these sections forming the limbic system, namely the hippocampus, amygdala, anterior thalamic nuclei, cingulate cortex, hypothalamus, and the limbic cortex, may result in autistic behavior. Initial qualitative analysis revealed abnormal cortical cytoarchitecture with increased cellular density in the limbic system of the autistic brain (4). This density enhancement did not seem to be universal to all areas of the brain, and may be dependent on the chronology of insulting events taking place during gestation (11).

Comparatively, recent studies have shown increased emphasis on the quantitative and qualitative study of minicolumnopathy as a potential mechanism behind the observed increased cellular proliferation of brains of autistic patients. Minicolumns are characterized as collections of cellular elements with a consistent morphology that, in association with pyramidal neurons, form a fundamental unit of communicational systems seen in the normal brain. Hierarchical grouping of these basic units forms the cerebral neocortex (12). In the post-mortem brain tissue of autistic patients, the number of minicolumns appeared increased, while the spacing between neighboring columns, the neuropil space, is decreased. This finding has also been observed in the frontal regions of the post-mortem brains of autistic patients with the greatest difference in the dorsal and orbital regions (13). Similar morphological changes were observed in BA 44 (14), associated with the production of speech and the written word.

Several studies have found a concomitant reduction in neuronal cell size in the amygdala, entorhinal cortex, subiculum, mammillary bodies, and septum of the limbic system (10). Yet, another group noted no increased density of neurons in cortical layers of the posterior cingulate cortex and fusiform gyrus (11), suggesting that not all areas of the brain present the same aforementioned pathologic findings.

Additionally, two types of glial cell proliferation were increased in autistic patients – microglia and astrocytes. Glial cells play a key role in regulating and sustaining an ideal microenvironment for neurons and may contribute to both hyperplastic and hypoplastic changes in the brain. As previously mentioned, microglia descend from the same lineage as macrophages, and undertake key immune responses in the nervous system. Increased microglia density was seen in the fronto-insular region, as well as the visual cortex (BA 17) of the cerebrum, possibly contributing to the increased cortical thickness of autistic brains (7).

Due to their regulatory mechanisms, activation of these cells may promote hyperactivity of an otherwise balanced function, leading to synapse pruning and loss of Purkinje cells in the cerebellum. One study utilized the expression of ionized calcium binding adaptor molecule 1 (IBA1, also known as allograft inflammatory marker 1 [AIF1]) as a target molecule for staining. This cytoplasmic protein is specifically expressed in the activated microglia and is often up-regulated after neuronal injury. Additionally, the activated microglial cell body was found to be larger, slightly grainy, with less distinct visualization of the plasma membrane compared to the resting microglia in the control sample. Loss of cellular processes extending from microglial bodies were also observed in the brain of an adult autistic patient (8,9).

Another study examined the role of astrocytes. Normally, these cells perform regulatory functions in maintenance of the extracellular matrix in the central nervous system. Data obtained from post-mortem brain tissue of autistic patients have shown that proliferation of astrocytes in the subventricular zone of the lateral ventricles of the cerebrum was increased through co-localization of the immunofluorescent markers for KI67, a nuclear protein antigen marker for proliferating cells. This change was specifically seen in autistic children only and has not been observed in the brains of adult patients. At this time, it is unclear if the contributory role that increases in astrocyte number functions in abnormal neuronal growth and abnormal synapse formation.

Dysplasia and dysgenesis

Morphologically, focal dysplasias are defined as disorganized neurons within various areas of the cortex, often associated with changes in laminar patterning, calcification, and agglutination in the shape of nodules. They range from mild disruptions with little cellular abnormalities, to more progressive morphological aberrations composed of irregular neurons and glial cells, as well as improper laminar formation. Several areas were found to be involved, of which the frontal cortex (2), anterior cingulate gyrus (10), middle temporal gyrus, somatosensory association cortex (11), occipital lobes, and floculo-nodular lobe in the cerebellum (1) have been included.

Mutations in the filamin 1 (FLNA1) and double-cortin (DCX) genes, two crucial genes required for normal cellular architecture and migration, have been linked to defective neuronal migration (1). Mutations in these genes cause neurons to clump together in improper places throughout the brain, sending irregular circles and loops of dendrites and axons that intervene with normal circuitry. Such nodules, as found in the subependymal cell layer of tuberous sclerosis patients, as well as some autistic patients, could potentially alter the function of any location they reside in and cause a wide range of effects and behavioral presentations. These findings, with further study, may provide a link between the genetic and pathologic causes of autism spectrum disorders. Especially in the Purkinje cells of the cerebellum, dysgenetic CNS development apparently begins before 30 weeks of fetal life.

Within many of these regions, changes in laminar patterning have been suggested to play a role in the development of increased cortical thickness. These changes were most apparent in laminas V and VI, where many of the larger pyramidal cells are located. Similar, but smaller differences were reported in layers II and III, which contain smaller pyramidal cells and more supporting glial cells (14). Additional phenotypes have displayed disorganized lamina patterning with no clear demarcation between layers IV and V (11). Up-regulation of growth associated protein 43 (GAP-43) has been proposed as a possible mechanism for abnormal myelination (12).

Scientists hypothesize a possible link between white matter size and aberrant neuronal migration (11), as well as the previously discussed changes in minicolumns. Nonetheless, because these cells do not exist in random arrangements, it is important to consider that the abnormalities likely exist within the cell assemblies as a whole, rather than as a mutation or single-cell pathology (6). While the development of these changes has not been tied to a well-substantiated mechanism, the observed reorganization of the cortex may cause the neurological sequelae observed in autism, such as cognitive impairment and behavioral stereotypies.

Proposed mechanims

Assuming that the immature or abnormal development of neurons in association with improper synapses formation later in life is attributable to the genesis of autism, the question still remains as to what is the mechanism that provoked these changes and when did it take place. It is yet unclear as to whether the answer herein lies in the cellular overgrowth, undergrowth, or a combination of both, that ultimately causes these aberrations.

Taking this assumption further, it is also difficult to state which hypothesis or perspective for cellular hyperplasia, hypoplasia, or dysplasia holds the key. In light of ongoing research, it is important to note the progression of interpretation and re-interpretation of data that influence much of the studies put forth. Thus far, mini-columnopathy and microglial activation/ proliferation are two of several hypotheses that have gained increasing attention from the science community as a means to characterize cortical thickening commonly seen in macrocephalic brains of a subpopulation of symptomatic autistic patients.

Additionally, it is also important to address the challenges that scientists face in dissecting these heterogeneous findings through their methodology and the nature of the disorder. Due to overlap between some of the postulated theories pertaining the pathology of autism, such as brain regions presenting with both hyperplasia and hypoplasia, it is possible that many of these studies are simply describing features of a bigger phenomenon that presents with variable morphology across the brain.

Thus, it is conceivable that discrepancies between findings could be brought about simply by differences in definition, by subjective classification of primary and secondary findings, or by unconventional methods of measurement. Moreover, currently, there does not exist a checks-and-balances system or model of assessment to validate the accuracy of some scales used in these studies against accepted biomarkers (2). Other confounding factors and limitations include the age-dependent progression of the autism, the sample size per age and gender group, and technological tools available at the time of the study.

The age groups examined in the majority of these studies spanned on average from 2 to 50 years. Biopsy samples were age-matched by one or two control samples. Several studies even sought to break down their studies into age-specific cohorts, although many of the characteristic symptoms of autism simply do not present exclusively in a certain age group. Therefore, such possibly associated changes in cellular morphology may not be seen in one group or another.

Furthermore, given the already limited number of brain samples available and used for study from organizations from California to Harvard and Boston. With the majority of tissue samples from the Autism Tissue Program, the resultant cohort sample sizes had frequently been reduced to less than five per cohort. One group also utilized the same sample as a previously published body of work (13-17). While helpful in showcasing increased body of evidence with one patient group, this practice rather limits these findings to a specific population or subpopulation of patients and is not representative of all patients with ASD.

Autism is most common in approximately 4.5 males to every female patient (chapter 1C). Based on this gender skew, many researchers have focused primarily on studying morphologic changes in the male brain. Several studies have, however, utilized a mixed sample of both male and female brains. Conversely, it is possible that gender differentiation does not contribute significantly to the resultant trends and findings. It is, nevertheless, important to account for the inherent gender bias associated with this disorder and the sample populations contributing to scientific research. Therefore, without larger bodies of supportive evidence, these current findings may not be fully representative of the population of autistic patients.

One other limitation to the current data presented is the lack of differential distinction between primary (directly causing) and secondary (indirectly causing) findings. The majority of current studies have been conducted on a limited supply of post-mortem tissue obtained from donations from families of deceased patients. Due to the variegated nature of ASD, it is difficult to say which of these findings are specific for autism, and not due to shared morphological changes associated with comorbidities or cause of death. Larger sample sizes without the presence of other disorders such as epilepsy or mental retardation, or a precise method to cull out these confounding factors, would be necessary to support and substantiate the theories currently held by the science community.

With this said, technological advancements in staining and imaging could potentially help researchers attain this goal. Several decades ago, to examine biopsy samples, researchers had primarily used Nissl staining (11,13,14). In recent years, there has been a shift towards usage of new technology and staining techniques. One current focus of use is on MRI/PET imaging (chapter 3A). To visualize morphologic changes of the cell as well as in the tissue, it has become popular to use immuno-histochemistry and immuno-fluorescence tissue staining techniques, including cresyl violet.

Stereology is another such example of technological advances. With increasing spatial visualization and interpretative ability, scientists would be able to more accurately characterize potentially contributing factors such as neuronal cell size, mini-column neuropil spacing and density, as well as microglial proliferation. However, it will likely be many years before high accuracy, high precision three-dimensional imaging and data analysis tools will be available.

It is clear from the present studies that many key morphological changes take place within the first few years of life, with trends not necessarily persisting into adulthood. These findings strongly suggest that a possible window of time to focus on for further studies is during the period in which the brain is initially being formed through the migration and regulation of neural tube and crest cells. It would be important to examine all aspects of the development.

Conclusions

Future directions will look to expand upon current findings in potential immune system mediators, genetic aberrations, as well as biochemical pathways that may regulate the development, structure and proliferative processes of neurons in the autistic brain. Additionally, it would also be important to determine how the morphologic and cyto-architectural changes result in the characteristic tissue abnormalities and symptomology of autism. Thus, further examination to determine the root cause of this disorder is essential and should include the longitudinal study of morphological trends and patterns of micropathologic/macropathologic findings often seen in the post-mortem tissues of autistic patient.

Indeed, micropathology, as the first visual evidence of any underlying cellular dysfunctions or abnormalities, holds much potential as both a method and a set of evidence in determining the physiological effects of autism. With continued focus and the allocation of resources to pursue the study of the etiological basis for autism, the community – families impacted by this disorder, the sciences and medical communities – stand much to benefit from the wealth of knowledge and the key to successfully treating and curing those afflicted by ASD.

Glossary
ASD – autism spectrum disorder
ATP – adenosine triphosphate
CNS - central nervous system
BA – Brodmann area

GLI – gray level index
IGF – insulin-like growth factor
MC – minicolumn
NS – neuropil space

Chapter 3E – Neurotransmitter Imbalance

Karolina Siniakowicz, Brett Schupack, Jemima Akinsanya, Christa Patrick

[The roles of neurotransmitter and synaptic disturbances, especially those involving GABA and glutamate, are examined to define the parts played by such malfunctions in the overall theory of dysregulation pathobiology of autism. – Ed.]

Hypothesis

As with many complex disorders, the hypotheses of the origin of autism span environmental, behavioral, and genetic components. Yet, one of the most recently explored concepts deals with a neurotransmitter imbalance between the excitatory (glutamate) and inhibitory (gamma-aminobutyric acid: GABA) aspect within the cortical structures and the networks they create. In this section, we will explore the proposed neurochemical basis of autism, specifically, a model based on neural 'dysregulation'. This model has the potential to effectively elucidate the origins of the phenotypic manifestations (outward physical characteristics) of autism—especially the repetitive, stereotyped behaviors as well as the inability to recognize, appropriately adapt, and respond to social cues. Additionally, we will discuss some recent findings regarding the neural network between the anterior cingulate cortex (ACC) and the amygdala as dysfunctional features apparently responsible for the most debilitating phenotypic trains in autism.

The ACC, a region shown to play a role in empathy, decision-making, and emotional responses to social cues, has been heavily implicated in the development of the disease (chapters 3B-3D). In this specific region of the brain, it is the imbalance between the excitatory and inhibitory signals that potentially dictates autistic tendencies. This has led to a neurochemical model of autism based on 'dysregulated' inhibitory and excitatory cortical signals.

Observations

Recent evidence supports the hypothesis that the disparity may arise not only from a chemical imbalance, but also from aberrant neuronal connections within the delicate circuitry involved in cue processing and appropriate behavior modulation. The amygdala has also been implicated to play a role in behavior modulation in people with autism spectrum disorder (ASD). With its vast reciprocal connections to the limbic system and the ACC circuit, the amygdala has been shown to take part in emotional learning, reward behavior and memory modulation (chapters 3B-3D). Several studies have shown that the size of the amygdala is increased in autistic children, but that the number of neurons and their connections actually decrease as the children age, thus further supporting the theory of neurochemical imbalance.

Finally, the latest imaging, histological, and clinical studies also implicate neurotransmitter imbalance between unregulated hyper-excitability paired with the lack of inhibition as an important factor in ASD development and progression (1,2). It is well established that neuronal transmission and signaling requires a delicate, almost perfect, balance for the brain to successfully take in cues and produce appropriate behavior. The lack of cue assimilation and diminished social interaction are only two components of autism, but they are the two that greatly contribute to the debilitating nature of the disease and, thus, are worth exploring further in search for therapeutic targets.

The central nervous system (CNS), including the brain and spinal cord, receives sensory information from the body such as sight, hearing, touch, position, and visceral processes. It integrates and interprets information to produce a coordinated response given a sensory cue. The functional units of the CNS are neurons, which communicate via neurotransmitters released into synapses. Synapses are highly specialized sites of communication between presynaptic nerve terminals and postsynaptic neurons. They contain a large variety of molecules at very high densities that include neurotransmitters, receptors, and associated structural proteins. Each presynaptic or postsynaptic neurotransmitter can either be excitatory or inhibitory, continuing the communication to the adjacent neuron or terminating the signal transmission, thus creating a complex network of reciprocal connectivity. The neurotransmitter receptors, however, will ultimately define the functionality of a synapse. By dynamically changing the strengths of their connections, synapses give our nervous system the ability to learn and respond to our environment accordingly to a perceived or sensed stimulus (1).

The CNS relies on a careful balance of inhibitory and excitatory neurotransmitters to produce appropriately coordinated thoughts and actions. Current molecular and neurochemical evidence suggests that the signs and symptoms of autism are related to an imbalance of inhibitory and excitatory neurotransmitters in the CNS (2).

GABA is the chief inhibitory neurotransmitter in the brain responsible for regulating neuronal excitability in local circuits, as well as inhibiting long-range synapses. GABA works by binding to its receptors: post-synaptic structures that mediate the effect of GABA, i.e., inhibition of further neuronal action. It is this process that reduces excitability in the CNS (3).

There are several GABA receptors subunits known to date:

1) $GABA_A$ receptor (responsible for fast synaptic inhibition), and
2) $GABA_B$ receptor (for prolonged, long range synaptic inhibition) (3).

$GABA_A$ receptors are ligand-gated chloride channels; inotropic receptors that are opened after GABA released from the presynaptic neuron travels across the synaptic cleft and binds to the postsynaptic receptor. A fully functional $GABA_A$ receptor contains an α, β, and at least one other subunit such as γ, δ, or ϵ. $GABA_A$ receptors are selectively modulated pharmacologically by benzodiazapines, steroids, and barbiturates.

GABA$_B$ receptors are metabotropic transmembrane receptors that trigger second messenger systems phospholipase C and adenylyl cyclase, and activate K^+ and Ca^{2+} ion channels via G-coupled proteins. GABA$_B$ receptors produce slow, prolonged inhibitory signals and function to modulate the release of neurotransmitters (4).

Dysregulation of the inhibitory GABA system in the autistic brain, specifically in the ACC, provides the neurochemical basis for the stereotyped behaviors seen in ASD. Dysregulation refers to an increase in excitation or disproportionately weak inhibition in neural circuits that mediate language and behavior (2). It is hypothesized that a dysregulated GABAergic system would lead to uninhibited, excitatory glutaminergic transmission producing excess "noise" in the CNS. It is now hypothesized that the developing autistic child is unable to grasp social cues and learn appropriate behaviors due to elevated cortical noise, secondary to lack of inhibitory signals.

Glutamate is the classic excitatory neurotransmitter found in virtually every region of the CNS. Glutamate receptors are classified as ionotropic N-methyl-D-aspartate (NMDA) ion channels or metabotropic G protein-coupled receptors (2). The balance of excitation and inhibition in the cerebral cortex is controlled by the relative numbers and activities of glutamatergic and GABAergic neurons. Disruptions in GABAergic signaling would lead to uninhibited glutamate-mediated excitatory transmission in the CNS. Over-excitation would result in uninhibited signaling that manifests as inappropriate cue processing and modulation, classic to ASD.

In the human brain, constantly receiving and processing stimuli from its surroundings, GABA serves to inhibit irrelevant processes, remove excess noise from the cortex, and give it the ability to maintain focus and attention on only the pertinent cues. This unique feature of the developing brain becomes essential for learning to "pick and choose" relevant stimuli in order to form an appropriate response (2).

Immunohistochemical studies involving the autistic brain have revealed decreased binding density of GABA receptors indicating a decreased overall density of GABA receptors. In these studies, a receptor binding technique was employed to radiolabeled GABA receptors in ACCs from fresh frozen brain tissue obtained from The Autism Research Foundation and Harvard Brain Tissue Resource Center. The studies reveal a significant quantifiable decrease in GABA receptor density in areas of the brain important for socio-behavioral processes (5). Decreased GABA receptor density in these regions provides evidence for the neurochemical basis for a dysregulated, hyperexcitable autistic brain where facial processing and emotional-behavioral responses are affected. These studies reveal a clear defect in the anterior cingulate cortex (ACC), a region known for its critical function in behaviorally demanding tasks.

Recently, R. Lunján et al. reviewed the role of GABA and glutamate in proliferation, migration, differentiation, and survival processes during neural development (1). They found several striking points regarding the role of GABA in neuronal development and regulation of excitatory synapse formation.

1- GABA and glutamate play an important role in the proliferation of neuronal progenitor cells, a fundamental developmental process responsible for generating the correct number of cells of each type in the correct sequence in the developing brain (1).

2- Activation of neurotransmitter receptors, including $GABA_B$, plays a role in controlling the migration of neurons, independent of brain area or neuronal phenotype (1).

3- $GABA_A$ receptor activation has been shown to promote neurite (axon & dendrite) outgrowth and maturation of GABAergic interneurons. It is also thought to regulate the morphologic development of cortical interneurons through membrane depolarization and increases in $[Ca^{2+}]$ (1).

4- Finally, evidence in mammalian models shows that GABAergic inputs onto the newborn neuron permits the development of glutamatergic synapses. Thus, the balance between excitation and inhibition is ensured from the beginning of synaptogenesis (6).

The evidence for the role of GABA on the developing CNS combined with the fact that the autistic brain shows a deficiency in GABA receptors in the ACC makes a striking case for the dysregulated CNS seen in ASD (2). While the dysregulated CNS model is still considered theoretical, research revolving implementing therapies that aim to alleviate the imbalance of excitation/inhibition to reduce cortical noise should be considered for future clinical trials. Furthermore, therapies that improve GABAeric expression in the developing brain could be used to improve synaptogenesis and reduce overt excitation.

Processes that disrupt the major inhibitory circuits in the brain can produce a noisy, hyper-excitable state as observed in the autistic brain (2). It is known that autistic individuals are hypersensitive to auditory and tactile stimuli. Developmental studies on non-human mammals have shown that genetic, physiologic, or environmental processes that generate a high level of noise in the cortex disrupt the formation of normal cortical 'maps' and thus leading to developmental sequelae that could contribute to brain dysfunction seen in autism. Evidence also shows that the basis for the dysregulated GABAergic systems can be due to decreased GABA receptor density in cortical areas involved in socio-emotional and face processing behaviors— notably the ACC and the amygdale (chapter 3D) (5).

The anterior cingulate cortex becomes activated when engaging in attention-demanding tasks. It is a key area in the integration of ostensibly disparate processes involving affect, cognition, behavior, and face processing. The ACC is also implicated in higher-level voluntary control of responses, specifically their selection and preparation (7). With its vast connections to the frontal cortex and other subcortical structures such as the amygdala, the ACC is thought to receive information pertaining to fear-related cues as well a significant role in monitoring performance and adjusting behavior to optimize reward (8). In the next section of this chapter we will discuss excitation-inhibition dysregulation on the level of the ACC and amygdala and their neuronal networks.

The cingulate cortex is a large structure positioned medially in the cerebral hemisphere that surrounds the corpus callosum (chapter 3D). By convention it has been divided into anterior (ACC), posterior, and retrosplenial regions, with multiple functionally and structurally specialized subdivisions. The precise location of the ACC region has been designated as encompassing Broadman areas 25, 24 and 33. Its neurons have been shown to form network connections with the amygdala, hypothalamus and brainstem periaqueductal gray, thus further elucidating its importance in information processing and cue integration. Because of the heterogeneity of the ACC, revealing its single function has been a challenge amongst the scientific community. Yet, over the years there has been a significant body of evidence pointing to the ACC's role in assessment of motivational valence of external stimuli or events, and integration of cognitive and affective responses to those stimuli.

The ACC has been implicated in processing of higher order sensory information as well as its function in emotion-related responses and attention of behaviorally demanding cognitive tasks. Additionally, ACC activation has been linked to play an integral role in the mechanism supporting awareness of self (7). The pathway that modulates self-awareness has been heavily implicated in the mechanism underlying understanding mental states of others and thus generating empathic responses. The abovementioned deficits are only a few of the signs classically attributed to early autistic behaviors. Children exhibiting early signs of ASD typically show difficulty with comforting others, recognizing their own emotional state, and comforting themselves. Often, such behavior in the early years is described as "inconsolable" or "colicky," but as the child matures it becomes more evident that the behavior is something more than a transient element of developmental maturation. This lack of self-awareness and empathy is also evident in autistic children as they find themselves in complex social situations requiring their active involvement or initiative. During times of engaged play with their peers, autistic children will either respond to social cues but take very little social initiative, or will not show the ability to proceed to further their friendships (9).

The physiological and neural responses that modulate the social component of human behavior have been supported by several fMRI studies; many of them showing a significant ACC and insular activation during self-related integrated processing (chapter 3A). Briefly, the studies focused on monitoring the ACC and insular regions via fMRI as the subject was being shown photos of their own face or body parts. The investigation showed a significant difference between the activation seen in subjects viewing their own body part versus the same subject viewing a randomized stimulus. It is thus reasonable to remark on the importance of the ACC and its neuronal circuit in the processing and integration of sensory stimuli and generating appropriate responses based on self-awareness.

Finally, increased ACC neuronal circuit activation has been shown in patients with Tourette syndrome who exhibit lack of self-regulation and impulse suppression (10). This finding further elucidates the importance of an intact and fully developed ACC circuit in behavior modulation and impulse suppression. It can perhaps be used to explain a set of behaviors which, although not classically associated with ASD, have been shown to be the most debilitating and difficult to control. At around two years of age, some autistic children may develop characteristic episodes frequently referred to as "meltdowns." They are defined as "aggressive and sometimes self-injurious behaviors brought on by some changes in routine" (9). Oftentimes the behaviors are stereotyped, repetitive, and adherent to a similar sequence regardless of the precipitating event. The origin of such repetitive behaviors is unclear, their onset is frequently insidious, and their character ranges from simple motions like licking or touching a surface to complex rituals that have to be completed in times of distress.

Structural and functional studies of the ACC have shown it to be composed of large dopamine rich, spindle-shaped neurons with long distance dendrites (8). Their morphology implies that these particular cells have the capacity for creating widespread cortical connections to other parts of the brain with functional consequences. These spindle cells cannot be distinguished at birth and first appear at four months of age at which time they resemble migratory neurons with heavily branched and elongated dendrites. The timing of appearance of these distinguishable cells correlates with the infant's ability to hold its head, smile spontaneously, track and reach for objects while maintaining attentive gaze. The presence of spindle cells and their active features at the time of when an infant is reaching behavioral social milestones only further suggests at their function related to focus, attentiveness, and complex emotional expression. As the cells appear postnatally, and their growth seems to follow the pattern of developmental milestones reached by maturing infants, it is important to note the plastic nature of this circuitry. As a child matures, the neuronal networks gather and consolidate sensory inputs and modify their outputs accordingly. In 30% of children with ASD a typical "regressive" phenotype can be observed often after the child reaches one year of age.

Their speech development halts, they become more withdrawn, unable to engage in make-believe play, and show difficulty with maintaining eye contact and focused gaze (chapter 2C) (9). As the child matures, the neuronal networks gather and consolidate sensory inputs and modify the outputs accordingly. Additionally since the circuit resembles migratory neurons, it is likely that environmental cues and learned behaviors heavily influence the physical connectivity and development. Thus, it is likely that along with genetic predisposition, sensory stimulation, parental care and stress may all affect spindle cell migration and further influence the neural network development (11).

Through various immunohistological studies, the ACC and its connections have been shown to receive one of the richest dopaminergic innervations of any cortical area in the brain (8). Activation of this neuronal network thus relies on dopamine (DA) and its excitatory input in circuit modulation and responsiveness. This finding holds vast implications in linking emotional maturity, social development, and sense of self with the reward-based mechanism of DA. The dopaminergic cell bodies in the ventral midbrain modulate not only reward-driven responses, but also cue the response when the anticipated reward is not received.

This conclusion was initially drawn from an original positron emission tomography (PET) study, in which healthy subjects were compared to subjects with Parkinson's disease (chapter 3A). In this study, subjects were presented with a motivational monetary reward upon task completion. In healthy subjects, ACC activation was clearly elevated during receipt of the reward. In the Parkinson's group, such activation was absent. This implied that, along with the DA neuronal loss, the reward-related activity was also lost, strengthening the association of the DA network with the ACC's function in reward behavior. It is postulated that attention towards social stimuli is associated and often driven by feelings of pleasure or reward. Such a mechanism may aid in memory consolidation of social experiences and thus further shape future responses to such stimuli (12). Thus, if the memory of social interaction is not associated with a positive experience, an individual is less likely to further engage in such behavior resulting in overall fewer experiences.

A recent study attempted to elucidate the nature of reward processing in subjects with autism by examining their response to an incentive delay task (12). Briefly, the task focused on completing a task after which the subject was given a reward of monetary or social nature (photos of happy faces). Upon task completion, autistic patients showed a marked hyperactivation in left midfrontal and anterior cingulate during monetary outcomes, and bilaterally in the amygdala during face anticipation. These findings point at the possibility that dysfunction in the ACC may decrease the motivation to engage in multifaceted social interaction, while a defect in the functional amygdala may lead to impaired detection, decoding and interpretation of social signals conveyed through the face.

This unique ability to interpret others' behavior in regards to mental states (desires, beliefs, thoughts, and intentions), as well as interact in complex social groups and relationships, has been described by scientists as social intelligence. Social intelligence includes the ability to predict how others will act, think or feel, and also empathize with others' mind states. It is believed that autism involves deficiencies in social intelligence as autistic children exhibit difficulty interacting with others, problems interpreting nonverbal communication, and difficulty establishing relationships. Individuals with ASD experience difficulty in understanding others' feelings and forming appropriate responses. It has been proposed that social intelligence is a function of three regions of the brain: the amygdala, the superior temporal sulcus and gyrus, and the orbito-frontal cortex (14). Thus, altered neural input to the amygdala may be a feasible mechanism by which the social deficits associated with ASD manifest themselves phenotypically.

The amygdala is comprised of an almond shaped group of nuclei that have a central role in emotional responses. As part of the limbic system, it plays an important role in memory and emotional responses. It receives information regarding sights, sounds, touch, smell, and taste, information regarding ones emotional and physical well-being, and also visceral sensory inputs (chapter 3B).

Due to its role in memory and learning, it is necessary that the amygdala maintain a certain level of plasticity to reorganize information, and form new neuronal connections (16). Social memory requires an even higher level of plasticity in order to organize varying stimuli and their accompanying temporal meanings (20). Studies have shown that neurogenesis, especially in the amygdala and hippocampus, are an important factor in learning emotional tasks. In contrast, the amygdala does not seem to be involved in learning visual and special learning tasks (17).

Long-term potentiation, particularly in mature neurons, seems to decrease in the presence of GABAergic stimulation. GABA however does not block new neurons. Researchers have hypothesized that this is the reason why new neurons are recruited for learning when the level of GABA is increased (18). This indicates that GABA regulates the amygdala's ability to process new experiences, and this process requires new or non-mature neurons (20). A decrease in GABA is associated with ASD (19); this altered regulation of GABA may be one of the factors that influence the social impairment seen in autistic individuals. This may also impact the amygdala's ability to process new emotional experiences and regulate corticostriatal connections (20).

Neurochemical differences in the amygdalae of autistic individuals also extend to its ability to habituate. Habituation was defined as decreased neural response upon repeated presentation of a stimulus, and sensitization was defined as an increase in response to faces (15). Brain imaging studies have shown that when autistic individuals are shown faces repeatedly; their amygdalae fail to habituate. This defect in habituation may be one mechanism by which deficiencies in social behavior develop and are maintained. It is theorized that the increased neuronal activity to the amygdala seen in autistic individuals may be caused by this failure to habituate and generate appropriate responses to faces. While non-autistic controls were found to have amygdalae that quickly habituated to faces, adults with ASD were found to become sensitized to faces. This increase in amygdala activity in response to faces may be a reason why previous studies have noted overstimulation of the amygdala in Autistic individuals (15).

Amygdala habituation may be affected by certain genetic factors, namely the serotonin transporter-linked polymorphic region variant (5-HTTLPR). Low genetic expression of 5-HTTLPR is associated with increased amygdala activation, and evidence suggests that behavioral symptoms are worse in individuals with both ASD and low expressing 5-HTTLPR genotype (15). Another notable discovery about the 5-HTTLPR genotype is how it changes the amygdala response to sad vs. happy or neutral faces. This may be due to the greater amygdala activation to sad faces observed in ASD patients.

Several studies involving the amygdala, including temporal lobe damage and reduced amygdala volume, have also implicated evidence of an amygdala abnormality in ASD. Human lesion studies conducted on the amygdala and hippocampus have suggested a relationship between damage to these temporal lobe structures and the pathophysiology of autism in both humans and animals. The development of autistic signs and symptoms has followed the infliction of severe temporal lobe damage in children. In cases of viral encephalitis and tuberous sclerosis, both of which affect the temporal lobe, there has been increased incidence of autism development in case patients (21) (chapters 6B,6C).

Postmortem neuroanatomical studies of approximately 30 autistic brains have turned up pathologic increases in the amygdala's cell density, while the amygdala is of either increased or normal size. There were observed decreased neuronal size, reduced myelination (chapter 6B), and large increases in the cell packing density in the amygdala nuclei, most prominently in the central, cortical, and medial nuclei. Abnormalities were also noted in the **hippocampal fields CA1 – CA4, the subiculum, entorhinal cortex, mammillary bodies, medial septal nucleus, and anterior cingulate gyrus** of all the brains studied (21).

Conclusions

In this chapter, we attempted to consolidate the vast body of evidence surrounding the theory of dysregulation within the discrete sub-cortical structures, mainly the ACC and the amygdala, as it pertains to possible origins and manifestations of autism. We have seen that the characteristic autistic phenotype consists mainly of stereotypical behaviors and inability to grasp social cues, implicating a dysfunction in the anterior cingulate and the amygdala respectively. Additionally we expanded on the neurochemical model of autism, as it is based on imbalance between excitatory and inhibitory stimuli, notably within those two discrete structures.

GABA and glutamate transmission in the developing brain appear to have a significant part in neural development such as proliferation, migration, maturation, and neuronal synapse formation. The current model of neurochemical dysregulation predicts a potential defect in any, or all, of the aforementioned developmental processes. These defects may include weakened or absent neuronal migration during times of embryologic, fetal, and even postnatal development as the brain matures and learns to process and integrate external cues.

Furthermore, considering the current body of evidence on the involvement of the amygdala, it is feasible to state that there is a correlation between lesions in the amygdala and the clinical symptoms observed in individuals with ASD. In the future, it is possible that brain imaging studies could become a useful diagnostic tool for autism. Further research efforts should focus on elucidating the parts of the amygdala that are hyper- or hypo-active in the presentation of ASD symptoms and their association with symptomatic presentation. The current concept of impaired communication between parts of the brain may be based on reduced myelination due to depressed insulin-like growth factor (IGF) *in utero* or at birth (chapters 6B,6E).

In conclusion, within this chapter we attempted to reveal a clear role of the ACC and amygdala in autism development and phenotypic manifestations. By carefully examining original publications and review articles on the subject, we have gathered a comprehensive body of evidence in support of the proposal of neurotransmitter and neural network dysregulation in autism. Lack of balance between the inhibitory and excitatory signals in the anerior cingulate cortex was shown to cause lack of motivation to engage in social encounters, decreased spontaneity of behaviors and decreased ability to self-control and problem solve.

Furthermore, deregulation of signaling within the amygdala, and changes within its neuronal connectivity and feedback to the ACC may be responsible for the decrease in social intelligence, empathy, memory formation and learning guided by positive reinforcement. The theory of deregulated neuronal networks between the ACC and the amygdala seems to explain some, but not all, of the behavioral manifestations associated with autism. Additional focused research is needed to explore further neuronal connectivity and other neurotransmitters involved in this pathway, as it could shed more light on the true nature of the origins of ASD as well as potential therapeutic targets.

Chapter 3F - Synaptic Pathology

Ruslan Banai, Brian Pritchard, Matthew Rosner

[Malfunction of impulse conveyance because of synaptic impairments has been proposed to be at the center of defective autistic neural transmissions. Observations supporting this hypo- thesis are discussed, especially those involving the MET gene and transmitter proteins. – Ed.]

<u>Hypothesis</u>

Although the mechanism leading to autistic spectrum disorder (ASD) is unknown, there have been several hypotheses proposed. The increased neuronal connections formed early in brain development may prime autistic patients to remain in a state of hypersensitivity to non-social stimuli. The lack of proper social processing in early development induces further deficits as the patient ages due to a failure to build upon the basic early neuronal activation. These pathologies can explain why people suffering from ASD have difficulty reacting to social stimuli and often get bogged down processing simple environmental messages.

Possible *in utero* disturbances such as the malformation of synapses and dendritic spines, synthesis of proteins, and an imbalance in excitatory-inhibitory networks in the brain cortex and hippocampus can also lead to the onset of ASD (1) (chapter 3E). These excitatory-inhibitory neurological imbalances modify cortical function, neural networking, and altered behavior associated with ASD (2). Appreciation of synaptic pathology and defects in neuronal network activity in the brain may help to explain the pathogenesis of ASD.

The synapse is the basis for all impulse transmission in the brain and its components include neurotransmitters and their receptors, ion channels, neuronal migration, synaptic scaffolding, autoantibodies, and growth factors. Autoimmunity is thought to play a vital role in the pathogenesis of the synapse in ASD, specifically the MHC I, glutamatergic, and GABAergic receptors. Contributing to this autoimmunity are cytokines (TNF-alpha, IL-6, IL-8, IFN-gamma, and GM-CSF) that induce a chronic neuroinflammatory state (3) (chapter 6C). Transmembrane proteins and efficient protein synthesis also affect the formation and maintenance of healthy synapses, which are typically deficient in those suffering from ASD. Genetics and epigenetics can modify synaptic functioning in the developing brain. These factors include mutations in the MET tyrosine kinase as well as the LIS1 gene (chapter 4E,8A). These mutations result in the failure to maintain effective dendrites and axons as well as the inability to make new connections during childhood development (4).

Observations

The α,β-heterodimeric, transmembrane MET receptor tyrosine kinase is responsible for synaptopathology *in utero* (5). It determines hyper- and hypo-connectivity in various parts of the brain, most importantly involving the dendrites in microcircuits of the forebrain. Although many neuropsychiatric disorders exhibit microstructural changes at the dendritic spine (6), there is long-range 'under-connectivity' between cortical areas and short range 'over-connectivity,' seen in autism spectrum disorder (ASD). Changes most typically occur in the frontal and temporal cortex (7) (chapters 3B-3E). These connections undermine the pathogenesis of ASD; they limit the integration of information (5). The malformation of synapses by MET-signaling the neuropil and long projecting axons of the cerebral cortex, hippocampus, septum and amygdala also suggest aberrant connections between these parts of the brain (8). This would also result in the expected deficiencies of ASD; in emotion, learning, and speech as well as the social and emotional dimensions of behavior (5).

Embryonic cell growth and development are governed by the involvement of MET. The maturity of the neocortical and hippocampal pyramidal neurons, as well as the formation, differentiation, and function of the forebrain neuronal synaptic connections neurons, are specifically influenced by MET activation. These same cortical areas have decreased synchronicity in those with ASD, particularly during the performance of various social and intellectual tasks (7). The degree of reduced cortical activity positively correlates with the severity of the ASD phenotype (8).

Autopsies of ASD individuals displayed at least a 50% reduction in MET protein expression (9). Recent transcript and protein mapping studies in the developing mouse forebrain have established a clearer pathology of MET's involvement with ASD. The striatum and dorsal thalamus, two major targets of these excitatory projections, express MET protein during the first fourteen weeks of life, potentiating terminal axon growth and development. Specifically, MET expression increases with the rapid growth of neuropil elements that form synapses and excitatory projection neurons during development from postnatal weeks seven to twenty one (8). It is during the second post-natal week that rates of dendritogenesis and synaptogenesis are highest (7). MET signaling feeds into PI3 kinase and ERK biochemical pathways, which are involved in neurodevelopmental events such as axon guidance and synaptogenesis. This results in the typical finding of the corticostriatal neurons in ASD; the presence of large, voluminous dendritic spines, premature gains in postsynaptic density size and thickness (5). The downstream targets of MET signaling, the PI3 kinase and ERK biochemical pathways, are directly implicated in ASD (10,11).

These alterations in the MET gene can be appreciated morphologically. In one study, MET-mutant mice displayed changes in neocortical pyramidal neuron dendritic appearance in layers two and three of the brain cortex. The pathway from layer two/three to layer five of the corticostriatal neurons was determined to be the primary source of interlaminar input to these neurons (7). Alterations in MET, manifested with hyperconnectivity between synaptic inputs, resulted in larger amplitudes of synaptic activity. This hyperconnectivity can be morphologically appreciated by the excessive ratio of excitation to inhibition at the synapse, leading to the generation of 'noise' in cortical signaling and sensory representations. Comparatively, layer five neurons that did not express MET exhibited morphologically and functionally normal synapses.

An alteration in MET resulted in an increase in branching of the basal dendrites, with a reduction in apical dendrites in the forebrain. This produced a 20% decrease in the volume of the dendritic tree leading to synaptic hypoconnectivity, similar to the type seen in ASD. This reduction helps to explain the significant loss of information processing at the circuit-level of the somatosensory cortex (5). Such apical dendrites are an important convergence point of ascending thalamic and descending cortical information, suggesting functional outcomes in autistic individuals.

The local hyperconnectivity in the cortico-striatal neurons of the forebrain demonstrated an increase in both probability and amplitude of synaptic connections. The increase in dendritic arbor volume implies that they are capable of receiving more broadly distributed striatal afferent input. However, since there is an increase in basal dendrites and a decrease in apical dendrites, this leads to patch-matrix compartmental organization of the striatum. This might result in atypical mixing of afferent sensorimotor and limbic information that is routed through this matrix amalgamation (5).

The expression of MET remains relatively constant between species and alterations to the gene have been observed in other mammals. The temporal and occipital lobe circuits, including the brain pathway for processing complex visual stimuli, were routinely damaged in primates and mice with altered MET expression. The anterior commissure, sublenticular internal capsule and the posterior corpus callosum all carry axons to the temporal and occipital cortical areas; all were positive for MET immunoreactivity. The MET deficiencies observed in other species are consistent with those perceived in ASD.

Mutations in the LIS1 gene also contribute to the pathogenesis of the synapse in the cerebral cortex, particularly in the hippocampus. *In vivo* imaging of the hippocampus with a mutation in LIS1 revealed reductions in elimination and turnover rates of dendritic protrusions in Layer V pyramidal neurons. These immature hippocampal neurons exhibited reduced density and length. Interestingly, LIS1 has been identified as one of the hub proteins in the functional interaction network of high-risk ASD genes that act in the synapse, suggesting that relatively minor alterations in LIS1 may impact synaptic function. However, it is unclear how LIS1 might participate in such complex neurobehavioral disorders (12).

LIS1 insufficiency is associated with the regulation of the RhoA family GTPases and has specific implications in the hippocampus. RhoA is part of the RAS superfamily, regulating proteins and timing of cell division (13). RhoA inactivation decreases dendritic spine density and neck length while RhoA activation inhibits spine formation while also blocking spine head growth and stability. The mechanism for LIS1's effect on RhoA is incompletely understood.

However, mice subjected to LIS1 downregulation suffered from similar attributes as ASD; deficits in social interactions due to a delay in synaptic cluster formation and reduced spine density. Since LIS1 is involved in multiple protein-protein interactions, it could modulate a number of signaling events important for synapse formation and maintenance. This bears a striking resemblance to the hypoconnectivity exhibited in MET expression and demonstrates LIS1's essential role in the development of the synapse and behavior via the growth of dendritic spines and protein migration.

However, LIS1 is also very different from the expression of MET in the pathogenesis of the synapse in ASD. While MET was vital to the development of synapses postnatally, LIS1 is implicated in the maintenance of dendrite spines. LIS1 haploinsufficient neurons are impaired in the pruning of dendritic spines throughout adolescent development. By the time neurons reach adulthood, neural plasticity is lost due to an 'overstabilization' of the synapse leading to dysfunctional synapses and abnormal social behavior (12).

ASD is defined by its disturbances in local networks. LIS1 activation plays a pivotal rule in cortical circuit assembly by regulating dendritic spine turnover to establish correct connections and promote synaptic plasticity, an element that is lacking in ASD. This distinctive phenotype makes LIS1 an attractive model for developing therapeutic treatments targeted to social aspects of behavioral disorders, particularly ASD. However, a study involving Chinese Han children diagnosed with ASD and their families concluded that LIS1 gene mutations were prevalent in <1% of those with ASD. Conversely, the study only focused on a specific ethnicity; significant genetic drift has been noted in the causes and manifestations of ASD among ethnicities. More significant research is required before LIS1 can be introduced as a therapy for ASD (14).

Transmembrane proteins known as neurexins play a vital role in the synaptic pathology of ASD. They are located presynaptically and interact with post-synaptic neuroligins. The neuroligins then interact with several postsynaptic proteins (known as the postsynaptic density: GABA-R, gephyrin, AMPAR, NMDAR) to localize and increase the number of receptors and channels, thus regulating the synaptic response. Five types of neuroligins have been classified. Mutations in neuroligin 3 and 4 have been exclusively studied and result in defective trafficking and accumulation of the protein in the endoplasmic reticulum. Knockout mice lacking neurexin and neuroligins display abnormalities in synaptic communication and maturation, showing increased inhibitory signals (15). Interestingly, the number of synapses in the brain was normal. Neurexins and neuroligins are imperative in maintaining the synaptic connections between neurons. However, they are not involved with the initial stimulus for the formation of synaptic connections in the young brain. Defective binding to neurexin may occur which results in an increase in the ratio of inhibitory signals to excitatory signals (16). The deficiency in neurexins and neuroligins phenotypically manifests at age three and is more involved in synapse pruning and maintenance rather than in the initial formation of synapses. It is not coincidental that this correlates with the average age of ASD diagnosis.

Mutations in contactin associated protein 2 (CNTNAP2), a neurexin, increase the chance of ASD development. These abnormalities result in the failure of language formation and seizures. CNTNAP2 is found in the frontotemporal-subcortical circuits, specifically in the frontal and temporal lobes, dorsal thalamus, and the striatum. These areas of the brain are important for cognitive functioning, including executive thinking, joint attention, and language, which may be abnormal in ASD (17).

A specific study in CNTNAP2 mutations in an isolated Amish family demonstrated the classic symptoms of ASD, including seizures and language disabilities [18]. All of the patients suffering from this rare and recessive mutation suffered from similar symptoms. Each of these patients showed diminished social skills, delayed language development, and two-thirds of them were diagnosed with ASD. These patients also suffered from seizures as a result of abnormal subcortical circuits in the temporal and frontal lobes. (In general, the overall prevalence of autism is lower in the Amish than in the general American population.)

Synapses are very adaptable and are changing all the time. This feature of synapses is termed synaptic plasticity. It is integral to memory formation and the ability to form new memories, code for new experiences, and learn new skills. It can also be thought of as a pruning process in those older less used pathways and synapses can be modified or even regress. Through a process called long term potentiation, strong NMDA receptor activation can lead to increased AMPA receptor placement in the post synaptic membrane. Opposing this process is long term depression, where diminished NMDA receptor activation leads to decreased AMPA receptors in the post-synaptic membrane. The AMPA receptor is important in modulating the strength of the synapse and is a key regulator in synaptic plasticity. This synaptic plasticity is determined by the dendritic spines of neurons (19).

SHANK 2 and SHANK 3 proteins are part of the postsynaptic scaffolding and plasticity, which are believed to contribute to early synaptogenesis. These proteins play a role in helping form and stabilize dendritic spines. SHANK 3 is an important component of the post synaptic density and recruits excitatory receptors such as iGluR and mGluR. SHANK 3 knockout studies show a reduced AMPA receptor function and diminished LTP in the hippocampus. SHANK 3 mutations have been found in autistic patients, causing decreased formation of dendritic spines and reduced size of formed spines (20). These mutations have a low prevalence rate in as much as 1% of ASD cases; and were extrapolated from multiple studies of ASD (21). Each individual gene mutation is estimated to impact 10-20% of those diagnosed with the condition. However, more investigation is needed since the correlation in SHANK 3 mutations and siblings with ASD is unclear. Uncertainty remains whether SHANK 3 mutations directly cause ASD or if their mutations are part of a cascade result of ASD (22).

Additional studies used knock-in mice to observe mutations involving Nlgn3R451C (human neuroligin-3 mutation). In this particular study, giant depolarizing potentials (GDPs) were observed. GDPs represent a primordial form of synchrony between neurons, thought to be essential for proper circuit migration. They are generated by the synergistic action of glutamate and GABA, both of which are depolarizing and excitatory at early development stages (23). In these transgenic mice, GDPs were increased. This increased the frequency but not the amplitude of hippocampal GABAergic events in principal cells. This synaptic imbalance may result in malformation of neuronal circuits. Tabuchi et al. proposed that these neuroligin 3 mutations may lead to enhanced spatial learning abilities but deficits in social interactions; both of which may be seen in patients with ASD (24). However, the prevalence rate of these neuroligin mutations may be extremely low in patients with ASD. One study in 2003, screened 96 individuals affected with ASD and found zero patients neuroligin (3,4) mutations. If these mutations do cause autism it may be an extremely low number in the total population with ASD (25).

The relationship of neurochemicals to ASD is not well understood, however mutations in the glutamate receptor have been implicated as a cause (26). During post-natal development, glutamate receptors are negatively controlled by the presence of major histocompatibility complex (MHC)-I molecules on both the axons and dendrites of cortical neurons during synapse formation, particularly in the second post-natal week in the hippocampus. MHC-I downregulates glutamatergic and GABAergic connection and controls the balance of cortical excitation and inhibition. Resultantly, any changes in MHC-I can be expected to alter glutamatergic and GABAergic receptors at the synapse. These reflections manifested in temporal and visual shifts in every experimental knockout mouse, similar to the temporal and visual shifts seen in those suffering from ASD. MHC-I is vital to restricting synapse establishment in cortical circuitry during the first weeks of post-natal life. Therefore, any chronic decrease in MHC-I would cause increased cortical connections and hyperconnectivity, similar to those seen in ASD (27). Autoimmune dysfunctions, such as those affecting the MHC-I receptor, have been proven to play a role in approximately 40% of those diagnosed with ASD (28).

Further research is needed to clarify the degree of influence of MHC-I on presynaptic release and its consequences on cortical network formation and plasticity (27). However, if MHC-I were to be manipulated in post-natal life, it could be utilized as a treatment for ASD. Limiting the formation of too many synapses in proximal dendrites, while permitting synapse formation in more distal growing dendritic regions, is a potential for treatment in ASD. This could maximize the number of neurons and their neural connections, restricting both hypoconnectivity and hyperconnectivity. Immune dysregulation is quickly becoming a viable hypothesis for the pathogenesis and treatment of ASD.

Another potential mechanism for ASD could be due to chronic neuroinflammation (chapters 6C, 6D). Pardo et al. confirmed the presence of activated microglial and astrocyte cells in the brain, along with inflammatory cytokines and interleukins such as TNF-alpha, IL-6, IL-8, IFN-gamma, and GM-CSF (3). Morgan et al. confirmed the presence of increased microglial density in autistic patients, preferentially in the dorsolateral prefrontal cortex. The increase in microglial activation and density contributes to a chronic neuroinflammatory state. This abnormal status leads to decreased formation and wasting of synaptic connections, leading to neuronal cell loss particularly in the cerebellum (27). Studies have shown that IL-6 may be increased up to five-fold in the cerebellum of autistic patients (29).

There are additional correlations between microglial activation and ASD. Kovacs et al. proposed that microglial cell release of nitric oxide (NO) enhances synaptic transmission and results in the seizures. Seizures occur in 20-30% of autistic patients (30).

Dendritic spines are crucial for learning and memory; they contain many glutamate receptors with excitatory function and post-synaptic densities. Overexpression of IL-6 in mice caused an increase in the length of dendritic spines with no increase in overall number of spines. Increased spine length is correlated with a decrease in maturation of the synapse and its involved structures. Abnormal mushroom shaped dendritic spines also develop; these are known to establish connections with excitatory synapses through glutamate receptors and larger post-synaptic densities (29). It is unclear whether abnormal dendritic spines and ASD are directly linked. However, mice with Fragile X syndrome typically have increased dendritic spine lengths.

Maternal IgG may cross the placenta and pass through the undeveloped blood brain barrier of the child up to the first six months of development. Recent hypotheses have concluded that these maternal autoantibodies may attack neural development proteins and play a role in the pathogenesis of ASD. Two important examples of these neural growth factors include cypin and collapsin response mediator protein (CRMP). Cypin plays an important role in normal neurite branching. CRMP proteins are critical for neuron and axon development. During this study, rat model recipients of brain reactive IgG showed offspring with impaired motor and sensory development as well as increased anxiety (26). Recognition of these factors in a pregnant mother may allow for early diagnosis and treatment. This is being developed as the MAR (maternal autoantibody-related) diagnostic ASD test (31).

Mutations, neuroinflammation, and autoimmunity can affect the normal circuitry of the developing brain. Insulin-like growth factor-1 affects the rate at which oligodendrocytes promote myelination in the brain and defects are linked to ASD. Decreased myelination may result in weakened or absent synapses. Myelination commonly begins around the 24-25th prenatal week and peaks at about 1 year of age. During this time, IGF-1 also promotes axonal regeneration, astrocyte proliferation, and neurite sprouting by motor neurons (32). Placental growth hormone promotes placental proliferation of IGF-1 in the fetus. As described earlier, IGF-1 is vital to the connectivity expressed in neurons in the brain.

Another proposed mechanism of ASD is exaggerated protein synthesis due to changes in translation. Research has found mutations and variation in the eukaryotic translation initiation factor 4D (EIF4E) locus of chromosome 4q. Santini et al showed that an increase in eIF4E caused ASD-like behaviors in mice. The mice also had difficulty adapting to new environments and situations, lagging behind their wild type peers. Lastly, the eIF4E transgenic mice showed less interaction with a stranger mouse. The transgenic mice had deviations in synaptic function in the medial prefrontal cortex, striatum, and the hippocampus. There was also a 12% increase in dendritic spine density compared to wild types. Researchers used an inhibitor of eIF4E, stopping its expression from having any effect on the synapse in the brain and thus the behavior of the mouse. Treatment with the inhibitor decreased symptoms of ASD in the mice (33).

Conclusions

The underlying pathogenesis of the synapse is complex and multi-factorial. There is not just one universal problem but a combination of many influences, some occurring *in utero* and others postnatally. While it is during the second postnatal week that MET affects dendritogenesis and synaptogenesis, the deficiency in neurexins and neuroligins phenotypically manifests itself by age three years. These dates are important for further research and to provide a timeline to assist in the diagnosis and treatment of ASD.

In ASD there is an imbalance in hypo- and hyper-connectivity in the brain leading to abnormal synapses. Whether due to genetic mutations, receptor modifications, immune factors, or structural deficiency, the overt manifestation of autism presents with similar symptomology. The prevalence of autism patients with these genetic mutations is low, disputing the theory of a single mutation as the lone cause. However, modern genetic techniques are allowing researchers to explore a number of new genes, DNA copy number variations, and point mutations. Further research of these pathologies may provide ideas into the levels of expression in those with ASD. However, further subtyping of these pathologies may provide ideas into the levels of expression in those with ASD.

Animal studies may provide a narrowed focus into the functions of scaffolding proteins. Although a few studies were noted in the observations, further knock-out mice utilizing differing combinations of neuroligins, neurexins, and SHANK proteins may contribute to determining the etiology of ASD.

Mutations in the LIS1 gene result in the reduction in elimination and turnover rates of dendritic protrusions in Layer 5 of the pyramidal neurons. LIS1 insufficiency also impacts the downstream signaling of RhoA, resulting in the inhibition of dendritic spine formation and growth. Deficient MET tyrosine kinase and MHC-I receptors lead to extensive voluminous dendritic spines as well a 20% decrease of the volume of the dendritic tree leading to abnormal communication of neurons.

Autoimmune factors, such as cytokines and dysfunctional MHC-I receptors, may lead to aberrant synapses in autism. Specific cytokines (TNF-alpha, IL-6, IL-8, IFN-gamma, and GM-CSF) play a direct role in neural and cortical inflammation, which may be a contributing factor to the abnormal synapse in autism (3) (chapters 3E,6D). Consistent measurement of IL-6 in proposed autistic children may provide critical insight into the development of the disorder (chapter 6B).

New research on maternal antibodies crossing the placenta and preventing normal neuronal growth has indications that need to be further explored in future studies. Diagnosis using immunohistochemistry may provide key evidence into this potential subtype of ASD. This test may eventually be combined with other diagnostic tests to provide a comprehensive outlook for a pregnant mother. A meta-analysis on this specific hypothesis of molecular mimicry is crucial in determining the cause of autoreactivity of IgG.

The synapse is apparently always altered in autism. These high activity synapses are all permanently damaged by the eighth week of human development (34). However, it is not known to what the extent any one gene contributes to the destruction of the synapse or whether these genes act alone or jointly (1). ASD results from various combinations of very different pathological mechanisms at the synapse. It remains indistinguishable whether ASD is the cause of many of these irregular synapses or arose as a result of them. The future of autism research should focus on attempting to link the seemingly disjointed variety of pathologies that accompany autism into a global picture of the disorder.

Glossary

ASD – autism spectrum disorder
CNTNAP2 – contactin associated protein 2
CRMP – collapsin response mediator protein
EIF4E – eukaryotic translation initiation factor 4E
ERK – extracellular signal-regulated kinase
GTP – guanosine triphosphate
IL - interleukin
LIS1 - lissencephaly protein
LTP - long-term potentiation
MET – mesenchymal-epithelial transition factor
MHC - major histocompatibility complex
MRI – magnetic resonance imaging
PIK3 - phosphatidylinositol-4,5-bisphosphate 3-kinase
SHANK - multidomain scaffold proteins of the postsynaptic density
TNF - tumor necrosis factor

Chapter 3G - Hypoxia

Clover Youn, Laura Schiraldi

[Hypoxic events, especially before and during delivery, are examined as possible environmental triggers promoting the subsequent development of autism.- Ed]

Hypothesis

Autism spectrum disorders (ASD) are thought to have both genetic and environmental factors. In the scope of developmental ailments, environmental factors that are particularly important to consider are prenatal and perinatal maternal and fetal conditions. Of these, one that has been extensively researched in connection with ASD is hypoxia (1). Hypoxia, simply defined as an insufficiency of oxygen within or to a certain part of the body, may starve tissues of much needed oxygen. This is particularly significant for the fetus, for whom both oxygen and nutrients are provided only by the placenta via the umbilical cord. Any obstruction of this flow or decrease in perfusion of the placenta can significantly affect fetal development. In this chapter, we explore hypoxia as an important factor that can create a suboptimal environment and subsequently predispose the fetus to developmental syndromes such as ASD.

Hypoxia is often seen in pathological situations. Hypoxic injury may occur for many reasons (2). Occlusion of arteries, corporal injury, or low cardiac output can result in decreased rate of blood flow, leading to hypo-perfusion of tissues and an ischemic hypoxia. Alternatively, hypoxia can occur due to a decrease in the oxygen content of arterial blood. Causes of this include hypoventilation, hypoxemia, or diminished oxygen (O_2) in inspired air. Hypoxia can also be caused by anemias, such as those resulting from thalassemias, sickle cell disease, iron deficiency, and glucose-6-phosphate (G6PD) deficiency, among others, due to a decrease in the oxygen-carrying capacity of blood. In some cases, a decrease in the physical ability of red blood cells (RBCs) to accommodate O_2 can result in hypoxia. For example, in carbon monoxide (CO) poisoning, O_2 is displaced because hemoglobin has a higher affinity for CO and preferentially forms carboxyhemoglobin, resulting in a net decreased oxygenation of tissues Finally, hypoxia can also occur due to decreased oxygen supply, which may be seen with umbilical cord compression, or due to ineffective aerobic respiration, which can occur due to a defect in the electron transport chain, resulting in decreased ATP production. A familiar cause of this is cyanide poisoning.

Hypoxia affects different tissues to varying degrees. Cells of the hair, nails, and vascular smooth muscle are able to endure hypoxic conditions for up to a few days. In contrast, cells of nervous tissue can only tolerate hypoxia for a few *minutes* before succumbing to serious injury (3). This is true in both the adult and the developing fetus.

Previous studies have postulated a connection between decreased perfusion of the nervous system and changes in behavioral and neural development (1). This is in part because hypoxia is a fairly common occurrence and is thus both an important and easy subject to investigate. It would seem that hypoxia affects mostly components of the limbic system, and that it is hypoxic alteration of these areas that accounts for the behavioral modifications seen in maladies such as ASD.

In the following section, we will discuss the areas of the brain most sensitive to hypoxic injury, how hypoxic injury may influence the genesis of ASD, and the maternal and obstetric conditions that may alter oxygen delivery to the fetus and neonate.

Observations

Though hypoxia can be globally detrimental to the central nervous system, certain areas of the brain tend to be more sensitive to its effects than others. These areas include the hippocampus, Purkinje cells of the cerebellum, pyramidal neurons within the cerebral cortex, as well as the amygdala and basal ganglia (4). The localization of hypoxic sensitivity becomes particularly significant when one considers the general behavioral characteristics of patients with ASD. It has been speculated that injury to the limbic system (a group of neural structures which together regulate emotional behavior), neocortex (or neocortical connections), and striatum may underlie, respectively, the autistic characteristics of social withdrawal, difficulties with communication, and stereotypical, repetitive behavior (5-7) (chapters 3B-3D). Let us turn our attention to the function and significance of the areas implicated in ASD.

The hippocampus is the chief structure of the central nervous system (CNS) for the creation and storage of declarative memory, which is the ability to remember concrete material such as facts and events (8). The human fetal hippocampus begins development in the temporal lobe around 10-11 weeks of gestational age, and only begins to take on a more adult-like form around 18-21 weeks (9). During this time, the hippocampus organizes itself into distinct areas: CA1, CA2, and CA3. Area CA1 functions as the major output system from the hippocampus, and has also been implicated in the contextualization of memory for later retrieval (10-12). It is also this area that is most susceptible to hypoxic injury. Cell death can occur after only a few minutes of oxygen deprivation (8).

More extensive damage, such as bilateral hippocampal ischemia, broadens the injury from affecting learning and memory to affecting the limbic system as well (8). The limbic system defines a group of structures in the brain that manage emotional and behavioral functions, with connections to the neocortex and striatum. These connections are illustrated via the Papez circuit, which extends between the hippocampus, fornix, anterior thalamic nuclei, mammillary bodies, entorhinal cortex and parahippocampal gyrus. Additionally, the amygdala acts as a source of afferents to the nucleus accumbens and the caudate nucleus and also communicates with the temporal and prefrontal cortices. The ventral hippocampus in particular has strong connections to the amygdala, hypothalamus, and prefrontal cortex (13). Damage to any of these areas, as well as parts of the basal ganglia and cerebellum, may play a role in the dysfunction or dysregulation of emotional behavior (8,14,15).

The neocortex consists of layers of cell bodies and cortical connections over the cerebral cortex. Damage to the neocortex can have wide variability in physical manifestation, depending on the area of injury. The amygdala, as well as hippocampus, is located in the temporal lobe, which most notably consists of the area for comprehension of language (Wernicke's area) on the left, with connections to Broca's area of expression of language nearby in the inferior frontal cortex, as well as to areas that determine tonal expression on the right (8). Due to the functional significance of this region, it may be a worthwhile area of further investigation regarding any association to communication difficulties that may be found in some cases of ASD.

The prefrontal cortex is an association area with extensive cortical connections, particularly with the amygdala and the dorso-medial nucleus of the thalamus. These connections have been found to modify reactions to current situations based on emotional reactions to past experiences (8). Along with the rest of the frontal cortex, the prefrontal cortex also has roles in higher executive functions, such as judgment, decision-making, attention, and foresight. The cerebral cortex also has large areas of motor cortex dedicated to the generation and processing of intentional movement. Ischemic and hypoxic injuries have the potential to cause any number of lesions and resulting dysfunction of the abovementioned processes in the developing neocortex.

The basal ganglia function as a unit in regulation of movement via excitatory and inhibitory pathways and have extensive connections to the motor cortex as well as to the cerebellum (8). The striatum, a major part of the basal ganglia, consists of the caudate nucleus, nucleus accumbens, and putamen. The amygdala is located at the very end of the tail of the caudate nucleus and provides input to the caudate nucleus and nucleus accumbens. Striatal output is inhibitory, mainly to the pallidum of the basal ganglia. Disruption of these circuits results in dyskinesias such as Parkinson's, Huntington's chorea, and hyperballismus. Dysregulation of the inhibitory pathway has also been shown in a mouse model to result in stereotyped motor behaviors, similar to those found in developmental disorders such as autism (16). As the basal ganglia are significantly affected by hypoxia, this region is also an important area to include when investigating the effects of hypoxia.

The localization of oxygen deprivation is an important consideration because hypoxic damage to the areas mentioned above has the potential to manifest in certain aspects of behavior frequently seen in ASD. Of the above-described areas, the region most sensitive to hypoxic damage remains the limbic system, in particular area CA1 of the hippocampus.

Imaging and postmortem studies of the autistic brain have consistently shown changes in the major areas that make up the limbic system (chapter 3A). Sections of the amygdala, hippocampal formations, and entorhinal cortex show neurons that are smaller and more tightly clustered in infantile autism, compared to the typical brain, and the Purkinje cells of the cerebellum, which project into deep cerebellar nuclei, were fewer in number in infantile autism (17). The researchers who carried out these studies concluded that the histology of the autistic brain suggested a prenatal interruption during development of these areas (17, 18). Because of the localization observed in these studies, hypoxia must be considered as a potential cause of this prenatal interruption of normal neurogenesis.

Considering the abovementioned significance of oxygen delivery in the neural development of the fetus, we must now examine maternal and obstetrical conditions that can alter oxygen homeostasis.

Smoking

It is a commonly known fact that smoking during pregnancy is detrimental to the health of both the mother and the fetus. The most recent data by the Pregnancy Risk Assessment and Monitoring System (PRAMS), an assessment sector of the CDC, revealed that in 2008, "approximately 13% of women reported smoking during the last three months of pregnancy" (19). Multitudes of studies have investigated the various effects of smoking on the fetus, from growth retardation and behavioral changes to developmental delay (20). Our scrutiny here will focus on the hypoxic environment that smoking can create for both mother and child.

The act of smoking itself involves the partial combustion of organic compounds (such as tobacco). Complete combustion of organic compounds yields carbon dioxide and water. In the simplest form (using methane), the reaction is:

$$CH_4 + 2O_2 \rightarrow CO_2 + 2H_2O$$

In partial combustion, there is not enough oxygen, so in addition to carbon dioxide and water, carbon monoxide (CO) is also produced. Carbon monoxide, as discussed previously, binds with high affinity to hemoglobin in red blood cells and causes an anemic hypoxia by reducing the amount of binding sites available for oxygen. In this way, smoking can cause hypoxia in the mother. Hypoxia in the mother can then lead to decreased oxygen transfer to the fetus via the placenta.

Decreased blood flow to the placenta will also diminish both oxygen and nutrients to the fetus. CO not only diffuses freely across the fetoplacental barrier into the fetal blood supply, but levels of carboxyhemoglobin in the fetus may even accumulate to reach slightly higher levels than those found in maternal blood (21). This signifies that, in addition to decreased blood flow to the placenta, CO build-up may cause less off-loading of oxygen in the fetus, further decreasing subsequent perfusion of the placenta and fetal tissues. Without an adequate oxygen supply, fetal tissues can shift from aerobic to anaerobic respiration. The latter is far less efficient and leads to lactic acid build-up, which may cause acidosis and a pH imbalance in the fetus. This creates a suboptimal environment that can be further detrimental to the metabolism, health, and development of the fetus. Many studies have reported the association between maternal smoking during pregnancy and ASD, but the exact mechanism remains unknown (22, 23, 24, 25). What is known is that smoking can have many global detrimental effects on mother and fetus, and here we present one potential mechanism of injury.

Maternal hypertension and gestational diabetes
Two closely linked conditions that can significantly affect both maternal and fetal health are maternal hypertension and gestational diabetes (chapters 3H,3I). Though there is some debate regarding the correlation between gestation diabetes mellitus (GDM) and ASD, a pediatric study found a slightly increased incidence of children with ASD being born to women with these conditions, though the study did not find these differences to be significant (26). Clearly maternal hypertension and GDM can affect fetal development negatively through various mechanisms. However, in this section we will specifically explore possible mechanisms through which these conditions could affect the fetus by inducing a hypoxic state.

Hypertension is a general health problem worldwide for both men and women, however during pregnancy, women can develop gestational hypertension, which can have several adverse effects on the pregnancy. Gestational hypertension can present in several ways. Maternal or gestational hypertension is seen more commonly in women with pre-existing high blood pressure, but can develop during pregnancy for unknown reasons, often in the second half of gestation. Gestational hypertension can be extremely detrimental to the mother and fetus, impacting blood flow to organs such the brain, liver, kidney and placenta (27). Complications of gestational hypertension, particularly with chronic hypertension of pregnancy, include placental abruption (especially if there is a superimposed preeclampsia), intrauterine growth restriction, increased risk of premature birth, and even stillbirth (28,30). Chronic hypertension, which predates the pregnancy, can affect approximately 5% of pregnancies (29). Preeclampsia, which is defined as high blood pressure and proteinuria after the 20th week of gestation, is proposed to be caused by abnormalities in placental perfusion. The risk of developing preeclampsia can be increased with diabetes, chronic hypertension, previous preeclampsia, and obesity (BMI ≥35) (28). The high blood pressure in preeclampsia may be due to the vasoconstrictive effects of increased sympathetic activity. This resulting hypertension can lead to a hypoxic environment for the fetus.

The factors in the mother affecting blood pressure include cardiac output and total peripheral resistance. Due to the direct relationship each of these factors has on blood pressure, if one of them increases, blood pressure elevation will follow. Cardiac output can be increased due to retention of water and salt as well as a rise in total blood volume during pregnancy, whereas the total peripheral resistance can be raised due to anything that reduces the radius of the blood vessel, such as arteriosclerosis in chronic hypertension. Using a rat model, it was found that chronic arterial hypertension during pregnancy may result in reduced fetal motor coordination and learning performances (31). Inadequate blood flow was also found to cause placental ischemia, which triggers the release of bioactive factors (cytokines and reactive oxygen species) that can lead to damage of vasculature lining and vascular smooth muscle dysfunction, resulting in increased resistance in the vascular system (chapters 4A,8B). Ultimately, this sequence of events can lead to dysregulation of the renin-angiotensin-aldosterone system. This produces an increase in angiotensin II (a vasoconstricting substance) and aldosterone (raising the serum sodium level) (31). This can result in inadequate blood flow to the placenta, resulting in decreased oxygenation of the fetus and potentially lead to a hypoxic environment for the fetus.

Gestational diabetes mellitus (GDM) must also be taken into consideration as a potential factor for hypoxic injury (chapter 3I). Aside from the potential to cause macrosomia and polyhydramnios in the fetus, maternal diabetes can disrupt the establishment of proper nutrient and oxygen exchange from mother to baby. Increased blood glucose levels in the mother results in the prolonged exposure of hyperglycemia in the fetus. To compensate for the hyperglycemia, the fetus produces excessive amounts of insulin. This can result in the familiar post-partum complication of hypoglycemia in the fetus, as well as an increase in fetal oxygen consumption and metabolism, which can ultimately lead to chronic intrauterine tissue hypoxia (26).

Increased blood glucose levels also increases intracellular glucose and its metabolites, which can then react with endothelial proteins and lipids, causing glycosylated proteins to build up on the walls of the vessels (32). These glycosylated biochemicals are referred to as Advanced Glycosylated End-Products (AGEs). AGEs can react with several components of blood vessels, resulting in a decreased vessel radius. They can form cross-links with the basement membrane, inhibit monocyte migration, increase endothelial permeability to macromolecules, produce reactive oxygen species, accumulate in the blood vessel walls, and block nitric oxide activity in endothelium (33). This final point is particularly instructive in understanding why AGEs can lead to atherosclerosis, given that nitric oxide relaxes smooth muscle and inhibits the mechanisms contributing to atherosclerosis in diabetic patients, such as leukocyte adhesion to vessel walls, vascular smooth muscle growth and platelet adhesion (33). If a pregnant woman has elevated glucose in her bloodstream, the presence of AGEs has the potential to become much more prominent. This could ultimately lead to damage of the vasculature of the mother, which then affects blood flow to the placenta.

Because of the decreased blood flow, a major concern for these patients is placental injury, which would contribute to reduced oxygen delivery to the fetus. Such placental injuries include fibrinoid necrosis and villous immaturity (34). In fibrinoid necrosis, tissue death occurs in the villi, which are essential in establishing transplacental supply of oxygen and nutrients to the fetus. When damage occurs, there is an accumulation of basic proteinacous material in the tissue matrix, impeding on oxygen exchange from the mother to the fetus. In addition, villous immaturity can increase the distance between the villi and the fetal capillaries, which increases the distance across which oxygen must diffuse and decreases the efficiency of oxygen exchange (34).

An additional finding in placentas of women with GDM is significantly elevated levels of nucleated fetal red blood cells (NFRBCs) when compared with women without GDM (34). NFRBCs are immature fetal red blood cells. An increased level of NFRBCs thus implies that the body is producing more progenitor red blood cell to compensate for a deficit and can thus serve as an indicator of chronic hypoxia in the fetus.

Umbilical cord blood taken from women with subclinical pre-GDM also shows an increased level of red blood cells, potentially a result of trying to increase the amount of oxygen being exchanged, as well as acidemia due to higher lactate concentration (35). Another observation found significantly lower oxygen saturation and oxygen content in the umbilical veins of GDM fetuses, but not in the umbilical artery. In this situation, there is often increased branching seen in the villi, perhaps as a compensatory mechanism to try to maximize oxygen exchange between maternal and fetal blood (35).

Perinatal Hypoxia

Thus far we have discussed several prenatal conditions that may increase the fetal risk for hypoxia. However, there are numerous significant perinatal considerations for this issue as well. Of note are complications pertaining to the umbilical cord and placenta, which can be perinatal causes of fetal asphyxia. Asphyxia is a state in which oxygen delivery is compromised due to a physical impediment. Several clinical parameters have been established by the American Academy of Pediatrics and the American College of Obstetrics and Gynecology to diagnose birth asphyxia, including but not limited to a persistently low APGAR score (0-3 for longer than 5 minutes), neurologic sequelae, and significant acidemia in umbilical artery sample (pH<7.00) (36). Perinatal causes of asphyxia can include compression, prolapse, or nuchal strangulation of or by the umbilical cord (37). The cord is the circulatory connection between mother and fetus. Via the placenta, the umbilical cord provides a route for transport of oxygen and nutrients to the fetus, while removing waste products. Anything that compromises blood flow through the umbilical cord or its structural integrity can impinge upon its function.

Umbilical cord compression can occur when pressure is placed on the umbilical cord, obstructing proper circulation through it. Cord entanglement around fetal body parts can occur *in utero* idiopathically. This risk can be increased with abnormal positioning of the fetus in the uterus, such as in breech position, or with monoamniotic twin pregnancies (37, 38). Also, cord prolapse, though a rare complication, can also cause asphyxia when the cord drops through the cervix prior to the body of the neonate during labor. This may happen prior to or during delivery (Stage I or Stage II), leading to the baby's body compressing the cord and compromising placental oxygen supply to the fetus (39).

Previously, we discussed the potential prenatal causes of placental injury, in particular as a consequence of gestational diabetes. However, perinatal injury must be considered as well in order to properly examine placental pathology as a potential source of birth hypoxia. The placenta is the connection between the developing fetus and the maternal uterine wall, allowing for exchange of substances between mother and baby. The placenta begins to develop once the blastocyst implants in the uterine endometrium of the mother. Around the second week of gestation, lacunar spaces develop within the placenta (37). Maternal blood from the uterine lining flows into and pools in the lacunar spaces. By the end of the second week, the arteriovenous network of the umbilical cord forms from primary chorionic villi. By the end of the third week, embryonic blood begins to circulate through the blood vessels, and by the end of the fourth week, gas and nutrient exchange is fully established between the mother and fetus (37). From then until term, the surface area of the placenta continues to expand to meet the needs of the maturing fetus. The thickness of the placenta, however, decreases with gestational age, which allows for greater facility in the transfer of substances and more rapid diffusion of oxygen across the placenta (37). Because the placenta is essential to maintain the growth of both itself and the fetus, placental function requires a high level of energy production. Thus, any cause of placental insufficiency can result in a failure of placental functions.

The placenta is typically examined immediately upon delivery, and there are several potential placental abnormalities that can affect the efficacy of gas exchange. One is arteriopathy, which can restrict maternal perfusion of the intervillous space and thus restrict oxygen exchange with fetal blood. Another may be perivillous fibrin, which restricts gas exchange between mother and fetus by coating the villous trophoblast, adding an additional barrier to effective gas exchange (37). One serious cause of placental pathology that can result in perinatal hypoxia is premature rupture of placental membranes near or during the onset of labor (37). These membranes usually rupture spontaneously, but in certain cases they can rupture prematurely, often due to an increase in luminal pressure or weakened structural integrity of the membranes. Some causes of increased pressure include premature contractions, cervical dilation, dystocia and polyhydramnios (38). Some causes of weakening in structural integrity of the membranes include trauma, inflammation, and ischemic necrosis caused by premature placental separation (*abruptio placentae*) (37, 38).

Perinatal hypoxia has clearly been shown to have significant effects on neural function (36), and here we have touched upon a few mechanisms by which birth hypoxia could occur due to adverse obstetric conditions. Though studies have found a higher prevalence of obstetric complications upon review of ASD cases, the mechanism behind these effects are in all likelihood multifactorial (40, 41). The interplay between genetic predisposition and environmental (prenatal, perinatal or obstetric) conditions is intricate, and a concrete correlation between the two remains to be determined.

Conclusions

Just a few minutes of acute oxygen deprivation, or chronic oxygen deprivation, can produce significant damage to the central nervous system. As discussed above, some areas of the brain are more sensitive to hypoxia than others. In particular, hypoxia can affect the hippocampus and limbic system, as well as the basal ganglia, Purkinje cells of the cerebellum, and neocortical areas. These areas, when functioning appropriately, allow for proper regulation and control over cortical processes, such as those moderating social and emotional behaviors. Any dysregulation of these processes can potentially lead to clinical manifestations commonly seen in ASD. Thus, hypoxic conditions, both during pregnancy and at birth, should be considered as factors that may be associated with the subsequent development of ASD.

A hypoxic environment is often detrimental to proper fetal development. Hypoxia may significantly affect the proper genesis of the nervous system. Further investigation must be done to determine whether there is a conclusive, significant connection between a hypoxic effect on these neural areas and the typical patterns seen in autism. Essential to these considerations is the study into hypoxia as a chronic insult (here explored as prenatal injury) versus hypoxia during acute injury (such as that which can occur during delivery). As a pervasive developmental disorder, prenatal and perinatal composition must be considered as well as the environment during infancy.

Autism spectrum disorders are generally thought to have both genetic and environmental factors (see Prologue). However, the extent of genetic predisposition, the presence of environmental triggers, and the effect and interplay between the two are not fully understood. No one element at this point can or should be considered causational for autism. Due to the multifactorial nature of the disease, each research study likely shows but a portion of the overall solution.

Chapter 3H –Perinatal Complications

Matan Elami-Suzin

[A number of perinatal complications, such as hypoxia, hypertension, diabetes, twinning, and growth restriction could conceivable serve as environmental triggers to promote the development of autism – Ed.]

Introduction

In recent years, there is growing evidence that perinatal complications have a potential associative role in the pathogenesis of autism and autism spectrum disorder (ASD). The aim of this chapter is to survey the current evidence regarding the contribution of these complications as etiological factors in ASD.

Observations

Obstetric suboptimality

This is a general term used in many studies and refers to a wide range of prenatal and perinatal complications. Obstetric suboptimality is measured as a scale or score that sums a range of complications in a single value (1). In general, there is an association between "pregnancy complications", as a whole, and ASD, as well as many more behavioral and neurological disorders, and the risk escalates with increasing number of complications (2,3). In the Nurses' Health Study II cohort, women with preeclampsia, pregnancy-induced hypertension and/or gestational diabetes, had an odds ratio of 1.49 of having an offspring with ASD compared to women without these complications. In the same cohort, women with four complications or more had 2.76 times the odds of having an offspring with ASD compared to participants without complications (3).

Other studies of obstetrical suboptimality have reached similar conclusions (1,4,5) or found clusters of multiple perinatal complications in mothers of children with ASD (6).
In addition, there have been few studies that did not find an increased incidence of ASD with higher suboptimality scores (7) or have suggested that after correcting for factors like birth order, parity and maternal age, there is no association between perinatal complications and ASD (8,9). These investigations are limited, however, by small sample size, resulting in low power. Many studies tried to assess the contribution of individual prenatal and perinatal complications, and have shown some significant associations with ASD (10-13). However, as will be discussed further, associations of ASD with individual complications are less consistent compared to suboptimality scores.

Multiple pregnancy

Multiple pregnancy has been studied for being an increased risk of developing ASD. In Gardener's meta-analysis, inconsistencies were found in the results from 10 studies that examined multiple pregnancy as a risk factor for ASD (2). Five reports that did not find such an association were limited by very small sample size and/or assessed only crude associations. Two Norwegian studies found no association in unadjusted analyses (10,12), while two other larger studies did find increased risk of autism with multiple pregnancies as compared to singletons, in adjusted analyses (6,14).

Another large study reported higher prevalence of multiple births in the autism group, but did not address potential confounders (15). The meta-analysis summary estimate suggested a significant 77% increased risk of autism among multiple births (OR = 1.77, 95% CI 1.23-2.55).

Another investigation not included in this meta-analysis also noted a significant positive association of ASD with multiple birth in adjusted analyses (16).

The mechanisms underlying the relation between multiple births and autism could be linked to the twinning process, sharing of the *in utero* environment, or other elements that often are consequences of multiple births and are associated with autism. For example, multiple gestation is associated with a higher risk for pregnancy complications such as small for gestational age neonates and prematurity, as well as poorer neonatal outcomes in general (17). Thus, while most of the available evidence to date from large studies suggest that autism is slightly more common in multiple pregnancies, the question remains whether it is the twinning process itself that increases autism risk, or, rather, the association is mediated through other perinatal complications, which are more prevalent in these multifetal pregnancies.

Growth restriction and preterm birth

Babies with low birth weight (less than 2,500 gram) have a higher risk for later neurological, psychiatric, and neuropsychological problems (18). Low birth weight has been associated with a variety of cognitive difficulties and psychiatric outcomes in children, including speech and language, internalization, attention and social problems, hyperactivity, and learning disabilities (19). However, newborns with low birth weight are a heterogeneous group in terms of etiology, and low birth weight is often an indicator of earlier, intrauterine pathology. The birth weight of premature babies is usually low. Thus, it may be more informative to consider gestational age and ASD. Similar to low birth weight, gestational age, and in particular, short gestation (birth before 37 weeks), has also been associated with adverse health outcomes including developmental delays and later intellectual impairments in childhood and adolescence (20-22). Compared to birth weight, gestational age is less accurately measured and is often undocumented, thereby necessitating more careful data evaluation. Despite being studied frequently (19), research results that relate birth weight, gestational age, and risk of ASD from individual studies are mixed, and the strength of any association is disputed (23).

A meta-analysis examining the association between indicators of growth restriction and preterm birth and risk of ASD supports an association between growth restriction and risk of ASD (24). After adjustment for potential confounding factors including paternal age, maternal age, sex, and parental socio-demographic characteristics, the random-effect pooled estimate of the risk of ASD in low- (< 2,500 grams) birth-weight individuals compared with individuals born at normal birth weight (≥ 2,500 grams) was 1.5 (95% confidence intervals: 1.0– 2.5). For individuals born preterm (before week 37) the random-effect pooled estimate of the risk of ASD was 1.5 (95% confidence intervals: 1.3–1.9). Fetal growth restriction (being born small for gestational age) was also associated with increased risk of ASD. The random-effect pooled estimate of the risk of ASD in individuals born small for gestational age was 1.4 (95% confidence intervals: 1.1–1.8).

Birth weight is affected by multiple genetic and environmental factors, as well as the duration of the pregnancy and rate of fetal growth. Maternal and prenatal conditions associated with low birth weight and preterm birth are likely to be heterogeneous in etiology. Thus, it remains obscured whether the intrauterine disturbances may directly compromise the fetus and result in ASD, or whether they reflect the effects of a fetus compromised by other factors. One study that examined the relationship between perinatal complications and ASD showed increased perinatal complications in siblings of individuals with ASD, and concluded that perinatal complications in ASD reflect the effects of a fetus compromised by other factors, most likely underlying genetic factors or their interaction with the environment (11).

Preterm birth has been linked with maternal infections, high blood pressure, maternal diabetes, and preeclampsia. Nevertheless, in almost half of all instances of preterm birth, the causes cannot be ascertained. A number of prenatal conditions are known to be associated with growth restriction. Placental problems can reduce blood flow and nutrients to the fetus, limiting growth. Maternal nutritional problems during pregnancy may also effect in utero growth. Finally, infections in the fetus have also been linked with abnormal growth. Maternal infections (13) (chapter 6C), maternal diabetes (chapter 6A), hypertension (10), and placental abnormalities (11) have been only sporadically examined in relation to ASD, and it is therefore unclear whether they could explain the association between growth restriction and ASD.

Gestational bleeding

Hemorrhage during pregnancy may be the result of, or an indicator for, various pregnancy complications, especially placental problems, especially when the bleeding occurs in the third trimester. Almost every study that has examined the association has suggested a slight to moderate increase in autism with maternal gestational bleeding, though only few achieved statistical significance (2). In a large Swedish case-control study (10), the risk of autism after gestational bleeding was non-significantly elevated, though analyses included adjustment for potentially downstream factors, including birth weight and mode of delivery, thereby potentially biasing results.

Two case-control studies reported strong increases in risk associated with bleeding (4,6), but neither adjusted for potential confounding factors, and both were based on comparison to population rates. Three other larger studies, including a population-based registry study and two case-control investigations, found no significant association in adjusted analyses (11). Another large case-control study also found no association; however, the group of reference was sibling controls, which may not be appropriate given the genetics of ASD.

In the meta-analysis of prenatal risk factors for autism, which included the studies described earlier, the summary estimate suggested a significant 81 % increase in risk of autism in offspring of mothers who experienced gestational bleeding (2). However, the results from Juul-Dam and colleagues (4), which suggested an OR > 10, may have unduly influenced the summary estimate. More recently, a large investigation found no significant association after adjusting for potentially confounding factors. The observed associations between gestational bleeding and autism in some studies may be related to fetal hypoxia, which has been purported to influence brain development.

Gestational diabetes mellitus

A recent large population-based case control study found a significant increase in autism risk in children of mothers with any of the following metabolic conditions during pregnancy: obesity, type 2 diabetes, gestational diabetes, or hypertension (chapter 6A). In addition, the Nurses' Health Study II identified nearly a doubling in risk of autism in offspring of mothers having gestational diabetes, as did a meta-analysis (2,3). Some studies have found no such association (10).

The mechanisms relating gestational diabetes to autism have not been distinctly determined, though some have hypothesized a metabolic pathway, by which hyperinsulinemia in the fetus may lead to increased oxygen metabolism and chronic hypoxia that affects the developing brain. This mechanism is consistent with some literature on other potential hypoxia-related conditions. Other hypothesized pathways are through nutritional status related to diabetes, including decreased micronutrient availability, or possible associations with hormone levels, which have also been suggested as relevant in autism (3,30). In addition, gestational diabetes is often associated with Cesarean sections and low infant blood sugar at birth (31) perinatal risk factors that could play a mediating role in the association.

Obesity

Higher prepregnancy weight was associated with autism in one study, as was increased weight gain during pregnancy (28) (chapter 6A). Weight gain remained significant in adjusted analyses taking into account prepregnancy weight, suggesting each factor may contribute independently to autism risk. In a large population-based case control study, maternal prepregnancy obesity (defined as a BMI of 30 or higher) was associated with a 70% increase in odds of autism when compared to typically developing controls (29). An additional study found an association with high maternal BMI during late adolescence (age 18), rather than at a time closer to pregnancy, in association with risk of having a child with autism (3). Associations with BMI or weight may be due to increased insulin resistance, or perhaps alterations in hormone levels, nutrition, or some other unknown mechanism.

Other perinatal complications

Obstetric variables with the strongest evidence for no association with autism, according Gardener's review of prenatal factors through 2009, include prior fetal loss, maternal hypertension, edema, and preeclampsia (2). However, the meta-analysis did not exclude studies based on methodologic weakness, and since factors like study heterogeneity, small sample sizes, use of control groups affected by another condition, and analyses that did not take into account potential confounders may have limited prior findings, some of these factors may require further study. More recently, aninvestigation including 87,677 births from South Carolina Medicaid data (472 children diagnosed with autism) nevertheless suggested a significant association between preeclampsia and increased risk of autism (32). The association was slightly attenuated after adjustments for birth weight but remained statistically significant for a moderate increase in risk;

however, such adjustment for a factor downstream of preeclampsia might introduce bias. These newer results suggest that additional methodologically rigorous studies are required to confirm whether preeclampsia puts one in danger for autism.

Other prenatal and perinatal obstetric complications appear to have been tested in only one study, which reported no association with ASD. These factors include chronic maternal diseases, venous thrombosis, frequency of intercourse during pregnancy, exposure to X-rays, amniocentesis, chorionic villus sampling, and month of initiation of prenatal care (2,28). Additionally, these factors have been found to have no association with autism in two studies to date: prenatal ultrasound (28,30), maternal oral contraceptive use, maternal menstrual cycle characteristics , and prior stillbirths or spontaneous abortions (2,3,28). Nevertheless, at this time, the research has been insufficient to draw conclusions about these factors. For some, (e.g ., prenatal ultrasound), further development of methodology for measurement or estimation of exposure may be required before definitive work can be undertaken.

Conclusions
Presumed mechanisms

Associations between obstetric complications and autism could arise from:

1) a causal association, that is, the complications act biologically to directly increase risk of autism;

2) a common upstream cause of both complications and autism, perhaps by genetic/ familial factors;

3) the result of the underlying pathology of autism, rather than a cause of it; or

4) interactions between genetic or other environmental factors and the complications lead to autism (in a type of two-hit model).

Each of these explanations has plausibility, and different explanations likely apply to different complications, subgroups of individuals with autism, or surveys. With regard to confounding, birth order and maternal age should be taken into account in studies of obstetric factors, because some complications occur more frequently firstborns, others in those of higher birth order, and some are more common among elderly mothers.

There is a lack of direct evidence of the mechanisms explaining associations between perinatal complications and autism. However, insights about potential pathways can be derived from certain investigations of familial factors. One study found that increased number of prenatal, perinatal and neonatal complications in autistic probands, was associated with a greater number of unaffected family members having the broader autism phenotype (i.e., milder autistic symptoms) (34). A similar association between familial broader autism phenotype and obstetric complications was also noted in another study (35). These findings may be consistent with a number of the explanations provided above, but suggest overlap between family history of obstetric complications and either autism or even perhaps tendency to developmental problems in general. In particular, it is worth stressing that obstetric complications have been associated with other psychiatric and neurodevelopmental disorders (10-13). Thus, complications in the prenatal, perinatal, and neonatal periods may be general markers of or predictors for vulnerabilities to a broad range of neurodevelopmental problems.

Chapter 3I – Gestational Diabetes; Obesity

Tova Chein

[The combination of gestational diabetes and obesity may act to lower insulin-like growth factor production, thereby adversely affecting axonal myelination in the developing fetus. – Ed.]

Hypothesis

For more than twenty years, members of the scientific community as well the general public have been puzzled by the unexplained apparent increase in the prevalence of autism and related conditions (chapter 1C). Many hypotheses have been proposed to explain this phenomenon and to understand the etiology of autism. None of the hypotheses has been able to withstand the rigorous requirements to be proven accurate and descriptive of the primary cause of this disease as yet.

Research findings point to the involvement of genetics (chapters 5A,8A) as well as environmental trigger factors (chapters 4B,8C). Such factors may have an effect through maternal exposure during gestation or directly via the baby early in infancy. Studies also suggest that the pathogenesis of autism is likely to begin *in utero* (1). (This information is discussed further in other chapters of this book as well.)

One of the more recent hypotheses describes several maternal metabolic conditions during gestation as risk factors for the development of autism and developmental delays in the infant. These include metabolic syndrome, which is characterized by insulin resistance, obesity, hypertension, and lipid imbalance (2). The present chapter will discuss the ways these metabolic conditions may pertain to the development of autism.

Observations

In recent years, the prevalence of obesity, diabetes type 2 (adult onset), and gestational (pregnancy-related) diabetes has increased dramatically, especially in women of child-bearing age. Today, these three conditions are among the most common complications during pregnancies. This is largely due to the relationship between obesity and diabetes type 2 (3). Obese patients commonly suffer from peripheral insulin resistance which often leads to full-blown maternal diabetes later in life. Overt diabetes is sometimes present before the start of the pregnancy. Although being obese may enhance the tendency to develop this condition, it is important to mention that not all women with type 2 diabetes or gestational diabetes are overweight.

These pregnancy-related complications carry with them inherent risks for both the mother and the unborn child. Such pregnancies are problematic especially if there is underlying renal or vascular disease in the mother, in addition to poor control of blood glucose levels. The fetal risks of overt diabetes with poor glycemic control include miscarriage, fetal macrosomia, preterm delivery, unexplained fetal demise, and excess fluid retention. Inadequate control of blood glucose can expose the developing fetus to hyperglycemia early in its development and may be associated with congenital anomalies such as cardiac, skeletal, or central nervous system malformations. The risk for fetal congenital malformations of the cardiovascular system in particular is increased 2-3 fold in pregnancies complicated with (overt) diabetes, relative to the general population (3).

In particular, the coexistence of diabetes during pregnancy poses threats to maternal vascular and neurological health and function as well. Persistent hyperglycemia may have a negative effect on blood circulation in target organs as well as peripheral tissue due to vascular plaque formation. Persistent hyperglycemia damages the large and medium muscular arteries, causing reduction in vascular patency. Significant harm occurs also to the small vessels and capillaries. As a result, common complications of long-term, poorly controlled diabetes include gangrene of the lower extremities, poor wound healing, renal failure, nerve damage, cardio-vascular disease, and blindness. In fact, diabetes is the leading cause of blindness and end-stage renal disease in the Western World.

Diabetes may also be associated with artherosclerosis, high blood pressure, and cardiac insufficiency. These conditions result from poor blood flow related to constriction of blood vessel endothelium from persistent hyperglycemia. An inflammatory response damages blood vessels and other tissues from deposition of glycosylate plasma proteins by macrophages, endothelial cells, and mesangial cells (4). Vascular injury causes poor wound healing by decreased potential for angiogenesis and repair.

Damage to small vessels supplying nerves in particular may induce loss of excitability and function. Due to injury to nerves of the extremities, patients do not sense cuts and minor harm to their skin. In particular, maternal hyperglycemia may lead to glucose deposition on the interior of blood vessels which narrows their lumen and decreases blood flow.

Diminished maternal circulation also reduces delivery of nutrients and metabolites to and from fetal tissues via the placenta, resulting in increased oxidative stress and fetal tissue hypoxia (chapters 3G,4B). Macrosomic fetuses in diabetic pregnancies are at higher risk for birth injury and prenatal/neonatal mortality and morbidity. Some involve traumatic birth injuries due to their large size, most commonly shoulder dystocia (obstruction), which may injure the nerves controlling arm function. Other causes of perinatal complications can be prolonged labor and fetal asphyxia/hypoxia plus amniotic fluid aspiration (5). Some of the conditions associated with these complications in diabetic pregnancies may affect the baby for short periods, while others may have lasting effects

A recent study provides evidence that maternal metabolic conditions such as diabetes and obesity during pregnancy may affect the occurrence of ASD (autism spectrum disorder) in the child (2). The study examined a large number of young autistic children, as well as youngsters with developmental delays, and compared them to children with normal development. The review compared the number of mothers who suffered from metabolic conditions during the gestation periods with the enrolled infants in both groups. Diabetes was more prevalent among mothers of children subsequently diagnosed with autism, where 9.3 % of the mothers in the affected group had had diagnosed diabetes during the pregnancy. On the other hand, in the group of children with neurologically normal postpartum development, only 6.4% of the mothers had gestational diabetes. In other words, the mothers with diabetes during pregnancy were more likely to have a child who subsequently exhibited the characteristics of autism.

With regard to obesity in particular, which is defined as BMI >30.0 (body mass index), the risk of having a child with autism was found to be significantly higher than in the general population. Among the group of children diagnosed with autism, more than 20% of the mothers were obese during the gestation period, compared with only 14.3 % obese mothers giving birth to unaffected children. Overall, the prevalence of all maternal metabolic conditions such as diabetes and obesity is higher among the group mothering children with autism. Among a set of children with autism 28.6% of mothers had one of the metabolic conditions mentioned earlier during the pregnancy. Only 19.4 % of the mothers of unaffected children had one of these conditions during the pregnancy (2).

Development of autism in these children has been linked to certain prenatal and perinatal problems. Poor regulation of maternal glucose during gestation may result in abnormal fetal development. Oxygen deprivation and oxidative stress are known to have negative effect on the neural tissue and the central nervous system (see chapter 5B). Some studies report that obese mothers are less likely to breast-feed (3).

Hyperglycemic conditions *in utero* commonly lead to high insulin levels in the fetal blood, which in turn increases the demand for oxygen and iron in the fetal cells. When the higher-than-normal demand cannot be met, the fetus develops hypoxia (6) and iron deficiency (7). These conditions are known to have injurious effects on nerve cells in particular (8). Pregnancies complicated with diabetes experience recurrent maternal and intrauterine hyperglycemia. As a result, the fetus's higher levels of insulin result in increased oxygen demand and metabolic rate. This can be the reason for chronic intrauterine hypoxia, oxidative stress, and injury to fetal tissue. Such cellular effects might explain some of the fetal anomalies such as congenital cardiac, skeletal and neurological abnormalities that are associated with these conditions during pregnancy, including the postpartum development of autism. (This subject is further discussed in great details in the chapter 5B about oxidative stress.) These circumstances can alter myelination and cortical connectivity (chapter 3D), as well as lead to aberration of neurons of the hippocampus. Iron deficiency in the fetus is also associated with reduction in recognition memory, behavioral, and developmental problems (9).

Finally, breast milk is especially important to the proper growth and development of infants. This tendency places neonates of obese females at a further disadvantage for proper development. In particular, prolonged breast-feeding is associated with the reduction in the incidence of autism (chapter 9A).

Conclusions

With the apparently rising prevalence of obesity and diabetes among women of child bearing age, evidence linking these controllable conditions with the development of autism in the child becomes a major concern. If the frequency of such metabolic conditions continues to increase, it could have further public health consequence in the next generation, namely, additional neurodevelopmental problems in the children born to mothers with metabolic conditions during the pregnancy (2). As noted, obesity and diabetes place the baby at a risk for development of neurological disorders such as ASD. Persistent hyperglycemic conditions may damage maternal blood vessels and decrease delivery of oxygen and nutrients to the fetus.

A very exciting, new study published late in 2012 describes intracellular events that occur due to persistent intrauterine hyperglycemic conditions in a pregnant diabetic female. The study reports epigenetic modifications to the IGF (insulin-like growth factor) gene. Modification of this gene occurs as a result of hyperglycemic conditions in the uterus of a pregnant diabetic female (10). [Epigenetic modification of a gene is a process by which on/off switch molecules are added to the external surface of the DNA molecule without changing the DNA sequence itself.] Usually these signal modification of gene expression. Such changes at the IGF gene segment decrease the access of transcription protein to the modified gene segment, thereby decreasing the expression of that particular gene. A child born to a mother at the end of a diabetic pregnancy may suffer from decreased IGF levels not only at birth but early in infancy as well.

A recent hypothesis regarding the etiology of autism describes decreased levels of IGF or IGF expression during fetal development as well as early in infancy as associated with the development of autism early in childhood (chapter 6D). This hypothesis considers several maternal conditions that deprive the developing fetus of placental IGF and the subsequent development of autism in these children (11). Should this factor prove to be central in defining the mechanism leading to autism, it might also shed some light on a more precise process by which diabetes and obesity can enhance the development of autism in the child in particular.

ENVIRONMENTAL TRIGGERS

Chapter 4A - Heavy Metals
Elina Davydov, Mary Ann Joseph

[Environmental toxins, especially heavy metals, have been frequently cited as possible instigators of the overt characteristics of autism. Although found in many affected children, a cause-and-effect relationship remains to be discerned. – Ed.]

Hypothesis

Since the Industrial Revolution there have been rising levels of toxic heavy metals (any metallic chemical element that can cause adverse effects in the body). The exposure to heavy metals has been suggested to be associated with the development of Autistic Spectrum Disorder (1). Toxic heavy metals include aluminum, arsenic, mercury, cadmium, chromium, and nickel. Trace elements that are commonly found with heavy metals include zinc, magnesium, calcium, selenium, and iron. The developing brain is significantly more susceptible to injury than is the mature adult brain. During the growth of the fetus, the placenta is not an effective barrier against many harmful environment pollutants. This allows some metals to freely cross the placenta and cause the concentration of such elements to be significantly higher in the umbilical cord than in the maternal blood. This chapter will examine the hypothesis that increased levels of toxic heavy metals in the environment may have a role in triggering the development of autism.

The initial discussion will review how exposure to neurotoxic metals occurs and what causes some children to be more susceptible to metal accumulation than others. Industrialization, burning of fossil fuels and domestic waste production increase the levels of heavy metals in the environment. Neurotoxic metals may seep into the soil and oceans then accumulate in animals, fish and plants, and finally enter the food chain (1). Daily exposure of these pollutants involves consumption of contaminated drinking and food, inhalation of fouled air, and exposure to industrial waste or soil (2).

Observations

Passage to the fetus occurs through the placenta. Three layers that make up the placental barrier are syncyctiotrophoblast, cytotrophoblast, and fetal endothelial cells. The presence of membrane transport mechanisms and the thickness of the placental layers are important in determining the permeability and transfer of heavy metals from mother to fetus. An example is Cadmium , a heavy metal in which placental levels correlate with maternal levels. (2).

The fetus synthesizes amniotic fluid, which functions in preventing mechanical insults, wetting the developing lungs, and providing nutrients for the fetus. From 10-20 weeks of gestation, amniotic fluid becomes similar in composition to fetal plasma due to the free diffusion bilaterally that occurs between the amniotic fluid and the fetus across fetal skin. Amniotic fluid is, in fact a product of fetal urine excretion. Kosanovic et al, in 2002, conducted a study determining the amniotic fluid concentration of cadmium and selenium in 37 nonhypertensive and 23 hypertensive pregnant women in relation to their smoking status. Tobacco smoking caused an increase in cadmium and a decrease in selenium in both hypertensive and nonhypertensive women. Even though amniotic fluid is considered an important marker for fetal exposure and placental barrier function, there are insufficient data on environmental and dietary impact on the composition of the amniotic fluid (2).

A proposal that was suggested for the susceptibility of heavy metal accumulation is that children who later develop autism have a defect in processing heavy metals (3). These individuals have difficulty exporting metals, which leads to toxic accumulations. The Holmes study examined the first baby hair preserved by families of autistic children and compared heavy metal levels with that of first baby hair of non-autistic children. Using coupled-mass spectroscopy, the finding was that the children who later developed severe autism had the lowest levels of mercury in hair. Mercury levels were affected by maternal fish consumption, medication use containing mercury, and dental amalgams. In normal children, mercury levels coincided with the known mercury exposure. Hair concentration of mercury in control children was found to be 3.63 ug/g, while in severely autistic children, mercury level was found to be 0.21 ug/g. This finding proposes that toxic metal accumulation can occur by low-level exposure affecting children with a defect in metal excretion or by high- level exposure affecting children with no defect in metal export. It has been suggested that mercury export is low in the first year of life and that export and detoxification mechanisms are very different in babies and older children. Elimination defects could extend to other heavy metals and may cause accumulation leading to toxicity. However, there is little research on the levels of other heavy metals in first baby hair.

The reason for this defect is believed to be due to a genetic predisposition. One such defect is in the methylene tetrahydrofolate reductase (MTHFR) enzyme, which is responsible for efficient metal export (chapter 5A). C677T allele differs from the MTHR in the 677 position, where cysteine is replaced by threonine. This causes the enzyme to become unstable and not fully functional. This unstable enzyme causes increases sensitivity to heavy metal toxic (3).

Another enzyme that may be mutated in an autistic child is metallothionein (MT), which is responsible for binding and mobilizing heavy metals. However, the specific role of the MT genotype in autism has not been discovered (3).

The next question that arises is methods with which levels of biologically imbedded heavy metals and genetic susceptibility are examined. These include analysis of hair and nails, blood levels, and urine. Hair and nails are useful means of quantifying heavy metal exposure because they are easily sampled and significant amount of metals from the bloodstream are deposited into hair and nails. However, interpretation of hair samples needs to be done with caution since previous studies have shown that first baby hair of autistic children has lower levels of mercury due to export defects than non-autistic children (3).

Analysis of blood can involve examining direct plasma concentration or transcription of metallothionein in blood leukocytes. Metallothionein (MT), a non-enzymatic antioxidant, was found to have increased expression in autistic children. This antioxidant functions in detoxifying the body of toxic metals and free radicals. Humans express four major isoforms which include MT-1 and MT-2, MT-3 which are specific to the brain, and MT-4 which is specific to squamous epithelium. Twenty-eight children with autism and thirty- two healthy children were included in the study that showed autistic children showed higher mRNA expression of MT isoforms in peripheral blood mononuclear cells. Levels in autistic children of MT-1A, MT-2A, and MT-1E mRNA were 5-fold, 35-fold, and 301-fold, respectively, higher than children in the control group. Significant p-values indicate that a compensatory mechanism is in place that increases antioxidant activity in response to increased oxidative stress (4) (chapter 4B).

Urine is another method of assessing levels of heavy metals. They can be directly measured from urine samples or level of porphyrins (intermediates in heme synthesis) can be used as an indirect measure. Higher levels of heavy metals increase the concentration of porphyrins and can be detected in the urine (3).

Aluminum

Industrial emission of toxic metals has been a concerning source of contamination and threat to human life. However, one seemingly overlooked route of exposure is the amount of experimentally demonstrated neurotoxin added to the vaccine to increase the body's immune response as an adjuvant. Aluminum is one of the most commonly used vaccine adjuvants and has been shown to correlate with increased prevalence of autism spectrum disorders (5). Although very little has been proven about the pharmacokinetics and toxicology of aluminum compounds in children, the method by which this demonstrated neurotoxin impacts the nervous system has been sufficiently supported. An article in *The New England Journal of Medicine* presents key evidence that preterm infant exposure to a miniscule amount of aluminum, such as 20 micrograms/kilogram for a period greater than ten days has the ability to cause significant neurodevelopmental delays (6). However, the use of aluminum as an adjuvant has become widespread due to its strength as a potent stimulator of the immune system (5) (chapter 7A).

Through experimental means supported by the University of British Columbia, it has been suggested that a correlation exists between the rising prevalence of autism spectrum disorders and the amount of aluminum administered to children in various age groups through means of pediatric vaccination (5). In this specific study, the licensed vaccines that were studied included DTaP, HA, HB, Hib, and PCV which all contain a form of an aluminum adjuvant. According to the U.S. vaccination schedule provided by the Center for Disease Control (CDC.gov) for administering pediatric vaccines, U.S. infants receive the greatest amount of aluminum per body weight at two months of age from all vaccines mentioned above except for Hepatitis A vaccine (chapter 7B).

The period between two and fourth months of age tends to be a major contributor in the development of sleep, temperature regulation, and brain wave patterns-many of which are known to be impaired in autism. This bio-behavioral system is regulated by the neuroendocrine network through hormonal regulation and neurotransmission. While the Food and Drug Administration (FDA) has set an upper limit for aluminum content in vaccines at 850 micrograms per dose, this margin was set based on the efficacy of the drug rather than from a toxicological standpoint (7). The main finding supports a correlation between the prevalence of autism spectrum disorder and aluminum adjuvant exposure that presents at its greatest at three to four months of age.

Though research confirms the regular exposure of children to greater relative amounts of aluminum adjuvants than adults, it is commonly misconstrued that children obtain more aluminum from their diet than from potential vaccinations. However, on average, 0.25% of dietary aluminum is absorbed into the systemic circulation (8), whereas, the common adjuvant, aluminum hydroxide can be absorbed at nearly 100% when injected intramuscularly over a period of time. With an average half-life of diet-absorbed aluminum of less than 24 hours, the aluminum adjuvant is expected to have a longer elimination period from a renal excretion standpoint and can potentially cause oxidative stress within brain tissue. From this perspective, the aluminum source from vaccination represents a significant toxicological risk factor to the nervous system.

Though the validity of these results from such an ecological study remain to be confirmed, aluminum is portrayed as a potential toxin poorly associated with biobehavioral transitions commonly involved in the pathogenesis of autism. Further speculation rises from the correlation between the period of three to four months of age and critical stages of brain development that are impaired in autism spectrum disorders: the onset of amygdala maturation, onset of synaptogensis, maximal growth velocity of the hippocampus, and brain-wave and sleeping pattern (9). Thus, further study is warranted to determine the influence that is available during the postnatal period by such an adjuvant and neurotoxin such as aluminum.

Arsenic

As reported by the Occupational Safety & Health Administration (OSHA), arsenic occurs naturally in the environment. However, higher-than-average levels of arsenic occur in workplaces near hazardous waste sites and in soil, rock, and water. The same study that analyzed transcription of metallothionein also examined plasma levels of heavy metals in these children(11). Arsenic was shown to be significantly increased in autistic children with a mean of 80.55 ng/g (SD ± 22.95), versus 13.72 ng/g (SD ± 6.57) in non-autistic children (10). Metal analysis of hair also showed a significantly elevated arsenic level in autistic children, with nearly absent levels in non-autistic children (11).

Another study which examined children from Jeddah, Kingdom of Saudi Arabia also showed higher levels of arsenic in autistic children, with a mean value of 2.94 mg/kg and a reference range for non-autistic children with 0.7 mg/kg (12). However, when correlating arsenic levels with the Autism Childhood Rating Scale, there was insignificant proof (p>.05) that the high levels of arsenic correlated with symptoms such as relating to people, imitation, emotional response, and object use. Urine samples were also taken from autistic Arab children and non-autistic Arab children, and did not show higher levels of arsenic in autistic children as the blood analysis did (13). Even though higher levels of arsenic were found in the blood of autistic children, there is no evident association with this heavy metal and specific autistic symptoms.

Cadmium

Cadmium is a white metal found in batteries, alloys, solar cells, pigments, and used in nuclear reactors. Exposure to cadmium occurs in the manufacturing sector, construction, transportation, and trade. The toxicities of cadmium include alteration of trophoblast cell migration, induction of early decidualization of human endometrial stroma cells, and alteration of endocrine hormone synthesis (2). Cadmium also increases expression of placental metallothionein, which retains cadmium, reducing its passage to the fetus. Plasma levels of cadmium were significantly ($p < 0.01$) higher in autistic children than in non-autistic children (10). As with arsenic, there is no significance in associating high levels of arsenic with symptoms such as relating to people, auditory response and visual response (12). The urine analysis for cadmium did not show higher levels in autistic children as plasma analysis did (13). This suggests that high levels of cadmium and arsenic are more likely due to heavy metal elimination defect than a pathogenic heavy metal effect on autism.

Calcium; Iron

Unlike heavy metals, trace elements in the environment such as calcium and iron were found to be deficient in autistic children with a reported 5.8% and 0.9% deficiency, respectively (4). The mean value of calcium from hair of autistic children is 43.98 mg/kg, while the 95% confidence interval of nonautistic children is 200-850 mg/kg (12). The mean value of iron from hair of autistic children is reported to be 5.7 mg/kg, while the 95% confidence interval of unaffected children is found to be 7.7-15 mg/kg. However, no correlation was found between the deficiency in calcium and iron, and symptoms of autism in imitation, body use, and adaptation to change or visual response (12). Another study measuring plasma levels showed increased levels of calcium with an 11% increase in autistic children and a $p < .001$ compared to nonautistic children.

Plasma levels of iron in autistic children showed 218% increase, with a $p < .001$ compared with no neurologically normal children (10). This indicates a discrepancy between plasma levels and hair sample levels that may be due to a difference in the deposition of metals in plasma and hair.

Chromium; Nickel

One of the major sources of environmental pollution includes the emission of heavy metals from contaminated soils and air around industrial centers such as cement factories. An investigation into the toxicological implications of heavy metal concentrations in cement dust from U.S. and Nigeria samples was completed in 2012 by the University of Texas Medical Branch. Samples of cement dust were analyzed using absorption spectrophotometry with appropriate wavelengths. Concentrations of nine elements were determined, two of which included chromium and nickel. Of note, the level of nickel in the U.S. dust sample was higher than the average published concentration of the element in cement dust (14) and also was twice the concentration in Nigerian cement dust (15). Similarly, the level of chromium in the U.S. sample was higher than the previously published average concentration.

More surprisingly, the concentration of chromium was 13.4 folds greater in U.S. cement dust than in that of Nigeria. These elevated levels expose workers and the environment of toxic effects of these metals. Major sources of chromium in cement dust are kiln-fed raw materials and refractory brick in mills. Interestingly, it has been shown that absorption of various species of chromium can occur through intact skin (16). Moreover, this 2012 study supports the concern that metals contained in cement dust can contribute to debilitating health conditions.

But despite the elevated level of chromium and nickel in various sources such as cement dust, the relationship toward autistic spectrum disorder is still in question. In blood samples obtained from autistic children by a 2011 study funded by the University of Genoa (10), thirteen metals including nickel and chromium were measured. Of the two metals mentioned, nickel was found to be elevated among autistic subjects in relation to healthy control groups. No significant difference was observed for chromium and several other metals among the two subject groups. The possibility of statistical significance warrants further investigation into the factors that cause elevation of such metals in plasma levels. The genetics behind expressed genes having a higher affinity for certain metal ions has been briefly researched and deserves further investigation. The critical dependence of the brain on a supply of natural heavy metals deserves to be investigated in the future as a source contributing to brain damage in autism spectrum disorders.

Magnesium

The level of the trace element magnesium was also significantly decreased in autistic children with $p<.001$ when analyzing hair samples (17). This study separated autistic children into low, medium, and high grades of severity according to the Childhood Autism Rating Scale with 15 children in each group and compared them to 50 nonautistic children. The study showed decreased levels of magnesium in hair samples in all grades of severity when compared to a control of 63.84 □g/g. The rate of magnesium deficiency in autistic children is found to be 17.6% when analyzing hair of 1,967 autistic children (4). Mean value of levels for autistic children is 12.38 mg/kg while the 95% reference range of nonautistic children is 20-115 mg/kg (12). However, there is no correlation between deficiency in magnesium and symptoms of autism previously mentioned.

Selenium

Selenium is another essential trace metal that, according to the National Institutes of Health Office of Dietary Supplements, is present in foods such as bread, poultry, fish, meat, grains and eggs (18). Selenoproteins have critical roles in thyroid hormone metabolism, reproduction, and DNA protection from oxidative damage. One of the most important selenoproteins is the glutathione peroxidases which are responsible for metal mobilization and preventing oxidative damage (3) (see chapter 4B). Selenoprotein P is a selenium transporter involved in binding and mobilizing metals such mercury and cadmium. Selenium deficiency increases neurodevelopmental damage caused by methylmercury since selenium is protective against mercury intoxication.

Serum selenium was found in unaffected controls to have a mean level of 3.37 µg/g (SD ± 0.4 µg/g), while the mean levels of low, medium, and high grade autistic children were 0.57 µg/g, 1.98 µg/g, and 2.55 µg/g, respectively (12). When correlating selenium levels in autistic children with symptoms, a deficiency in selenium was significantly associated with a disability to adapt to changes.

Zinc

As opposed to toxic levels of several of the metals and essential elements discussed in this chapter, the association between zinc levels in hair samples and the prevalence of autistic characteristics is most significant for a negative correlation (12). Statistics within the aforementioned study of 44 children with autism spectrum disorders based in Jeddah, Saudi Arabsia have shown that a decrease in hair zinc levels may be associated with an elevated level of fear and nervousness and difficulty with verbal communication, to which many individuals dealing with autism spectrum disorders can relate with varying severity.

However, contrastingly different from the stated 2012 study of hair samples, a study from the year prior noted an elevated concentration of zinc in plasma concentrations of 28 children diagnosed with autism based off the criteria of Diagnostic and Statistical Manual of Mental Disorders (10,19). Although there are earlier studies available with contrasting results, particularly higher levels of zinc observed both in hair (20) and in teeth samples (21) of autistic individuals, the results of various studies consider autism as multifactorial with an influence of genetic, environmental and immunological factors that may induce elevated levels of metals in plasma concentrations.

Conclusions

While certain sources may praise the use of chelation treatment to reduce heavy metal deposits especially lead (see chapter 4C), some sources have surveyed the public and found that 7.4% of parents reported the use of chelation in their child with ASD (22). However, when medical professionals were surveyed (23), a significant 26% reported they did not have sufficient knowledge to make a reliable recommendation in reference to chelation treatment. Though more systematic research may need to be considered for validation of its use, current evidence does approach chelation treatment for autistic spectrum disorders with a significant challenge.

According to Blaucok-Busch et al., the mean level of certain metals in hair samples in 44 autistic children were greater than the reference range observed in 146 non-autistic children (12). For the metal aluminum, hair levels in autistic children were found to hold a mean of 15.21 mg/kg which was significantly greater than the hair reference range of 8.0 mg/kg in non autistic children. With a standard deviation of 9.0, the results for aluminum held a large 95 percent confidence interval of +/- 2.66. Similarly, Arsenic was found to have a mean of 2.94 mg/kg in autistic children, still significantly greater than the reference of 0.7 mg/kg in non-autistic children hair samples. The article listed a large standard deviation of 4.05 with a confidence interval of +/- 1.2. Hair samples of the participating autistic children also contained an elevated level of nickel at an average of 2.37 mg/kg as compared to the reference range of 0.85 mg/kg in those who were non-autistic. This metal also held a significant standard deviation and confidence interval at 1.28 and +/-0.38, respectively. Less drastically, the metal cadmium also showed an elevated average in hair samples of those with autism at 0.62 mg/kg in comparison with a hair reference range of 0.32 mg/kg in the non-autistic participants. The authors listed a small standard deviation of 0.06 and confidence interval of +/-0.02. Finally, the article made note of a marked decrease in the mean hair level of chromium in autistic subjects: it was calculated to be 0.08 mg/kg which was clearly less than the listed reference of 0.53 mg/kg in hair samples of non-autistic children. (12) The analysis of hair samples of autistic children mentioned in the stated article provides a potential opportunity for early intervention and nutritional education.

Despite evidence that some heavy metals may be linked to autism spectrum disorder, there seems to be a lack of concrete evidence that the manifestation of autistic characteristics is a direct consequence of the elevated levels of these toxic metals, whether it is in hair, nail, or serum samples. Though the association between the two topics cannot be ignored, further testing is necessary.

For metals such as aluminum, its involvement in the pathogenesis of autism is crucial to understanding the reasoning behind bio-behavioral transitions in infants. Brain development can be impaired by elevated levels of aluminum by interfering with brain-wave and sleeping patterns as well as the growth of the hippocampus (9). Nevertheless, current studies remain inconclusive on the depth of influence of such a strong neurotoxin and vaccine adjuvant such as aluminum.

For other heavy metals such as cadmium and arsenic, even though the levels in the hair and plasma were higher than levels in nonautistic children, there was no correlation between symptoms of autism and increased levels. However, urine analysis did not correlate with the higher levels of cadmium in the hair. Similarly, with calcium, iron, and magnesium even though significant decrease levels were found in hair of autistic children versus non autistic children, there was no correlation found with symptoms. Further research should be done to determine whether accumulation of these heavy metals and trace elements is a result of autism development.

On the other hand, the association between autism manifestations and zinc deficiency has been well-recognized by multiple sources as a significant finding. The prevalence of low levels of zinc in individuals with verbal difficulty and heightened fear and nervousness warrants further investigation. This concept is additionally supported by an alteration in behavioral markers for hippocampal function that became evident in those with zinc deficiency during pregnancy. Such a deficiency produced a long-lasting behavioral deficit in a study that focused on animal subjects and its effect on hippocampal damage. Such a strong finding in animal models exacerbates the structural deficits in individuals dealing with zinc deficiency.

As with zinc, selenium deficiency was found in autistic children when compared to non autistic children. Selenium deficiency correlated with the symptom of the inability to adapt to change. Further research can be done comparing selenium deficiency in autistic children and non- autistic children to examine if the same symptoms were observed.

Despite the elevated levels of elements such as chromium and nickel in serum samples or cement dust, the correlation between autism spectrum disorder and natural metals is still in question. The briefly studied genetics behind the higher affinity of specific expressed genes for metal ions deserves further investigation to determine its validity. Since the crucial dependence of the brain on an available source of metals may be contributing to proposed brain damage in autism spectrum disorder, it may be arguable to suspect that a deficiency of some metals, rather than an excess, may be contributing to autistic characteristics.

Chapter 4B - Lead

Cassandre Marseille, Benjamin Steinman

[Lead has often been cited as an environmental toxin which is at the heart of autism. As a result, chelation has been applied to affected children, without significant benefit. – Ed.]

Hypothesis

Lead poisoning is one of the oldest known forms of heavy metal toxicity. First described in Egyptian papyrus as a homicidal agent, it is an intensely studied condition, and its many effects have been well documented. (1) Neurological, cognitive, and behavioral deficits have been linked to lead toxicity, with many of its mechanisms fully realized, while strong hypotheses are proposed to explain the etiology of other maladies. (2) The initial connection between lead and autism or ASD (autism spectrum disorder) cited is a 1976 paper that noted a markedly increased blood lead level in some autistic children in comparison to other developmentally delayed and normal peers (3). Several studies observing a higher rate of lead poisoning among autistic children were published (4,5), leading to the speculation that lead poisoning may in fact be a cause of autism. While this chapter analyzes the merits of those claims, it must be noted that there is a paucity of available research that analyzes the etiologic link between lead poisoning andSD.

Observations
Brain alterations

The first question we need to ask is what are the changes seen in the brain infiltrated with lead versus that of a child with autism. Many researchers have conducted studies that have documented that lead contamination has the following consequences, among others, on the developing brain:

1) Lead competes with calcium to interfere with neurotransmitter release in the developing brain (6,7) (chapter 3E).

2) At high levels of lead, it disrupts the function of the endothelial cell of the blood-brain-barrier, thereby not protecting the brain against the neurotoxins.

3) Lead interferes with excitatory neurotransmission by glutamate, which is the transmitter at more than half the synapses in the brain and is critical for learning (6) (chapter 3E).

4) By storing lead in the mitochondria of astrocytes and oligodendrocytes, it ends up damaging these important cells. This affects the brain energy metabolism essential for cellular and molecular processes; (7,8). Malformation of myelin is also observed (7) (chapter 6A).

5) Lead also causes inappropriate release of neurotransmitter at rest (7,9).

6) Lead affects protein kinase C (PKC), which participates in many important cellular functions, including proliferation and differentiation. In addition, PKC is also involved in long-term potentiation, a form of neuronal plasticity that may be implicated in memory and learning (6,7,10). Chronic lead administration *in vivo* reduces hippocampal PKC expression (11).

Very few papers have been published about the changes that seen in the autistic brains that are contaminated with lead. One publication that has gained notoriety is that of El-Ansary and his colleagues. These scientists conducted an experiment attempting to shed light on the relationship between blood Pb^{2+} concentration as a ubiquitous environmental pollutant, and plasma neurotransmitters as biochemical parameters that reflect brain function in autistic patients. To try to prove their theory, they measured the lead content of red blood cells as well as the plasma concentration of γ-aminobutyric acid (GABA), serotonin, and dopamine in 25 autistic patient and 16 age-matched control samples (chapters 3E,3F). The authors found that autistic patients had increased plasma levels of GABA, serotonin and dopamine. They also reported the lead plasma level to be more elevated in the autistic patients. According to the author, the high plasma level with reduced cerebral GABA could be attributed to a reduced number of neurons expressing this neurotransmitter. They supported their hypothesis with the results of other researchers, in which it was reported that inhibition of catabolic enzymes of GABA using divalproex (DVPX) was effective in treating autistic children due to the elevation of brain GABA. The high plasma level of serotonin indicates its decreased synthesis due to negative feedback. However, the small sample size questions the statistical validity of this claim. The researchers concluded that these finding could be linked to autism since such patients can be treated with drugs that increase serotonin availability in the brain (9). Elevated plasma levels and decreased brain levels of serotonin are apparently consistent with neurochemical change in autism. The authors were able to associate autism to the high plasma level of dopamine (DA) recorded. DA blockers (i.e., antipsychotics) have been observed to be effective in treating some aspects of autism. Antipsychotics appear to alleviate hyperactivity, stereotypes, aggression, and self-injury in autistic children.

Young conducted animal research showing that stereotypic behavior and hyperactivity can

155

be induced by increasing dopaminergic functioning, suggesting that such neurons could be overactive in autism (12). Additionally, the serum lead level was significantly elevated in affected children than the control group. This was thought to explain their attention deficits often recorded as an important autistic feature. The authors concluded by suggesting that postnatal lead toxicity could be an associative factor of autism.

Postnatally, blood levels of lead peak between 18 and 36 months of age, leading to neurobehavioral defects in exposed children (6). Similar symptoms are sometimes seen in autistic patients around the same time. This supports the contention of those advocated the point of view that lead and autism are linked. However, very few scientists have been able to successfully establish a convincing correlation between areas affected in the autistic brain and those of someone intoxicated with lead (chapters 3B-3D). Although lead poisoning has detrimental effects on the brain, there is not yet enough evidence proving it is the fundamental agent causing autism. We do not know enough about the autistic brain to be able to make that statement. It has not been demonstrated that all children affected by autism have been exposed to high level of lead at some point during their development and before three, the age when characacteristic symptoms appear in autistic patients. It remains to be proven that the neurotransmitters that are affected in these studies are always deregulated in all autistic patients. Furthermore, the decreased brain levels of serotonin, GABA and dopamine have been more commonly associated with other brain disorders such as schizophrenia (13,14).

Pica

An aspect of lead poisoning is the pica disorder, defined as "the persistent eating of non-nutritive substances for a period of at least one month, without an association with an aversion to food." (15) One of the first descriptions of a possible coexistence of pica and autism was in a 1976 paper, which depicted the symptoms of both as starting in early childhood (3). Other studies have identified pica as an observed behavior in autistic children (4,5). Additionally, the observation has been made that some autistic children have had prolonged exposure to lead through pica (16,17). It is not clear if this is a temporal co-morbid or cause-and-effect relationship. While there may be a relationship between the prevalence and severity of lead poisoning and autism, at this juncture that is all there is: a correlation. There are no prospective studies supporting this hypothesis. There is no research that demonstrates a distinct progression from a diagnosis of lead poisoning to a diagnosis of autism. The reported observations have only shown them to exist concurrently (4,18-20).

Another noteworthy point is that with the banning of lead paint in 1978 and the change from leaded to unleaded gasoline in 1996 with the Clean Air Act, blood lead levels in children have shown a precipitous decline from 1997 onwards, while the incidence of autism appears to rising steadily (chapter 1C) (19). Likewise, a recent study that enrolled autistic children to assess the risks of pica behavior and lead toxicity found blood lead levels to be well within acceptable limits typically (17). This merely indicates that autism may well have multiple associated factors. What emerges from the available research is that while there may be a correlation between lead poisoning and ASD, it may be an incidental relationship based on ASD-triggered behavior rather than lead inducing autism disorder.

Chelation therapy

Another development that arose out of the hypothesized connection between lead poisoning and autism was the application of chelation therapy. This technique is an effective therapy that binds to, and serves to reduce blood levels of, toxic metals by renally excreting the heavy metal complex. There are several different chelators. Their selection is determined by the severity of the metal exposure. In severe lead poisoning (>70 mcg/dl; recommended levels <10 mcg/dl), edetate calcium disodium ($CaNa_2EDTA$) is the drug of choice. It is often given with dimercaprol (British AntiLewisite, BAL) to avoid side effects. For treatment of moderate cases of lead poisoning, succimer (DMSA; 2,3-dimercaptosuccinic acid) is orally administered. Chelation therapy was suggested as a possible treatment for autism, given the apparent (but unsubstantiated) relationship between autism and heavy metal toxicity (21,22).Criticism and warning of chelation has being published in the medical literature as well as clinical studies being halted.

Conclusions

It is important to note in the studies discussed here that two phenomena may be associated and co-morbid, but do not define a cause-and-effect relationship. Thus, it would be tenuous to conclude from the reports cited here that postnatal lead toxicity is the central causative factor leading to autism. A review of the literature, however, is not promising. For one, as related above, other than elevated blood levels of toxic metals, a causative relationship between heavy metals such as lead and autism has not been established. Additionally, the available literature is extremely limited. The research which is available is often flawed in methodology, e.g. using parental reports requiring a 3-month recall to multiple variables that may correlate with improvement (e.g., home learning programs as well as nutritional supplementation) (23,24). Other positive reports of chelation therapy being beneficial are typically found in non-peer reviewed journals as well as parents self-reporting of improvement of symptoms (25).
One such paper claimed that autism was linked to lead poisoning, yet the authors admitted that the lead toxicity simply may have caused exacerbation of symptoms much like those found in autistic children. Similarly, another case study that showed behavioral improvements may have simply been due to the removal of the noxious stimulus (3,20,25,26). In some cases, despite showing improvements, symptoms returned after cessation of chelation treatment (25).

No neurodevelopmental improvements have been demonstrated with chelation therapy, which is consistent with findings in standard cases of lead poisoning (22, 27). Although one report does show some neurodevelopmental improvement, it is the first and only one thusfar to demonstrate positive changes; more research must be done (28). Additionally, there are dangerous side effects with the administration of chelators. In the absence of heavy metal poisoning, chelators may cause lasting cognitive impairments (28). A National Institute of

Mental Health (NIMH) study was commissioned to assess the efficacy of chelation therapy in autism and was cancelled after the study showed lasting cognitive deficits (29,30). Hence, the use of chelation therapy as an effective treatment for autism thus far has no basis in fact and its misuse can have tragic consequences.

Lead, being a neurotoxin, does have a significant effect on the brain, more specifically on the neurotransmitters. Although we see some similarity in the brain of a patient that has lead poisoning and that of an autistic patient, we need more research in that area before we are able to say that lead is or is not the cause of autism.

While lead may have devastating effects on the developing brain that are manifest in neurological, cognitive, and behavioral deficits, at this point it would be presumptuous to claim that lead is a specific environmental trigger of autism. More research must be done in order to make that determination.

Chapter 4C - Teratogenic Drug Classification

Matthew J. Fasullo, Qiuying Huang

[In anticipation of the discussion of mediations associated with the appearance of autism, the present chapter explains the system for classification of drugs based on the potential effect on developing fetuses in utero. – Ed.]

Hypothesis

There are many classes of drugs and potentially harmful medications, of which one is able to cross the placental barrier and affect the growing fetus. This class of drugs is the "Teratogens" and in some cases may have devastating effects on a growing fetus, leading to physical and mental disabilities. In addition to pregnancy, a mother must also be aware of the risk of newborn exposure to toxins (especially while breastfeeding), possibly inducing defects in physical and mental development (perhaps including autism).

Observations

The current government regulations provide that, unless a drug is not absorbed systemically and is not known to have a potential for indirect harm to a fetus, a ''Pregnancy'' subsection must be included within the ''Use in Specific Populations'' section of the labeling on the medication bottle. This "Pregnancy" subsection must contain the information on the drug's possible teratogenic effects on the fetus (1). In general, birth defects are routinely found in at least 5% of all newborns, half of which may be major. Some may be attributable to pharmaceuticals.

Over the years, there has been a multitude of systems for classifying proprietary drugs and medications. The drugs were first classified for possible side effects in 1978 in Sweden. In this system, medications were ranked in order of "A" through "D" according to their potential to cause significant injuries to the fetus (2).

Although we now use a nationally adopted system in the United States, there is some confusion concerning the array of classification systems, each with different criteria for categorical drug placement. One study has demonstrated that, when comparing individual classification systems, there was only an overlap between 26% of drugs considered. This suggests there is a dramatic need to unify and improve the class definitions to reduce possible confusion among physicians as well as consumers (3).

Since 1979, the United States has employed a single method for classifying drugs with potentially adverse effects on a growing fetus. In particular, this system includes a ranking from "A" through "D", plus a special Class "X." To be classed in **Category A**, there has been no identifiable harm caused by ingestion of a particular drug during all three trimesters of pregnancy. There are also no known animal studies that demonstrate the drug as having adverse side effects on a developing fetus. Well-documented case-control studies are cited to support this classification. Although Category A drugs have not been shown to cause any adverse effects on the fetus, this classification system cannot rule out the risk with absolute certainty. Two common examples of Category A drugs are folic acid and levothyroxine (4).

Category B drugs have not been reported to cause any adverse effect or harm to a developing fetus in both human and animal studies. The difference between Category A and Category B is that in Category B there are no case-control studies in humans to support this designation. Also, drugs may be classified as Category B if animal studies have reported adverse teratogenic effects. In addition, there is no known negative impact on human pregnancies. Some common drugs that fall into Category B are acetaminophen, amoxicillin, and metformin, as well as some forms of insulin (such as regular or NPH) for diabetes (4).

In **Category C**, animal studies have identified one or more adverse fetal effects, there are no reported well-controlled studies in humans, and the drug is acceptable for human since its benefit appears to outweigh potential risks. The medication container must state that, although there are no well-controlled studies in humans, there have been cases in animal species known to cause potential adverse effects to the fetus and should therefore only be used in clear necessity. In Class C, in at least one animal species the drug has been known to be a teratogen. Two examples of Class C drugs are rifaximin (an antibiotic) and diclofenac (a non-steroidal anti-inflammatory) (4).

With **Category D** drugs (such as aminoglycosides and benzodiazepines), there have been studies that demonstrated adverse effects in some developing human fetuses. These drugs should only be used if absolutely necessary, due to the clear evidence of impact. Patients who are pregnant or who are planning to become pregnant should be advised by their healthcare advisor to use alternate methods of treatment due to the risk of teratogenic effects, if an alternative medication can be found. Commonly used Class D drugs include tetracycline (a commonly prescribed antibiotic) and phenytoin (a drug for seizures).

In **Category X**, by contrast, there have been significant adverse effects in both animals and humans, as well as harmful reaction reports from marketing or investigational experience. It is essential to explain the medication risks to the patient who is pregnant or who plans on becoming pregnant. These drugs have been proven to have serious side effects in the fetus and should therefore be discontinued (unless absolutely necessary). The complications with Class X drugs should be made known to the patient, stating that they can cause potentially damaging effects on the growing baby. Common examples of such drugs include thalidomide, temazepam, and valproic acid (chapter 4E).

In all cases, the potential adverse effect of a given drug on an unborn baby or a breast-fed neonate must be stated.

Table 4.1: Examples of medications in Category Classes C, D, and X, and their known or potential teratogenic effects. (The selected illustrations in this table (based on ref. 5) exemplify the classification scheme and its relationship to potential birth defects.)

Category	Drug	Teratogenic Effects
C	Acamprostate calciurm	Malformed iris, retinal dysplasia, retroesophageal subclavian artery, and hydronephrosis
	Angiotensin-converting enzyme (ACE) inhibitors (first trimester)	Fetal and neonatal renal failure, bony malformations, intrauterine growth restriction (IUGR), and premature labor
	Corticosteroids (first trimester)	Increased risk of oral and lip clefts, reduced birth weight, and increased risk of preeclapsia
	Estradiol gel 0.06%	Decrease in the quality and quality of milk
	Fluconazole (single dose)	Craniofacial, cardiac, and skeletal effects
	Rifaximin	Cleft palate, brachygnathia, hemorrhage, and incomeplete ossification
D	Aminoglycosides	Hearing defects, inner ear damage
	Anticonvulsants, first-generation	Neurological hyperexcitability, facial dysmorphia, gingival hyperplasia, and multiple malformations
	Benzodiazepines	Oral cleft
	Phenytoin	Coarctation of the aorta, hand and foot defects, dermatoglyphic abnormalities, and growth retardation
	Potassium iodide	Goiter, and hypoplasia
	Tetracyclines	Dental staining
X	Acetohydroxamic acid (first, second, and third trimesters)	Atrial and ventricular septal defects, coccygeal hermivertebrae and fused coccygeal vertebrae, supernumerary vertebrae, and lumbar hemivertebrae
	Danazol	Virilization of the external genital organs, and pseudohermaphroditism
	Lenalidomide	Reduction in fetal body weight, increase in postimplantation losses, and fetal variations
	Retinoids	Hydrocephalus, craniofacial alterations, thymic aplasia, and psychological impairments
	Thalidomide	Hearing defects, absent ears, malformed intestines, and renal anormalies
	Warfarin	Hypoplastic nose, eye abnormalities, deformities of the axial and appendicular skeleton, and scoliosis

Although most of the drugs mentioned here may have serious implications in pregnant women, only a few are in the group of environmental triggers (see Conclusions section) which have been connected with the development of autism (chapter 4E). One particular illustration of such a drug is the anti-seizure medication, valproic acid (VPA). Mice exposed to this agent show delayed physical development, impaired olfactory discrimination, and dysfunctional pre-weaning social behavior (6). Another such drug is thalidomide, which was commonly used to control nausea in pregnancy during the 1950s and 1960s. This drug proved to be effective against leprosy in different regions in the world, but was also shown to have a link with autism in the developing neonate (most likely during days 20 through 26 of the pregnancy) (7).

Conclusions

In conclusion, there are a number of different teratogen classification systems now available. In the United States, the particular system most commonly employed uses the letters A, B, C, D, and X to denote the potential degree of impact a given drug may have on the developing fetus (chapter 4E). Women who are pregnant or who plan on becoming pregnant should be aware of the potential adverse effects any medication they are taking or going to take, including both prescription and over-the-counter drugs. The degree of potential harm to the fetus is different for any given class and the patient should proceed with great caution before consuming any of the potential teratogenic classes of drugs (C, D, and X).

Although any medication with possible serious side effects should have a label pertaining to the possible consequence of use, a lack of a specific label does not entirely indicate that it is safe for a pregnancy. It is in the mother's best interest to discuss with her healthcare provider all the medications and possible risks (if any) that can be applicable to her. The subsequent chapter will go into greater depth about the specific autism-related drugs.

Chapter 4D - Autism-associated Drugs

Nicholas DaPrano, Jonathon Marshall

[Prenatal exposure to valproic acid, misoprostol, and thalidomide, in particular, has been commonly associated with an increased incidence of infantile autism. Consequently, these environmental triggers and certain other pharmaceuticals are avoided in pregnancy. A common mechanism explaining this characteristic remains to be elucidated. – Ed.]

Hypothesis

Teratogenic drugs (chapter 4D) generally act and convey their most deleterious effects on the fetus within the first eight weeks after conception (1). Many pharmaceutical and recreational drugs have been prescribed or taken during pregnancy, with the resulting physical and cognitive defects revealing a new wave of possible mechanisms and hypotheses, including etiologies for autism spectrum disorder (ASD).

Valproic acid (VPA), thalidomide, misoprostol, and ethanol are teratogens that are linked to the alteration of early neural development and migration, changes to blood perfusion and angiogenesis in the developing brain, and alteration of regulatory genes and their expression in the growing embryo (2). These four drugs have different mechanisms of action, and their effects on the molecular biology and genetics of the embryo have not yet been completely elucidated. However, they show a positive correlation to the appearance of autism, possibly by affecting the neuronal development and vascular perfusion of the brain.

Observations

Valproic acid

Valproic acid is an anticonvulsant used in treating bipolar disorder and epilepsy. As a class D teratogen, it is not normally prescribed during pregnancy, but has been associated with a higher incidence of autism. It triggers the most detrimental effects when exposed during the closure of the neural tube, the third week of embryonic development (1). VPA disrupts the closing of the neural tube (3), which is the precursor to the human central nervous system, by antagonizing the synthesis of folic acid within the embryo. It can also cause an increase in oxidative stress (chapters 5A,8B) and concentrations of the inhibitory neurotransmitter, gamma-aminobutyric acid (GABA) (chapter 3E). It can inhibit angiogenesis and histone deacetylases (HDACs), thereby altering epigenetic mechanisms, which also can occur with ethanol, thalidomide, and misoprostol (2).

Experimentation on rats shows further support of its mechanistic changes in the brain, showing gross abnormalities that resemble those found in autistic humans. Following a VPA injection to an embryonic rat during its corresponding developmental period, a 50% increase in neuronal connections was observed within the somatosensory cortex (4), the area of the brain responsible for interpreting sensory stimuli. However, despite an increase neuronal linking, the quality of these connections is diminished when compared to normal neuronal connections. These data suggest the increase in neuronal connections may be compensating for a lack of signaling between neurons. Given their location in the somatosensory cortex, it could describe the difficulty in interpreting the environmental stimuli that are needed for social interaction.

Along with a change in physical connections, autism patients who undergo lab studies show an increase in serotonin in the brain, hyperserotonemia (5). Both VPA and thalidomide induce this increase. Additionally, there is an increase in dopamine to the frontal cortex, the area responsible for combining stimuli from other areas of the brain and a major component of a human's personality (chapters 3B-3D). Serotonin controls emotions, sleep cycles, food intake, and motor control. These changes could be clues into the biochemical disorders of ASD. However, more studies are needed to determine which changes are associated with learning and behavior in rats with this phenotype.

Thalidomide

Thalidomide, a synthetic glutamic acid derivative and Class X teratogen (chapter 4D), is an antiemetic previously prescribed for morning sickness in pregnant women. Thalidomide was determined to cause its harmful effects between days 20 and 36 post-fertilization (1). It is widely known for causing dysmelia, or stunted limb growth, along with ocular abnormalities, growth malformations, and angiogenesis inhibition, the normal process of creating new blood vessels in the body (6). Disruption of blood flow, primarily very early in development, initiates alterations within the brain, allowing disruptions to the natural blood-brain-barrier. The loss of immature blood vessels is believed to be the main cause for thalidomide's teratogenic effects. In addition, with these vascular changes, the brain's neural development cannot migrate and mature correctly, consistent with VPA causing changes to neuronal development (1,4).

A Swedish thalidomide study noted that out of 86 patients prenatally exposed, four were later discovered to have autism, reporting a fifty times greater incidence of autism when compared to the general population (1). However, the exact amount of thalidomide exposure is unknown, making it difficult to evaluate. These patients also expressed ocular and cranial nerve defects similar to those exposed to misoprostol.

Separate studies demonstrated other biochemical effects on the genetics within growing embryos. Monkey embryo gene expression profiles were altered via thalidomide doses, downregulating pathways for angiogenesis and inflammation, while upregulating cellular structural and signaling components (7).

Misoprostol

Another pharmaceutical drug, misoprostol, is a prostaglandin analog used to treat stomach and duodenal ulcers. It is a Class X teratogen, with side effects including limb defects similar to thalidomide, and an increase in Möbius Sequence, a usually spontaneous cranial nerve defect severely restricting eye abduction, and incorporating cranial nerve palsy (1). Notably, a Swedish study reported that out of 22 Möbius Sequence patients, six were diagnosed with autism and one with an autistic-like condition. Additionally, it was noted that early developmental hypoxic insults to the embryo from bleeding and uterine contractions was a common factor to all the clinical cases, consistent with etiologies of hypoperfusion and changes to vascular development (chapter 3C).

Misoprostol causes uterine contractions with secondary vaginal bleeding, which is the basis for its use as an abortifacient drug. Taking misoprostol has not always resulted in abortion when used alone, and if the embryo continues to term, the child may present with ocular and behavioral malformations. A Brazilian study examined 28 pregnancies based on exposure or non-exposure to misoprostol in early pregnancy, with 23 able to be evaluated for ASD. Out of the 23 patients, five patients were diagnosed with autism, and three had been exposed to misoprostol. Two patients were diagnosed with an autism-like disorder, one of whom was also exposed to the drug (8).

These numbers are not large enough to be statistically powerful in analysis, but they do need more cases for a thorough examination. A separate study reported that an effect of prenatal misoprostol exposure is a decrease in the length and number of neurite extensions in mice via changes in calcium fluctuations (9). Similarly, misoprostol was reported to modify gene expression. As previously discussed, changes in neuronal development and genetic expression may give some clues about the genesis of ASD.

Alcohol

Unlike the use of thalidomide and VPA, the consumption of ethanol during pregnancies is on the rise (2). Its teratogenic effects are not necessarily confined to a specific prenatal period, as pregnant mothers may be ingesting it at various times throughout gestation. Ethanol is a class D teratogen, and children who were exposed to ethanol during pregnancy can be grouped under the disease of fetal alcohol syndrome (FAS), an illness characterized by physical malformations and mental retardation. It is hypothesized that ethanol exerts its teratogenicity by limiting neuronal proliferation, migration, and apoptosis during the development of the fetal brain (2). Similar to thalidomide, ethanol also downregulates gene expression in the ubiquitin pathway, a method the cell uses for signaling and degradation that also controls neuronal protein concentration.

Prenatal exposure of mice to ethanol delays the migration and limits the total number of serotonergic neurons within the raphe nuclei and medial forebrain bundle (2). The raphe nuclei are responsible for serotonin found globally within the brain, while the median forebrain bundle is involved with social and reward systems. Based on their respective functions, it may explain many of the symptoms seen in FAS including mental retardation, learning disorders, short attention span, hyperactivity, anxiety, and overall developmental delays.

FAS is a distinctly different disease from ASD, which presents with more characteristic delays in the development of social interactions. While it is possible in some individuals to have both FAS and ASD as co-morbidities, they are classified as two separate diseases. Indeed, the mechanisms of malformation for both ASD and FAS continue to show overlap in the areas of gene regulation, angiogenesis, and inhibition of neuronal transmission.

Conclusions

Importantly, the label of "teratogen" creates moral and ethical boundaries for most studies on humans. Most data and conclusions are based on animal models, then compared to human anatomy and physiology, or their results were retrospectively obtained after pregnancy. However, in some very rare situations, such as thalidomide being used to treat leprosy or nausea of pregnancy, there could be opportunities for collecting new data. Moreover, while positive correlations with autism have been reported, the general use of the drugs during pregnancy, with the exception of ethanol, has essentially stopped, while the incidence of autism has apparently increased (2).

Despite the marked reduction in the use of these drugs in pregnancy due to the knowledge of their side effects, the incidence of autism has increased. This would suggest that other factors are the main etiologic agents. While ethanol may be a contributing factor and shares biochemical changes with other causative agents, its teratogenicity in the early embryonic window specific to autism has yet to be fully established. Additionally, given the moral and ethical boundaries of performing studies prospectively on pregnant women, as well as the current lack of clarity on the etiology of ASD, there may be additional mechanisms at work that are still unknown.

Evidence clearly relates the harmful effects of valproic acid, thalidomide, misoprostol, and ethanol on the fetus, and their varying degrees of involvement with ASD. However, one cannot draw the conclusion that they are the cause of the prevalence of autism today. Before the discovery of their deleterious effects, it is possible the use of these drugs contributed to an increase in autism. Today, the use of these drugs during pregnancy is negligible, and indicates another explanation for the apparent rise seen in ASD is more likely responsible. These teratogens may serve as environmental triggers for neonates that have a genetic predisposition for developing autism.

Much like environmental pollutants (chapter 4F), smoking (chapter 3G), and viral infections (chapter 6B), autism-promoting drugs are apparently most potent when maternal exposure occurs during the first trimester of pregnancy. This sensitivity may relate to fetal organogenesis, especially neurologic, such as completion of embryonic neural tube closure at 25 days of gestation (10). Such observations reinforce the need to emphasis to pregnant or potentially pregnant women to reduce exposure to such potential teratogens as alcohol, viral infections (by pre-pregnancy vaccination), air pollution, and smoking, especially in the early months of gestation.

Chapter 4E - Pesticides; Air/Traffic Pollution

Joslyn Joseph, Snaha Sanghvi

[In the search for environmental triggers which would activate genetic predispositions, the presence of toxins found in pesticides and air pollution are identified in locations where the incidence of neonatal autism is elevated – Ed.]

Hypothesis

Autism is a multifactorial neurological spectrum of disorders – varying in severity, population, and age of onset of development. Twin concordance studies indicate that despite a strong genetic contribution, environmental factors play an important role in its development (1). It is no secret that air pollution has been shown to be malignant to our health. A large number of research studies have been published demonstrating the toxic effects of air pollutants and their role in the development of asthma, cardiovascular disease, and cancer. This has led to many revisions in Environmental Protection Agency (EPA) governmental standards in air pollution and pesticide usage, from the US banning of the insecticide DDT in 1972 to the more recent reclassification of vehicle emissions standards in 2010.

Once a trend, living a "clean lifestyle" or "going green" by only purchasing pesticide-free, organic-certified produce and driving hybrid/electric cars have become the norm for millions of people across the United States. While the allergic, cardiopulmonary, and neoplastic effects of pollutants have preceded this "green" revolution and are well known to the public, the toxic effects of pesticides on neurological and cognitive development, including the possibility of an increased risk for autism development, are not as well known or understood. A bustling and recently developing field of research, this chapter will review the current findings on the possible association of pesticides and air pollution exposure with the development of autism spectrum disorder (ASD).

Observations

Whether living in a densely populated city or barren rural farmland, both prenatal and postnatal exposure to air pollutants may have neurotoxic effects on the developing fetus. From a rural perspective, many pesticides, such as organophosphates, have been used for years, for agricultural and household uses. More recently, they have been found to be associated with acute and subacute neuronal toxicity (2) (chapter 3F). Organophosphates (OPs), in particular, are well documented neurotoxicants. In large doses, OPs act as acetylcholinesterase inhibitors, preventing the breakdown of acetylcholine, a critical neurodevelopmental transmitter, at the synapse. Organophosphate poisoning causes cholinergic effects such as headache, hypersecretion, muscle twitching, nausea, diarrhea, vomits, tachycardia and bradycardia, bronchospasm, respiratory depression, seizures, and miosis. These effects can be so severe that antidotal reversal by atropine (and rescue of cholinesterase activity by pralidoxime) is often necessary. In fact, the potential for use of pesticides in biological warfare exists.

The association of OPs in autism development is suggested not only a direct result of the toxin on acetylcholine (Ach), but it is also believed to come from interference with ASD susceptibility genes (3). Although many distinct possibilities exist for exactly how this occurs, a single mechanism has yet to be defined. Due to the most basic role Ach plays in synaptic transmission and neurological signaling, current findings suggest that the likely that the mechanism of ASD development lies within the destruction of normal neuronal signaling and the depletion of functional synapses in the brain (chapter 3F). The interference of normal neuronal connectivity and synaptogenesis is a current convergent target of research in the risk factors for the development of ASD.

Interference with synapse formation is not unique to organophosphates and rural pesticide use (2,3). In fact, many distinct processes toxic to proper synapse formation and connectivity have been detailed in traffic-related air pollutant exposure. Whereas OPs mainly interfere with the neurotransmitter ACh, traffic-related air pollutants induce the mechanisms of both inflammation and oxidative stress in humans that produce the most variety of respiratory and cardiovascular diseases – such as asthma and chronic obstructive pulmonary disease (COPD) (chapter 8B). As discussed in chapter 6B, inflammatory processes and their effects on oxidative stress may well serve as significant environmental triggers in the overall generation of the autism phenomenon. However, to date there is little evidence that these irritants directly induce ASD.

These respiratory effects are well documented in animal studies and are the reasoning behind the reclassification of vehicle emission standards. Whether exposed to high or low doses of the pollutants NO_2 and particulate matter, two byproducts of automobile exhaust, a neurological toxicity is produced. The former pollutant is known to affect the cerebellum and coordination, and the latter shown to trigger cellular toxicity and alter immune function of lymphocytes [1].

While these mechanisms may induce neurological disorders in general, exposure to other exhaust pollutants, such as polycyclic aromatic hydrocarbons (PAHs), may indeed have a triggering effect on ASD development. One such PAH, benzo(a)pyrene (B(a)p), not only produces a toxic oxidative load that intensifies brain inflammation, but has been recently shown to directly interact with the *MET*, a plausibly ASD-related oncogene [4]. *MET* acts as a potent modulator of neurologic circuitry development, or synaptogenesis, in newborns.

In terms of timing, this process of synaptogenesis occurs late in pregnancy, in the second to third trimester, and well into the first year of post-natal life [4]. During this time, dendritic growth, myelination, and synaptogenesis occur (chapters 3F,6A). This period is believed to be the crucial point in time at which neurologic pathology may occur. This is supported by the fact that extensive formation and refinement of synaptic connections in the human brain are formed [3]. Interruptions with this process may result in behavioral and neurological deficits in both animal and human subjects, including decreased cognitive test performance due to PAH itself, and acute disease such as cerebral palsy from hypoxia and trauma during birth (chapters 3G) [5]. These disturbances, in general, interfere with the formation of important, meaningful networks that result in the deficits in functional connectivity such as those sometimes associated with ASD [3].

To review, abnormal neuronal connectivity and synaptic functioning are considered overall convergent processes related to ASD development. Exposure to air pollutants, such as pesticides in rural areas and auto exhaust byproducts in cities, has been shown to effect respiratory impairment via toxic metabolites and direct interference of synaptogenesis genes. Furthermore, the timing of exposure especially during the 2nd and 3rd trimesters of gestation, through early postnatal life, coexists with the development of ASD and is consistent with other known functional central nervous system (CNS) teratogens. Thus, maternal–fetal exposure to environmental air pollutants during gestation may increase the risk for development of ASD via toxic byproducts of organophosphates/PM. These factors are known to cause an array of pathologies, affecting synaptogenesis and normal neuronal signaling during a period of critical brain development.

Pesticides/Organophosphates - the Ach hypothesis

Organophosphates affect acetylcholinesterase by phosphorylating the enzyme and thereby inhibiting it from carrying out its synaptic action. This causes a buildup of acetylcholine at the neuronal junction. Ach is needed throughout the body for a variety of functions: At the neuromuscular junction it promotes muscle movements, is needed in secretory cells and autonomic ganglia, and is critical for signal transmission in the CNS.   At the neuromuscular junction, excess of Ach can cause muscle twitching, a side-effect seen from excess OP exposure. It may weaken or paralyze the end plate which can result in hypotonia and ataxia as seen in some cases of autism. This relaxation can also affect the respiratory diaphragm and cause other cholinergic symptoms seen in excess OP exposure. In the brain, ACh causes "sensory and behavioral disturbances, incoordination, depressed motor function and respiratory depression" (2).

Prolonged pesticide exposure during critical stages of brain development, even in low levels, may induce persistent neurodevelopmental, behavioral, and cognitive disorders (2). In these cases, the amount of toxin may be so low that no anticholinesterase activity is present, but the disease still develops. This might also be due to other factors such as GABA malfunction, oxidative stress, or a reduction in glutathione in the developing brain (chapters 3F,8B).

The relationship between the proximity of mothers to pesticide concentrations and the occurrence of autism was studied by Roberts et al. in a review of mothers in the California Central Valley. The highest correlation with neonatal autism was found between maternal exposures to pesticides at around 8 weeks post-neural tube closure (which usually occurs around 25 days). The closer the proximity of the gravidas to the pesticide application, the higher was the incidence of autism occurring within that population. (However, this conclusion should be accepted with caution since the main limitation of the published study was the misclassification of data.)

It has been shown by Canfield et al. that one-in-three pregnant women relocate during their pregnancy. There are also no data showing how much time these mothers spent at home to be exposed to these farming toxicants. It is possible, due to the proximity of these agricultural sites, that there are a disproportionately larger number employed in agriculture and, therefore, have a higher exposure to the chemicals due to occupational as well as household contacts.

Organochlorides (OCs) and GABA

Pesticides such as organochlorides (OCs) have been shown to affect GABA receptors (6). This neurotransmitter helps to balance the inhibitory and excitatory neuronal signals, and is critical in the developing brain (7) (chapter 3E). GABA is also involved in differentiation, migration and elongation of neural stem cell proliferation (8). Brannen et al. found that exposure to organochlorides prenatally reduces the affinity of GABAa receptor binding in the brainstem. This can be caused by alteration of the subunit amino acid composition of these receptors by OC exposure (9,10).

Although a symptom associated with autism, motor impairment such as hypotonia, ataxia, toe-walking, reduced ankle mobility, and gross motor delay has been studied by Ming et al. and could possibly be due to a decrease in affinity of GABA. Because of the lack of effect of GABA in these patients, this outcome can also cause a hyper-excitable state, resulting in seizures which are also sometimes co-morbid with some autism disorders (11,12).

Oxidative stress

Oxidative stress, through an increase in production of reactive oxygen species (chapter 8B.8C), could be caused by organophosphates and other pesticides. Some pathophysiological mechanisms that have been implicated in the development of autism are environmental pollutant exposures, immune dysregulation, faulty detoxification, redox regulation, inflammation, and oxidative stress, and mitochondrial dysfunction (13).

Pesticides could damage cells through oxidative stress causing autism-like behavior through the depletion of glutathione and impairing cellular signaling (13). This has been shown to cause apoptosis in the nervous system of zebrafish (14). There are three major consequences of mitochondrial dysfunction: decreased ATP production, increased ROS (reactive oxygen species) production and oxidative stress, and the induction of apoptosis. Any one or all three of these changes can be caused by pesticide exposure. This correlation is strengthened by the fact that only 8% of autistic patients versus 0.05% of general population exhibit mitochondrial dysfunction (15). However, when considering the cause of autism, it remains to be elucidated why this does not occur in 100% of the affected cases.

Traffic/air pollutants - toxic mechanisms of PAH and B(a)p

We have mentioned previously that polycyclic aromatic hydrocarbons (PAHs) are considered neurotoxic. These metabolites are directly destructive as mediators of oxidative stress and inflammation in the CNS. However, one PAH in particular, benzo(a)pyrene (B(a)p), demonstrates the most specific and well-defined correlation between air pollutants and ASD development. Maternal B(a)p exposure in pregnancy has shown direct neurological deficits in pregnant and breastfeeding mice, as well as in humans. In fact, B(a)p interferes with several mechanisms crucial to normal neurological developmental (15).

Since B(a)p levels in the brain cannot be monitored directly in children, studies in mice have provided useful data on the effects of the pollutant on both neuronal circuitry and genetic interference (4). In mice, prenatal exposure to high levels of B(a)p during middle and late gestation has demonstrated decreased neuronal plasticity and increased behavioral abnormalities in the offspring (16). It also appears to induce a decreased ability for long-term potentiation in the hippocampus and induced deficits in memory and learning (3). B(a)p exposure has also been shown to reduce in mice the expression of the serotonin receptor in breastfeeding, glutaminergic signaling, and N-methyl-D-aspartate (NMDA) subunit expression.

Studies in humans have shown that B(a)p exposure during the 2nd and 3rd trimester of gestation is correlated with an increase in the levels of pro-inflammatory cytokines in the fetus (5).

B(a)p and the MET hypothesis

In addition to the above mechanisms, the most promising explanation of B(a)p exposure as a risk factor for ASD development is its interference with the tyrosine kinase gene, *MET*. This gene plays an important role in establishing the plasticity of the brain and in generating excitatory synapses, including the formation of both dendritic and spinal neuronal growth (4). *MET* is expressed at moderate levels at birth, followed by a dramatic increase that coincides with the rapid onset of synapse formation (17) (chapters 3F,8A,8B).

In humans, a noteworthy association between the mutant *MET* promoter variant rs1858830C allele with ASD risk in humans has been observed, as well as significantly decreased *MET* transcripts and proteins in the post-mortem brains of autistic individuals. In 2008, a study of 367 families (92% having multiple children with diagnosed ASD) registered in the Autism Genetic Resource Exchange (AGRE) Consortium were pedigreed and genotyped to search for the *MET* C allele. The data were then correlated with three diagnostic functional phenotypic behavior analyses: a parent/teacher reported Social Responsiveness Scale (SRS), an Autism Diagnostic Interview-Revised (ADI-R), and an Autism Diagnostic Observation Schedule (ADOS).

Results showed a statistically significant association of the *MET* C allele in both additive ($p = 0.037$) and dominant ($p = 0.0008$) analyses of familial association with ASD diagnosis. A statistically significant relationship also exists between the *MET* C allele and two out of the three behavioral phenotypes – the SRS ($p < 0.005$ for social awareness, cognition, communication, motivation, and autistic mannerisms) in dominant familial associations, and the ADI-R for all analyses. Taken together, these data provide evidence for the putative role of *MET* C as an ASD-associated risk gene (18,19).

Furthermore, for those who are genotypically normal with respect to the *MET* gene, *MET* expression has been found to be highly sensitive to B(a)p and diesel exhaust particles, due to the inflammatory and oxidative stress effects mentioned above. PAHs have been shown to markedly reduce the expression of the *MET* receptor in autistic brains. In mice, *MET* gene expression has been shown to decrease greater than five-fold as a function of early postnatal B(a)p exposure of 24 hours ($p<0.05$). When these B(a)p-exposed mice were tested for behavioral deficits, they displayed significantly less time with novel objects during an object discrimination test, a known negative behavioral deficit exemplified in ASD [4]. Finally, mice with mutant *MET* genotypes demonstrate significantly altered dendritic morphology and abnormal dendritic spines (3) (chapters 3B-3F).

Traffic and air pollutants

In 2011, Volk et al. defined the possible relation of proximity to freeways during pregnancy and autism. Data from 304 autism cases and 259 non-autism cases were derived from the CHARGE (Childhood Autism Risks from Genetics and Environment) study. Neonatal participants ranged from 24 to 60 months old and were born in California with at least one English- or Spanish-speaking biological parent. Autism was defined in this study as a positive diagnosis via the ADI-R and ADOS psychological tests. Non-autism cases were defined as a Social Communication Questionnaire (SCQ) score of ≤15 and normal Mullen Scales of Early Learning and Vineland Adaptive Behavior Scales scores. Trimester-specific maternal residential addresses were obtained and geocoded to determine the distance of the mother's residence from major freeways to estimate exposure to residential traffic and air pollutants per trimester.

After correcting for confounding factors, it was determined that living less than 309 meters from a freeway at the time of birth is associated with increased odds of autism development relative to other cutoff points of exposure distances of 309-647 meters, 647-1,419 meters, and >1,419 meters (OR = 1.86; 95% CI = 1.04-3.45). In each trimester, living <309 meters from the freeway was associated with autism when compared with distances >1,419 meters. Statistical significance was only observed with exposure during the third trimester (OR = 1.96; 95% CI = 1.01-3.93). Finally, after restricting the sample to addresses within 309 meters to the freeway throughout all three trimesters and at birth, representing exposure to teratogen throughout the entire pregnancy up to and including birth (n = 485; 257 autism cases and 228 controls) the OR (odds ratio) doubled among those cases relative to distances of >1,419 meters (OR = 2.22; 95% CI = 1.16-4.42). Taking all of these data together, living close to a freeway (<309 meters) during pregnancy/early life is most strongly associated with increased odds of autism development relative to those that live far distances from freeways (>1,419 meters) (5).

To follow up on these results, a second study was conducted to estimate and quantify the levels of both traffic-related air pollutant exposure based on distance living from the freeway during each trimester and after birth, and regional air pollutant exposure. Traffic-related pollutants were estimated using a CALINE4 model, California average emission factors by year for freeway travel, roadway geometry, and meteorological data from 56 monitoring locations correlated positively to time and location. Regional air pollutant exposure was calculated via data from the US Environmental Protection Agency's Air Quality System data from monitoring stations within 50 km of the participant's residence.

Results showed that the likelihood of autism development increased three times for the highest traffic related pollutant exposure group (>31.8 ppb of PM - particulate matter) relative to the control group. All three trimesters of pregnancy showed a correlation of high exposure to increased autism development in the offspring. In general, the probability of autism increased relative to traffic-related air pollutants, plateauing around 25-30 ppb (parts per billion) during pregnancy and the first year of life. Regional air pollutant results showed similar results, with exposure to highest quantities of PM and NO_2 (nitrous oxide) corresponded to a two-fold increased likelihood of autism development. These effects were prevalent throughout all three trimesters. Taking all of these data together, children with autism were 3 times more likely to have been exposed to high levels of traffic pollutants, with a threshold of approximately 25-30 ppb for an increased level of risk. Furthermore, the effect of ambient air pollution preserves the hypothesis of late-pregnancy/early-postnatal life as the critical period of pollutant exposure to increase ASD development risk (20).

While an exact critical period of exposure to development has yet to be defined for traffic and air pollutants, data from these studies and the previously aforementioned B(a)p studies suggest that the late-pregnancy/early postnatal period is the critical period of exposure for ASD development. This stage correlates strongly with a surge of synaptogenesis and the establishment of excitatory networks. Interrupting the development of these pathways results in dysfunctional neuronal networks may result in behavioral and cognitive deficits.

Some studies suggest that autism is a disease resulting from prenatal insults at 20-24 days into gestation (21). When examining the effect of OP on chicken embryos, there was greater neurologic damage during the earlier stages of development versus the later (22). Another study determined that the risk of developing autism was higher in children born in December through March (conception March to June). Although not directly related, it is possible that since the heaviest pesticide use is typically in late spring to early summer that the pesticides may contribute to this increase (23).

Other factors influencing teratogen exposure and disease development

Although both organophsphates and air pollution have different mechanisms of pathogenesis leading to CNS dysfunction and autism-like behavior, the severity of both can be determined by proximity to exposure source and the gestational timing of exposure. These two factors have the potential to predict the increased likelihood of the development of autism relative to individuals not exposed to these pollutants.

Some shortcomings with studies analyzed here for both pesticides and air pollutants include defining exact periods of exposure with the amount of time physically spent in the residence. For example, in the California Valley study, no data were obtained for how many hours a day each woman physically spent inside her residence. Had the pregnant females been living at a different address at the time of their pregnancies, working long hours away from home, or traveling often, the effect of pollutants would be overestimated. The quantification of real-world exposure needs to be defined with organophosphates and replicated in future traffic pollution studies.

Conclusions

After reviewing the most current research available, it would appear that a correlation may exist between traffic and air pollutant exposure and the risk of a child developing ASD, especially when exposed during late pregnancy and early postnatal life. In particular, the negative effect of B(a)p exposure during this time on the function of the *MET* tyrosine kinase gene provides a possible mechanism for ASD development via altered synaptogenesis and dysfunctional neuronal circuitry formation. However, increased oxidative stress, inflammation, and interference with NMDA and serotonin receptors cannot be excluded as viable possibilities for a pathological mechanism. Overall, these findings point to a correlation between pollution and autism. Pollution and inflammation may be co-morbidities that contribute in some way to the development of autism. Whether this defines the cause of this disease remains to be established.

For organophosphates, however, the link may not be as clear. Although there have been many studies showing the strong effects of pesticides on neurodevelopment of a fetus, there are very few definitive reports that show that this impact can contribute to the genesis of autism.

The small group of cases reported thus far may not be enough to draw an authoritative conclusion on whether or not pesticides can cause autism. What is clear is that pesticides inhibit of acetylcholine esterase (AChE), decrease the affinity of γ-aminobutyric acid (GABA), and increase oxidative stress. As a result, these factors individually or as a group may induce some or all of the symptoms of autism.

Further investigations should simulate teratogen-exposed environments and account for time spent both within and outside of the residence in order to address exposure dosing and to simulate real environments. Such studies could be used to determine a more causal effect for both pesticides and traffic pollutants. Future surveys should also account more for the effects of postnatal exposure on autism development up to four years of age. To this point, most research has focused on gestational exposure and does not extend to exposure past birth. To better solidify a critical period for ASD development and narrow down this exposure window, analyses should continue for exposure up to at least one year postnatal – the period of most rapid synaptogenesis and dendritic growth. By coincidence, this is the period of greatest CNS myelination (chapter 6A).

Finally, future investigations need to determine the duration of exposure relative to the chance of formation of ASD – or rather, will switching residences and removing environmental exposure of pesticides/air pollution halfway through pregnancy diminish the damage done? How long does one need to be exposed before the effects of contact are irreversible? The main shortcomings of these studies are that humans may be less than candid or keen in their retrospective recall. Future studies should examine fathers preconception or follow prospectively newly pregnant mothers throughout their entire pregnancy and 2-3 years postnatally, while monitoring their blood levels of pesticides and pollutants, while correlating to environmental exposure data. These data would provide an overall look at mothers throughout their pregnancies. It would not only determine whether pesticides affect autism risk, but also define the causality, levels, and duration of exposure to air and traffic pollutants that may show a relationship with autistic behavior in the newborn.

Newly pregnant mothers should plan to avoid both air pollutants and pesticides throughout their pregnancies, if at all possible. Although there is not a certain cause-and-effect link between autism and pesticides, there is potential harm to the neurodevelopment of the fetus by either toxin type. Pregnant women can limit their exposure by increasing circulation of clean air inside the homes, using non-toxic pesticides in their home and garden, and having a "no-shoes" policy inside the home to avoid spreading outdoor pesticides around the house. "Going green" during pregnancy and while breastfeeding by consuming pesticide-free, certified organic (or well washed) produce may also cut down on ingested pesticides.

Avoiding air pollutant exposure is more difficult, as one individual working alone cannot dispel regional air and traffic pollution. However, if enough individuals choose to "go green" by driving a hybrid/electric vehicle, for example, the amount of air pollution in an area can theoretically be decreased over time. More practically, when choosing a location for a new residence, pregnant mothers, mothers with children below the age of three, and those women planning to become pregnant in the near future should avoid moving to a residence very close to a freeway or major highway, if possible. Finally, the avoidance of occupational exposure to vehicle exhaust and combustion, such as working on vehicles as a mechanic or in a garage during pregnancy, while breast-feeding, and during her child's first few postnatal years to avoid direct exposure to vehicle pollutants is recommended.

Chapter 4F - Television

Shelley Co, Samantha Mucha

[The occurrence of ADHD and autism may suggest a co-morbid influence of the extent of television watching among children, although a cause-and-effect relationship remains to be documented. – Ed.]

Hypothesis

In 2001, the American Academy of Pediatrics (AAP) released a policy statement, which recommended that television viewing by children younger than two years of age be redirected in favor of more interactive play like singing, reading, and talking to promote brain development (1). They also advocated that television use be limited to no more than one or two hours per day for older children. To support their recommendations, the AAP stated that research on television viewing by children has demonstrated "primary negative health effects". It was claimed that television viewing by children could have an impact on "behavior, sexuality, academic performance, body concept and self-image, nutrition, dieting, obesity, and substance use/abuse patterns".

At about the same time, one child in 150 was diagnosed with an autism spectrum disorder (2). The frequency became one in 110 in 2006; in 2008, it became one in 88, according to the Centers for Disease Control and Prevention (CDC). With the increasing number of diagnoses, parents, doctors, and scientists wanted to know what was going on and the reason for this increase.

Observations

It was in this backdrop that three economists in 2006, proposed a hypothesis stating that "too much or certain types" of television viewing during the early childhood years triggers autism in the fraction of the population who is vulnerable to developing the condition because of their genetic disposition (3). Such an association between autism and television viewing was introduced and explored by Michael Waldman of Cornell's Johnson Graduate School of Management, Sean Nicholson of Cornell University, and Nodir Adilov of Indiana University-Purdue University in the article, "Does Television Cause Autism?" While the study made an interesting connection, there were too many flaws, some which their article even mentions, with the study and its analyses, to say with any certainty that television does cause autism.

Waldman et al., in their article, first discussed the four reasons that led them to examine the relationship between television viewing and autism. This included their examination of autism data in California, the existing evidence that associates television and attention deficit hyperactivity disorder (ADHD), the behavior of so called "high risk" infants to autism and the Amish lifestyle (3). First, the authors focused on autism rates in California, a state that developed regional centers that worked with those affected with certain disabilities, including autism. From the data collected at these regional centers, the authors showed "that autism rates gradually rose during the 1970s and then the growth in autism rates accelerated starting around 1980." In addition, the autism rate, which was calculated using data from the regional centers, in 2005 was approximately thirty percent greater for individuals born in 1980 than for those born in 1970. The rate increased again twofold by 1986 and doubled again by 1992. (In chapters 1B and 1C, a distinction is made been *apparent* rate and *diagnosed* rate of autism because of varying diagnostic criteria.)

The authors claimed that the increase in autism rates matched the increase in early childhood television viewing during the 1970s and 1980s (3). According to Waldman et al., the increase in childhood television viewing could have been a result of the videocassette recorder (VCR) becoming a major consumer product in the late 1970s, growing access to cable television beginning in 1980, and the development of channels, like Nickelodeon® in 1979 and the Disney Channel® in 1983, aimed at children. Another reason for the rise in television viewing could have been the increase in households having multiple television sets at the time.

The second issue that prompted Waldman et al. to investigate the connection between autism and television was the possible relationship between childhood television viewing and ADHD (3). The authors referenced a 2004 Christakis et al. study where the investigators sought to prove that early television exposure "during the critical periods of synaptic development would be associated with subsequent attention problems," which is defined using the hyperactivity subscale of the Behavioral Problems Index (BPI) (4). As the report noted, this is not necessarily equivalent to a diagnosis of ADHD. To examine the relationship between television viewing and the onset of attention problems, the authors focused on observational data from 1278 children at age one and 1345 children at age three from the National Longitudinal Survey of Youth. They found that ten percent had attentional problems at seven years of age and determined in a logistic regression model that "hours of television viewed per day at both ages 1 and 3 was associated with attentional problems at age 7." Christakis et al. acknowledged, however, that they could not determine a causal relationship from this and "it could be that attentional problems lead to television viewing rather than vice versa."

Nevertheless, that a possible link between television viewing and ADHD might exist was enough for Waldman et al. to suggest that maybe television watching had an effect on autism rates. This is especially plausible since they portrayed autism and ADHD as related conditions, and they described autism as a "more severe attention disorder" (3). As discussed in the Christakis et al. study, because various types and degrees of environmental stimulation can influence "the number and the density of neuronal synapses," what children are exposed to and the "types and intensity of visual and auditory experiences" that they have may influence how their brain develops, something which also advanced Waldman et al. to pursue their study (3,4).

The third factor mentioned by Waldman et al. which inspired their thinking was that television and autism could be connected as in an article by Zwaigenbaum et al., published in 2005. It described their longitudinal study of high-risk infants, defined as having an older sibling with a diagnosed autism spectrum disorder. They focused on a group of high-risk infants and another group of low-risk infants from six months to twenty-four months of age. In one aspect of the study, they conducted a visual orienting task (5). This involved a child seated in dark room in front of a screen, on which colorful stimuli were presented. Once the child was engaged, a second stimulus was presented in the periphery and eye movement to the peripheral stimulus was observed. This eye movement is what the article refers to as "disengagement" from the primary stimuli. Zwaigenbaum et al. then proposed that an impaired disengagement mechanism "may underlie the early social orienting deficits in autism," meaning that there is a decreased ability to attend and respond to multiple stimuli.

In their study, Zwaigenbaum et al. did find that delayed disengagement within the high risk sample predicted later social and communication deficits (5). Some of the siblings of children with autism had difficulty disengaging at twelve months, which predicted "social-communicative impairments at 24 months of age." Although the report did not refer to television directly, Waldman et al. extrapolated from the Zwaigenbaum et al. results and rationalized that "high risk children have more difficulty disengaging from watching television once they begin watching" (3). Because of this, the Waldman et al. article states that the Zwaigenbaum et al. findings are consistent with the notion "that television has a more significant effect on infants at high risk of autism than others," further inspiring Waldman et al. to explore the link between childhood television watching and the onset of autism.

The autism rate among the Amish, a population that does not use electricity and is not exposed to television, was the fourth issue that prompted Waldman et al. to suspect the role of television in precipitating autism (3). The expected number of individuals with autism among the Amish should have been in the hundreds if one extrapolates the affected rate in the general population to the Amish population. The article referenced an informal investigation conducted by Dan Olmsted, a news reporter for United Press International, who studied this issue. Fewer than ten cases were identified, however, which would seem to verify the relationship between television and autism. Waldman et al. acknowledged that "this is far from definitive evidence for our hypothesis" and reiterated that the investigation was informal. They also posited several variables which could account for the low numbers of autism among the Amish. According to the report, it could be that the Amish lifestyle causes less exposure to some autism trigger than the non-Amish lifestyle or that because the Amish represent a small population, the genes responsible for autism might occur at a low frequency.

After laying out four reasons to suspect television, the investigators delved into an examination of the question of their paper, "Does Television Cause Autism?" To explore this, they studied three key relationships:

1) childhood television watching and precipitation levels;

2) autism rates and precipitation levels (3);

3) autism rates and the number of households with cable television subscriptions (chapter 1B).

They concluded that if their hypothesis that television viewing is a trigger for autism is correct, then there should be a positive correlation in the three relationships mentioned.

First, they explored the related hypothesis that television watching during the early childhood years is "positively correlated with precipitation for children under the age of three" (3). They used the Bureau of Labor Statistics' American Time Use Survey (ATUS) to investigate this possible connection. The survey asked adult respondents to record activities that are executed on a specific day. To extract the relevant data, Waldman et al. focused on adult respondents who watched television with a child under three years old present. The researchers acknowledged that this method did not measure total television watching for a child, but rather television exposure. Therefore, the number retrieved was just an estimate for total television watching time for a child.

To evaluate the precipitation variable, Waldman et al. looked at data from the National Climactic Data Center and the corresponding amount of precipitation that fell on a specific day (3). When applying a broad definition of television watching, "a young child watches about twenty seven more minutes of television" on a day when precipitation equals one inch, considered to be a "heavy day of rain," compared to a day with no precipitation. The investigators affirmed that "precipitation causes increases in early childhood television" and thus, should be used to test "the effect that early childhood television watching has on rates of autism." They hypothesized that "the autism rate itself should be positively correlated with precipitation," (3). They concentrated on data in California, Oregon, and Washington, three states which have variable amounts of precipitation from 1987 to 2001. They also looked at county level autism rates in 2005 for children between six and eighteen years of age. They concluded that a positive relationship existed between autism and precipitation in Oregon and Washington, but not California (3). They concluded that a positive relationship did exist "between autism and precipitation, as predicted by the television as trigger hypothesis."

Waldman et al. then examined the third relationship involving autism rates and the number of households with cable television, which they predicted would be positive (3). They concluded that there was a positive correlation between the percentages of households with cable and autism rates, asserting that "there is substantial evidence for exactly this type of positive relationship in the California data, in the Pennsylvania data" and in the data combined between the two states (3).

Even though the Waldman et al. article made such conclusions, the thought-provoking title of the article and the study's claims on the etiology of autism elicited strong sentiment among parents and the media, and as a result, efforts to squash the study were swift. The same week the study was released, the magazine, *Time,* published an article questioning the merit of three economists dabbling in scientific research. While it is true the Waldman et al. article makes some sort of sense, statistically speaking, does it make sense scientifically and medically speaking? Months after the Waldman et al. study, *The Wall Street Journal* published an article examining the infiltration of economists into previously unprecedented fields, specifically science and medicine, fields in which they are untrained to study (chapters 1A,2B) . The article states that a tool that has supported economists in performing such research is the called the "instrumental variable." (6).

The biggest concern of this method employed by economists was the use of one variable as a substitute for another. For example, Waldman et al. substituted rainfall patterns for television watching. Precipitation was their instrumental variable, because it randomly selected some children to watch more television than others. In fact, no television watching was ever directly measured. So how can we be sure what their results actually measure (5)?

The same week the Waldman et al. study was released, neurobiologist Levitt, in a study published by the *Proceedings of the National Academy of Science*, revealed that his team had found strong evidence for a genetic predisposition to autism. Their focus was a "chromosome 7q31 autism candidate gene region" and the gene coding "the pleiotropic MET receptor tyrosine kinase." They found that MET signaling is involved in "neocortical and cerebellar growth and maturation, immune function, and gastrointestinal repair," which is disrupted in some children with autism (chapter 8A). Furthermore, it was found that families that have more than one child diagnosed with autism also have the strongest allelic association. In his study, Levitt effectively provided evidence of a pathophysiological basis for autism, proposing that anywhere from five to twenty genes may underlie the vulnerability to autism, suspecting that there may be many routes to developing autism—involving a genetic basis, but also environmental influences (8).

The timing of Levitt's and Waldman's studies leaves us beg the question, could watching television be one such environmental influence? In response to Waldman et al.'s study, Levitt says, "you have to be very definitive about what you are looking at…how do you know, for instance, that it's not mold or mildew in the counties that have a lot of rain?" (9) Since precipitation is correlated with young children spending more time indoors, perhaps the unknown environmental trigger for autism could be poor indoor air quality, some unknown toxin—such as mold or mildew as Levitt postulates—rather than the correlated television watching (3).

An article in *The Wall Street Journal* suggested that, "the best way to figure out whether television triggers autism would be to do what medical researchers do: randomly select a group of susceptible babies at birth to refrain from television, then compare their autism rate to a similar group that watched normal amounts of TV."(6) Simply, a case-control study would be able to produce an odds ratio of developing autism—if the abstaining group has a lower odds of developing autism, it would point to television watching as the culprit.

Conclusions

At the end of their article, Waldman et al. admit that their results do not definitively prove that early childhood television viewing is a trigger for autism, but conclude that "until further research can be conducted, it might be prudent to act as if it were."(3) The scientific community as a whole has rejected their hypothesis; the AAP has neither made any such changes in its current recommendations on childhood television watching nor linked television watching with the precipitation of autism (10).

NUTRITION

Chapter 5A – Folic Acid

Kessiena Aya, Ekaterina Hossyn

[Decreased maternal periconceptional consumption of folic acid, as well as genetic mutations which affect production of active forms of folate, appear to be related to the incidence of autism in some infants. – Ed.]

Hypothesis

There is a growing movement in the study of neurobehavioral disorders, such as Alzheimer's and Parkinson's diseases, to elucidate the metabolic basis of the syndrome. The study of autism is no exception, as seen in the growing body of literature on the effect of numerous vitamins and minerals on the propagation and treatment of the autism spectrum disorders (ASD), or the prevention of this disorder in its entirety. Various nutrients and/or nutritional deficiencies have been proposed as either a contributory factor, or essential in the propagation of this disorder. Common examples readily seen in a standard search of published literature include casein, gluten (wheat protein), and various common vitamins and minerals such as vitamins A, C, and D.

One vitamin of particular scientific interest is folic acid (folate). The applications of current folic acid research findings in the modification of ASD are multifactorial. New studies show that select autistic children have altered folic acid metabolism, the inclusion of folic acid into the maternal diet may deter the development of autism, the pathological modification of its metabolism may propagate aspects of the ASD, and, lastly, supplementation of this vitamin in an autistic child may alleviate particular symptoms. Such findings make the study of folic acid helpful, and perhaps essential, to the better understanding of this disorder.

Observations

Folic acid is essential for the transfer of carbon fragments in biological reactions and the biosynthesis of several molecular compounds. The various manifestations of folic acid deficiency have been extensively studied. It is known that a deficiency of this vitamin is a primary cause of megaloblastic anemia, and has been correlated with the prevalence of neural tube defects. Common prenatal care protocols call for the supplementation of folate in the peri-conceptional and pre-natal diet, as pregnant patients are particularly susceptible to develop a deficiency. The proper growth and development of the fetus necessitate an increased consumption (1).

Folic acid and the amino acid methionine form a pathway that is essential for cellular redox balance, DNA synthesis, and DNA methylation. The biologically active form of folic acid is tetrahydrofolate (N^5-methyl-FH_4). This form is arguably the most stable and the structure most readily able to transfer one-carbon fragments to intermediates in the synthesis of components of both DNA and amino acids. However, for this carbon transfer to occur, the methyl group must first be removed from this molecule and contributed to various DNA synthesis reactions. Since the removal of the methyl group requires both the enzyme, methionine synthase, and vitamin B12 (cobalamine), the deficiency of either of these factors results in a sequestration of folic acid in the N^5-methyl form, and, hence, a functional shortage.

Methionine, a breakdown product during protein metabolism, is transformed into homocysteine via a series of reactions. As homocysteine has been implicated in various pathological processes, regulation of the steps involved in both its creation and removal are of particular interest. For example, increased homocysteine levels are associated with atherosclerosis and may affect proper brain functioning. There are two prominent ways by which serum homocysteine levels are decreased:

> 1) re-methylation of homocysteine to methionine (regulated by both folic acid and B12), and

> 2) transulfuration of homocysteine into cysteine (with vitamin B6 as a cofactor).

Consequently, though a host of various biological and clinical functions have been attributed to folic acid, for the purpose of this chapter we will focus on its role in the propagation and possible modification of the autism symptomology. (More information on the enzymatic regulation of folic acid will be provided in the relevant sections to follow.)

There is growing evidence that maternal supplementation with folic acid around the time of conception, and within the first three months of pregnancy, reduces the risk of developing fetal neural tube defects as well as other neurodevelopmental disorders in children including the autism (2). The following are several studies that have shown an association between prenatal folic acid intake and a reduced risk of autism:

Based on the most recent study conducted in Norway (Norwegian Mother and Child Cohort Study (MoBa) Autism Birth Cohort), there is evidence that maternal folic acid supplementation during pregnancy reduces the risk of autism. A follow-up study of over one hundred thousand children born from 1999 and 2009 was based on maternal consumption of folic acid from 4 weeks before to 8 weeks after the start of pregnancy. At the end of the follow-up in 2012, 270 children were diagnosed with ASDs, 114 of them with autism by DMS-IV-TR criteria (chapter 1D). However, in children whose mothers took prenatal vitamins with folic acid, 0.10% had developed an autistic disorder, in comparison to 0.21% in those unexposed to folic acid. The adjusted odds ratio (OR) in the study for autistic disorder in children of folic acid users was 0.61 (95% confidence interval (CI): 0.41-0.90) (3). Thus, the use of the prenatal folic acid around the time of conception was associated with a lower risk of autistic disorder in this cohort.

A second investigation of children in the Norwegian Mother and Child Cohort Study (MoBa) was conducted. The study reported that among 38,954 children, 204 (0.5%) had severe language delay. In the reference group – children whose mothers took no dietary supplements (n=9052 [24.0%]; 81 child had severe delay [0.9%]). Other adjusted ORs for 3 patterns of exposure to maternal dietary supplements were

(1) Other supplements, but no folic acid: In this group of 2480 children [6.6%], 22 children had severe language delay [0.9%]; OR, 1.04; 95% CI, 0.62-1.74);

(2) A second group studied mothers who took folic acid only (n=7127 [18.9%]: 28 children [0.4%] were found with language delay; OR, 0.55; 95% CI, 0.35-0.86); and

(3) Folic acid in combination with other supplements (n=19 005 [50.5%]: 73 children [0.4%] were diagnosed with severe language delay; OR, 0.55; 95% CI, 0.39-0.78).

Therefore, these studies demonstrated that maternal intake of folic acid supplements from 4 weeks before to 8 weeks after the start of pregnancy was associated with a lower risk of severe language delay at age 3 years (4).

These findings are not isolated in time and geographic location. Unlike studies done with other nutrients and minerals, findings on the relationship between autism and folate are consistent with results from other recent studies from Asia, Europe and North America. For example, an investigation conducted in Nepal found evidence that maternal prenatal supplementation with iron and folic acid was positively associated with higher intellectual ability, some aspects of executive function, and motor function, including fine motor control, in offspring at 7 to 9 years of age (5). Furthermore, a case control study from California on autism showed that maternal intake of folic acid and prenatal vitamins during the 3 months prior to pregnancy and the first month of pregnancy was associated with a lower risk of ASDs in the offspring. Complementary genetic analyses indicated that the association was modified by gene variants that determine the ability to utilize available folate (6,7).

These studies highlight an important concept: It is already known that periconceptional intake of folic acid will reduce a woman's risk of a neural tube defect in the baby (8-11). This knowledge has led to the recommendation in the US that women capable of becoming pregnant consume should 400 µg/day of folic acid. Recent reports on the possible effect of the folic acid on reducing the risk of autism may further motivate more women to consume vitamin supplements before and during early pregnancy.

Folic acid and the deterrence of autism

With the observed association of folate intake and autism came questions on the metabolic bases of the results. Research conducted from 2003–2009 in Northern California explored interaction effects with genetic variants involved in one-carbon metabolism as carried by either the mother or child. The results suggested that some polymorphic genes that are involved in maternal folic acid metabolism – methylenetetrahydrofolate reductase (MTHFR C677T), cystathionine beta-synthase (CBS rs234715 GT +TT), dihydrofolate reductase (19bp deletion-DHFR), and fetal catechol-O-methyltransferase (COMT 472 AA), are grouped together with increased risk for the future development autism, especially when mothers do not take such vitamins periconceptionally. Women who had either one of two gene variants associated with folic acid regulation had two to five times the risk of having a child with autism, especially if the mother did not take prenatal vitamins containing folic acid around the time of conception. Children who had one of these gene variants had seven times the normal risk of developing autism if the mother did not take prenatal vitamins around conception, but the normal risk if she did take them (12). The following mutations were analyzed in a context of increased risk of developing ASD:

1) MTHFR is a gene that encodes for the enzyme, methylenetetrahydrofolate reductase. It plays a role in processing amino acids which combine to form proteins. Methylenetetrahydrofolate reductase is involved in the folic acid cycle and is important for converting potentially toxic homocysteine to cysteine, and then back to methionine (13). On the other hand, CBS is a gene that encodes the enzyme, cystathionine beta-synthase, which converts homocysteine to cystathionine, which then is converted to cysteine (14). A deficiency of either MTHFR or CBS may be associated with an increase in plasma the plasma homocysteine, which in turn is sometimes associated with an increased risk of autism (15). Results of the study showed that homocysteine levels were significantly higher in children with autism as compare to healthy controls. The researchers speculated that in autism, high homocysteine levels could impair neuronal plasticity and promote nerve degeneration during development. Increased homocysteine levels are known to be associated not only with ASD, but also various neuropsychiatric disorders (15,16).

2) Dihydrofolate reductase (DHFR) is the sole enzyme maintaining the reduced state of dihydrofolic acid needed for de novo methionine and thymine synthesis, which is critical for DNA expression and elaboration. According to the researchers, the 19 bp-deletion polymorphism of DHFR is believed to be a significant risk factor for autism (17).

3) Another mutation that is often identified with an increased risk of developing ASD is catechol-O-methyltransferase (COMT), which is also linked to increased levels of homocysteine. COMT gene encodes a physiologically important enzyme in the metabolism of catecholamine neurotransmitters and catechol drugs. It is one of the enzymes that degrade dopamine, epinephrine, and norepinephrine by introducing a methyl group into the catecholamine (18). A common normal variant of COMT single nucleotide polymorphism results in valine-to-methionine replacement at position 158 (19). Homozygosity for COMT158met leads to a 3-4-fold reduction in enzymatic activity, compared with homozygotes for COMT158val (20). Due to the fact that the Met variant is overexpressed in the brain, resulting decrease in enzymatic activity increases dopamine levels and dopaminergic stimulation of the post-synaptic neurons. As COMT plays a role in prefrontal dopamine degradation, the Val158Met polymorphism is shown to affect cognitive tasks, such as set shifting, response inhibition, abstract thought, and the acquisition of rules or task structure (21).

Folic acid supplementation

It has long been noted that with autism comes an atypical feeding pattern, that may further contribution to ASD, mainly due to the challenge of ensuring adequate nutrition (22). Autistic children are generally 'picky' eaters, and thus restrict certain food groups since they only accept a limited range of food types. As this may lead to deficiencies in vitamins, minerals, and other essential nutrients, the supplementation of a child's diet has been a regular procedure in the care of autistic children. A recent meta-analysis on several studies supports this long held theory. It confirmed that children with ASD have a much greater risk of nutritional intake challenges (due to behavioral disorders like food selectivity and tantrums) versus their unaffected peers (22).

Although specific nutritional deficiencies or imbalances vary from child to child, it was noted by the Autism Research Institute that some children, on average, did better on specific supplements. By providing a "Treatment Effectiveness Survey questionnaire" to patients, they were able to rate various nutrient supplements on a score from "made better," "made worse," to "no effect," and from this make a "Better:Worse" ratio (B:W ratio). They found that folate provided a B:W ratio of 11:1, i.e., 11 children improved with folate supplementation for every 1 that did not (21). One hypothesis for this improvement given by the authors was that with increased folic acid comes reduced oxidative stress in the brain, leading to improved cognitive behavior (chapter 8B,8C).

Conclusions

This chapter gives a short overview of folic acid research in the study of autism. While much work is needed to conclusively prove a causal relationship between folic acid and ASD, this growing body of research work on the application of this vitamin to modify this disorder cannot be ignored. However, it remains unclear if the depressed level of folic acid is a co-morbidity or is causative. Much more prospective research needs to be done to settle this enigma, especially considering consumed dose versus effect.

Chapter 5B - Leaky Gut Syndrome (Opiate/Gluten/Casein)

Erica Mirigliani, Marlee Forte

[The concept of gastrointestinal malfunction as a precursor or co-morbidity to autism laid the foundation for spurious speculation on the putative etiologic relationship between the "leaky gut", vaccination, and this neurological disorder. – Ed.]

Hypothesis

The relevance of diet in relation to health and disease is gaining notoriety in several areas, and autism is no exception. Restricting certain foods, sometimes referred to as the

"Autism Diet," encompasses various meanings (1). In this section, we will focus on the gluten-free, casein-free (GFCF) diet and its implications with "leaky gut" syndrome as well as the opiate theory as possibly related to autism.

An association of gastrointestinal dysfunction and autism spectrum disorders is not a new concept. In fact, Leo Kanner, who first identified autistic children, wrote a paper in 1943 entitled "Autistic Disturbances of Affective Contact" (1). This paper included a description of dietary problems and pointed out that 6 of his first 11 autistic patients had issues with feeding and diet (2). A report in 1998 by Wakefield was among the first to describe inflammatory bowel disease as a co-morbidity to autism in some affected children (3). Specifically, lymphoid nodular hyperplasia (LNH) and autism were thought to coexist as a result of MMR vaccination, but this was later refuted (chapter 7A). Also, LNH has been found together with maladies other than autism as well (4).

The leaky gut opiate theory proposed by Reichelt and Knivsberg, however, did not emerge until the 1990's. Leaky gut or increased intestinal permeability starts at the level of the tight junctions. These microscopic structures, also known as zonula occludens, are the key component in the junctional complex between intestinal epithelial cells. As the major barrier within the paracellular pathway between intestinal epithelial cells, it is important that its structure and function are intact to prevent unwanted substances (proteins or pathogens) to pass from the intestines into the blood stream (5).

The source of digestive products that have become of possible interest in the autistic child are mainly gluten and casein. They are exorphins – structurally similar to endorphins – short chain peptides produced from incomplete digestion of dietary gluten and casein in the small intestine. The structure of these components makes them especially resistant to peptidase (6). Peptidase is an enzyme that assists in digesting proteins to amino acids. It is in the form of an amino acid that the body is able to construct needed proteins. Reichelt and Knivsberg found substances resembling opioid peptides in the urine of ASD children (1). Since the amount of peptides in the urine exceeds what the central nervous system could alone produce, these researchers thought the peptides originated from the defective breakdown of food as opposed to coming from the brain. Casein incompletely breaks down to casomorphins (7), and gluten to gluteomorphins (8). Both these substance groups have opiate activity (1,6). Their theory states that in children with autism, peptides can escape a permeable gut, cross the blood-brain barrier, and cause neurological manifestations.

In conjunction with the opiate theory is the GFCF diet. The GFCF diet has been studied, and claims exist that those children with autism benefit from such a diet. A child on this diet would avoid all foods containing casein and gluten. His/her diet would not consist of milk as casein is a protein in milk, or anything made of flour like breads or pastas, as they contain the protein, gluten. The diet would be similar to that of a person with a combination of lactose intolerance plus celiac disease. Also considered are many anecdotal assertions, but does the research back them up? As far as defining an etiology for ASD, we will see that current research does not link leaky gut syndrome to the cause of autism or to a commonly associated symptom. However, the hypothesis persists that children with autism may benefit from a GFCF diet.

Observations

Perhaps leaky gut syndrome has persisted as an autism-associated condition because the idea was introduced so long ago. As mentioned above, Dr. Kanner reported gastrointestinal dysfunctions from the beginning of the autism discussion in the 1940's. A decade later, in 1951, Prugh and colleagues noted autistic-like behaviors in children with gluten sensitivity. Continuing with the same notion in 1961, Crook found that elimination of certain foods improved behaviors (mood, concentration, less irritability) in autistic as well as schizophrenic people. In 1966, Dohan pointed out the increased consumption of processed grains after World War II paralleled a rise in autism and schizophrenia. Not long after, in 1971, Goodwin et al. published a paper on ASD children with diarrhea and loose stools (1). As time progressed, the consideration of gastrointestinal disturbances in autistic children continued.

More recently, patients with autism as well as their first degree relatives were tested for intestinal permeability (IPT) in order to investigate leaky gut hypothesis. Intestinal permeability is a protective function of the intestinal mucosa. When the barrier, i.e., the tight junctions, becomes compromised, the permeability can increase and allow unwanted substances (peptides, toxins, bacteria etc) to enter the body. The IPT measures how much peptide crosses the epithelial tight junction barrier. The hypothesis formed by this group of investigators stated that the lack of efficiency of these intestinal blockades might be a gateway in childhood developmental impairment, including autism (9). By studying the IPT level in first-degree relatives of subjects with ASD, the level of peptides could correlate with a genetic predisposition for leaky gut.

In order to test this hypothesis, the function of IPT was assessed by the lactulose/mannitol test in autistic patients and compared with unaffected adult and child controls. As mentioned before, IPT monitors mucosal damage of the small intestines. Fecal calprotectin (FC) was also measured in patients with autism and in their first-degree relatives with high IPT. FC was used to determine intestinal inflammation. The study results also substantiated no correlation between IPT and FC values. However, there was evidence to support that abnormal IPT has a genetic basis and is present in some people with ASD. The results showed that IPT was elevated in >20% of healthy genetically-connected relatives of children with autism (9). It was concluded that if IPT is abnormal in a subgroup of affected children could be used as a biomarker for those who might benefit from treatment aimed at the leaky gut. While there may be some correlation between IPT and ASD, it is not enough to conclusively say that the two demonstrate a cause-and-effect relationship.

The hypothesis of a link between leaky gut syndrome and autism involves not only intestinal permeability but also the nature of brain function. The gut-brain axis consists of the notion that components of the intestinal lumen can traverse an abnormally permeable mucosa, cross into the blood stream, and from there permeate the blood-brain-barrier (10). As a result, this might cause psychiatric, cognitive, and behavioral disturbances.

The investigation of childhood developmental disorders has focused on the gut-brain interaction and the role it plays in the abnormal neural development and ensuing expression of unusual behavior. Wakefield evaluated the gut-brain axis by reviewing several studies focused on primary gastrointestinal pathology possibly playing a role in the clinical expression of some childhood developmental disorders, including autism. He noted that gastrointestinal symptoms are a common finding in children with autism (10). Aberrations in opioid biochemistry are thought to play a central role in these gastrointestinal manifestations. Small studies have been conducted, but a large controlled investigation is lacking. Therefore, the solid evidence needed to make a conclusion has not been reported (chapter 7A).

Gut-to-brain relations have been proposed over the years. As a focus on whether or not autism necessarily correlates with a permeable gut, D'Eufemia et al. studied 21 autistic patients. Nine of the children (43%) were determined to have mucosal damage using the intestinal permeability test (11). None of the 40 control patients demonstrated intestinal damage. They reported that behavioral abnormalities may be due to elevated food peptides crossing the intestinal barrier as a result of the barrier being altered, or abnormal. Unfortunately, this review, among other similarly conducted studies, could not substantiate the claim that agluten-free, casein-free (GFCF) diet could benefit autistic children. However, for those who are autistic, leaky gut may exist as a co-morbidity, i.e., an additional disorder/disease that occurs along with the primary disease.

More specifically, gluteomorphin, the peptide from gluten, has been stated to be more common in children with autism (12). Researchers speculated that gluteomorphin in the blood stream "could" affect behavior. They also claimed that evidence supported the theory that blocking even some of the gluteomorphin actions improves the behavior of children with autism. Though this may have shown positive results, there exists no proven direct connection between gluteomorphin levels and autistic children's behavior.

In a more recent paper, the authors made supporting comments of the GFCF diet based on previous claims (13). For example, they said all who have autism have increased gut permeability, and therefore, gluten and casein should be removed from the diet in autistic children, when in fact the references this paper used did not indeed state that this is inclusive of all autistic children. Unfortunately, what the authors of this paper were claiming to be true was not actually validated through research. There exists no evidence that all autistic children consistently have increased gut permeability. To support the leaky gut hypothesis, it must first be demonstrated that the autistic population all have GI dysfunctions, namely, permeability to gluten and casein opiate compounds, in order for a GFCF diet to be effective. The attempts to correlate urine peptides with behavior have been successful in showing *some* autistic patients contain gluteomorphin and caseomorphin in the urine (14). It is by means of urine analysis to determine whether or not these peptides are elevated. Also, inheritance of this trait needs to be examined to see if it correlates with incidence of autism.

Other studies have focused on a population of autistic patients with urinary peptide abnormalities and investigated dietary intervention. In 2002, Knivsberg et al. examined 20 participants with ASD and abnormal urinary peptides. The goal was to see if a gluten and casein-free diet could improve learning. Children were paired and randomly selected to the diet group or the non-diet group (14). Background information included the presence of opioid-like peptides found in the CSF, urine, and serum of autistic children. Opioids from gluten and casein have an effect on the CNS such as the formation of communicating networks between neurons. The study assumed the children's behaviors were interferred with by opiates from gluten and casein, which led to diagnoses of autism in children with abnormal urinary peptides. The researchers hypothesized that on a GFCF diet the autistic traits would decrease. They used a single-blinded and randomized approach. Standardized tests were used to evaluate behavior, language, motor abilities and cognition at the beginning of the study and after one year. All participants showed aloofness, a characteristic autistic trait, at the beginning of the trial.

Significant improvements were found regarding aloofness, routines and rituals, and responses to learning in the GFCF diet group, whereas the control (untreated) group demonstrated no significant changes. The most marked difference was found in the social and emotional traits. The diet group showed improvement over the non-diet group. The results led to the claim that the children on the diet exhibited improvement over the children on the non-diet regimen. It is important to keep in mind the small study sample size (20 participants) who were split into two groups. However, this study was successful in checking the urinary peptide status of all participants, providing a uniform population. The results demonstrated improvement in behavior for a specific subgroup of autistic children - those with evidence of dysfunctional intestinal permeability.

A preliminary double-blinded clinical trial by Elder and colleagues evaluated 15 children with autism. Half of the children were put on a non-restricted diet containing gluten and casein, followed by restricted GFCF diets. The other half started on the restricted GFCF diet, followed by the non-restricted gluten and casein diet (15). Observations were made of the children's frequency of interaction and communication, parent behaviors, and urinary peptide levels. Results showed no significant differences between affected and normal subjects. However, the observations made by the researchers seemed to differ from that of the parents.

Another double-blinded trial by Hyman et al. studied 22 children who did not have a diagnosis of celiac disease or allergies to milk or wheat. The team examined the effects of a GFCF diet (16). Twelve of the children remained on the GFCF diet, while ten were on a common diet. The testing was not limited to children with urinary peptide deviations. Overall, this study showed no statistically significant difference among the children.

Besides the testing of a GFCF diet, there have been investigations of gut permeability and autism via endoscopy. According to Buie, who has performed over 2,000 endoscopies or colonoscopies on people with autism, patients frequently do report gastrointestinal issues. Therefore, he concluded that a GI history and workup should be part of every person's medical assessment with autism (2).

Conclusions

Some hypotheses suggest a correlation between leaky gut and autism, but the actual studies have not reported evidence that **all** children with autism have leaky gut syndrome. Also, there was no verification to suggest that leaky gut is a cause of autism, but rather appears to be a coinciding pathology. Many studies concluded that there is some gastrointestinal pathology that can be found in some autistic children, but it was never inclusive of all children with autism.

A major factor limiting the validity of these hypotheses was the small number of subjects in the studies. With only 10 or 20 children, it is hard to extrapolate the findings to a large population. More numerous, controlled, blind studies are needed in order to give statistical strength to these claims.

What can be concluded from these studies is that there may be a subset of autistic children who suffer from increased intestinal permeability. This appeared to be the case with the accumulation of gluten and casein peptide found in the urine of some affected patients. In this case, marked improvement in behavior was seen in a small group of subjects when placed on a gluten-free, casein-free diet, in comparison to those who were not. In contradistinction, this cannot be stated for all children who suffer from autism because the studies were limited by small test size. On the other hand, significant associations with the gut-brain axis (increased levels of peptides crossing from the intestine into the blood) seemed to be related in some patients with autism, warranting further investigation.

The approach to dealing with GI symptoms that are manifested in the autistic child should not be limited to a restricted diet. To fully understand the origin of this effect, it is imperative that a full GI workup be completed, as well as a urine analysis monitoring for abnormal peptide levels. The gluten-free, casein-free diet could be an option to improve behavior and functioning in autism if a child is presenting with suggestive digestive symptoms. At this point in time, there is not enough supporting evidence to claim gluten-free, casein-free, or any other special diet, as a "cure" for autistic behavior.

Chapter 5C - Vitamin D

Daniel Lefkowitz, Szymon Rus

[It remains to be determined if the vitamin D deficiency often found in cases of autism represents a causative or co-morbid association.. – Ed.]

Introduction

Vitamin D is the common name given to a group of fat-soluble sterols that behave like hormones, and control potassium/calcium levels within the body. While present naturally in a variety of foods such as fatty fish, egg yolk and liver, vitamin D is not an essential vitamin -- it can be synthesized from precursors buried in the skin with help of UV radiation from sunlight. Therefore, dietary vitamin D supplementation is only required in individuals with limited sun exposure such as people living in northern latitudes. Deficiency in vitamin D can lead to bone disorders such as rickets in younger individuals and osteomalacia in adults, and predispose them to fractures. However, high doses of vitamin D can also bring on deleterious side effects such as nausea, thirst, loss of appetite and stupor (1).

Two major forms of vitamin D exist in nature: Ergocalciferol (vitamin D_2) is found in plants and cholecalciferol (vitamin D_3) is found in animal tissues. These compounds are not biologically active and need to be transformed into an active form of vitamin D, calcitriol (1,25-dihydroxycalciferol, $1,25(OH)_2D$, or cholecalcitriol) through a series of enzymatic hydroxylation reactions. Nonetheless, the majority of vitamin D production is internal. Cholecalciferol is transformed in the skin from an intermediate compound (7-dehydrocholesterol) by ultraviolet rays of the sun and is transported to the liver, where it is hydroxylated to produce calcidiol (25-hydroxycalciferol, $25(OH)D$, or cholecalcidiol). Calcidiol is moved to the kidneys, where it is hydroxylated to produce calcitriol. The final transformation into the active compound is tightly controlled by parathyroid hormone, which is released in response to low calcium or phosphate concentrations (1).

Vitamin D's major function is to maintain proper levels of calcium and phosphate in the blood by increasing calcium and phosphate uptake in the intestines, minimizing calcium loss in the kidneys and if necessary, extracting calcium and phosphate from bone with help of parathyroid hormone. While vitamin D's most direct impact is on bone formation and strength, it has been found to play a role in various developmental processes such as aging, embryogenesis and neurodevelopment. Other roles such, as inflammation and brain homeostasis are suspected since vitamin D can bind thousands of gene sites and has been found to regulate more than 200 genes (2).

Autism is defined as a disorder of the central nervous system characterized by impairments in communication and social reciprocity (3). Although the etiopathogenesis of autism spectrum disorders (ASDs) remains unclear, there has been an apparent progressive increase in the prevalence of ASD since the 1980s (see chapter 1C). There are two groups of factors that contribute to autism: genetic and environmental, which includes vitamin D deficiency.

ASD is considered not only to be a psychiatric disorder, but also a neurologic disorder, as there is a functional and physical change in the size and structure of the brain. The change in brain morphology can be traced back to the embryological development of the central nervous system. Vitamin D is extremely neuroprotective. It stimulates the release of neurotropin, which has various protective effects in the brain (4). The brain is not completely developed at birth, and is therefore still vulnerable to developing the characteristics of ASD (3). Research findings support the necessity of vitamin D throughout neurodevelopment in utero and early infancy.

As noted above, Vitamin D can enter the body in three ways: it can be ingested through food, be converted from a precursor by UVB sunlight in the skin, or be synthesized in various tissues. The most important of these is from sunlight, as over 90 percent of the vitamin D stores come from skin production in most people (4). Additionally, a pregnant woman would have to drink more than 200 glasses of milk or take over 50 prenatal vitamins to produce the same serum vitamin D level attained from exposure to sunlight for 20 minutes. It has also been found that in rainy areas with fewer daily hours of sunlight, there are more children with autism (5), again supporting a putative link between ASDs and vitamin D levels.

Observations

There are multiple possible mechanisms linking vitamin D and its effects on ASD. Vitamin D deficiency causes an exaggerated immune response to infectious agents and toxins, and is a key regulator of self-tolerance (3). Also, vitamin D is a neuro-steroid hormone and binds at the nuclear level to regulate over 200 genes (4). It exerts its effects through binding to the vitamin D receptor (VDR). The vitamin D-VDR complex then binds to numerous sites of DNA, thus influencing gene expression (2). Developmental vitamin D deficiency has also been found to regulate brain development, oxidative phosphorylation, redox balance (glutathione levels), cytoskeleton maintenance, calcium homeostasis, chaperoning, post-translational modification, synaptic plasticity, and neurotransmitters (6-8), as well as neuronal differentiation, structure, and metabolism (2). Disturbances in any of these multiple functions may all contribute to the importance of vitamin D and development of disorders such as autism. However, no convincing evidence exists that such actions actually cause autism

Observations that support vitamin D's role in neurodevelopment include the fact that high levels of VDR in the brain are found very early on in development and increase with gestational age (8). Additionally, animal studies have shown that hypo-vitaminosis of vitamin D early in life leads to disruption and permanent changes in brain development similar to the changes in brain morphology seen in those with autism (larger ventricles, reduced nerve growth factor expression, reduced expression of numerous genes involved in neuronal structure or neurotransmission) (9). Therefore, it appears that vitamin D is required for normal brain function, morphology, development and homeostasis (10).

Because vitamin D can be synthesized and metabolized in the brain, it would seem that autocrine and paracrine pathways involved with this factor play an important part in brain functioning (10). Vitamin D has been noted to have an apparent role in brain cellular differentiation, as the VDR is localized in differentiating areas of the developing brain (11,12). Although causal correlation between the VDR and developing brain cannot be established at this time, a previous study found an increase in the VDR simultaneously with a decrease in cell proliferation and increase in cellular elimination. Therefore, this suggests a linkage between vitamin D via the VDR in the developing brain. Whether or not this link between a vitamin and its receptor has a direct or indirect role in brain development remains uncertain (13).

If low levels of vitamin D are contributing factors in developing autism during pregnancy and/or childhood, it is reasonable to postulate that low serum vitamin D levels (either calcidiol and/or calcitriol) would be more prevalent in mothers of children with autism or their offspring. In turn, a number of studies have investigated serum vitamin D levels in subjects diagnosed with ASD or their mothers. To date, there still no clear evidence to support the hypothesis that low vitamin D causes autism, but several studies do show that vitamin D levels are lower in children with autism compared to controls.

One finding of a significant link between vitamin D and ASD was made by Meguid et al. (2010), where 70 children with diagnosed autism were matched with 42 randomly selected healthy children of the same socioeconomic status and age in a case-controlled cross-sectional study that measured levels of calcitriol and calcidiol in all subjects. The investigators found that children with autism did have significantly lower calcidiol (28.5 ng/ml; $p<0.00001$) and calcitriol (27.1 ng/ml; $p<0.005$) levels compared to controls (calcidiol: 40.1ng/ml; calcitriol: 32.8ng/ml). Furthermore, there was no significant difference between the birth month and season of birth of children with autism and healthy controls since there are seasonal variations that accompany serum vitamin D levels. The results of the Meguid study show a significant association between low vitamin D levels and autism, but it is important to note that the small sample size puts great statistical limitations on extrapolating these conclusions as a reflection of the general pediatric population (14).

A similar study conducted by Mostafa et al (2012) also examined serum calcidiol levels in 50 autistic children (5-12 year old Saudi children diagnosed by the criteria in DSM-IV) compared to 30 healthy age- and sex-matched controls. The study found that children with autism had significantly lower serum calcidiol levels (18.5 ng/ml; $p< 0.001$) compared to controls (33ng/ml). Furthermore, 40% of the autistic children had deficient levels of serum vitamin D (<10ng/ml) compared to none of the controls. A total of 48% of the autistic children were vitamin D deficient (10-30ng/ml) compared to 20% of controls (15). Once again, a small sample size precludes the study from making any general conclusions about the role of vitamin D in development of autism.

The main question to be answered is whether these low vitamin D levels are causative or coincidental in autism. Autistic children may be predisposed to having low vitamin D levels based on their selective eating habits (16), so hypo-vitaminosis D may be a coincidental finding. A larger study is also required to give greater support to the link between vitamin D and autism since previous studies had a regional component as well as a small sample size.

A conflicting report by Molloy et al., 2010, that measured plasma calcidiol levels in 49 Caucasian males (aged 4 to 8 years) with diagnosed ASD with a control group of 40 age-matched normally-developing boys found no significant differences between the groups (p=0.4) (17). However, in addition to a small sample size, the study did have some important limitations. Specifically, the control group consisted of children that had intravenous catheters placed for outpatient tonsillectomies. The acute inflammation that they were exhibiting could have affected the plasma vitamin D levels. Interestingly, while no significant link between levels of vitamin D and autism was found, 61% of children with ASD had low plasma calcidiol levels (<20 ng/ml).

Reduced serum vitamin D in patients with autism has also been found in a cross-sectional study by Humble et al. in 2010 (18). In it, a chart review of 117 European adult white males and females suffering from psychiatric disorders, including autism, found significantly lower levels of calcidiol (12.6 ng/ml) in patients with autism or schizophrenia than in other groups. Since there was no control group and a range of other psychiatric disorders was being investigated, the study has serious limitations, but may support a potential link between vitamin D and autism.

Another area of research into a possible link between vitamin D and autism has focused on maternal vitamin D levels during pregnancy. Support for low maternal vitamin D and autism has come from several epidemiological studies summarized by a review by Dealberto (2011) (19). It found that dark-skinned immigrant mothers (especially those that immigrated to higher latitude areas) were at a higher risk for having children with autism. Since a main source of vitamin D comes from sun exposure, dark-skinned individuals need longer sun exposure than light-skinned subjects and are consequently at a higher risk of vitamin D deficiency or insufficiency. This problem is compounded by living in communities at higher geographical latitudes that receive low levels of UV radiation required for vitamin D conversions in the skin (20). While these factors would predispose the mothers to low vitamin D levels, none of the studies reported by Dealberto (2011) included maternal serum vitamin D levels during pregnancy or offspring serum levels after birth (19).

In one study by Fernell et al. (2010) mothers of Somali origin were compared with a control group of Swedish mothers. To account for differences in vitamin D bioavailability throughout the year, two blood samples were collected from each subject (autumn and spring). The results of the study did find that Somali mothers did have significantly lower levels of calcidiol compared to Swedish mothers in both autumn and spring. However, a comparison of calcidiol levels between mothers of Somali origin with and without an autistic child was not statistically significant, although the lowest calcidiol values were found in mothers with a child with ASD (21). The small sample size limits the scope of the study. Furthermore, several years had passed since pregnancy for all mothers (range: 4.3 to 7.1 years) and it is not known what the levels of calcidiol were during pregnancy. With these considerations in mind, it is difficult to draw any definite conclusions.

A larger study by Whitehouse et al. (2013) examined serum calcidiol levels of 929 Australian women at 18 weeks of pregnancy and followed the offspring of 406 mothers into early offspring adulthood. Children were assessed at ages of 5, 8, 10, 14 and 17 for autism and autistic-like traits. In the study, 3 offspring out of 929 did develop ASD, but the maternal levels of calcidiol at 18 weeks pregnancy (78, 63, and 65 nmol/L) were above the sample mean (58 nmol/L). There was no significant correlation between maternal calcidiol levels and offspring risk for autism and autistic-like traits. While these results largely dismiss low levels of maternal vitamin D during pregnancy as a cause of developing autism, parts of the study do find show a positive correlation (22). Specifically, offspring of low calcidiol (<49 nmol/L) mothers were at a higher risk for exhibiting autistic behavior (≥2 SD above mean) on one of 5 subscales testing for an autism phenotype, which was the Attention Switching subscale ('I enjoy doing things spontaneously'). Therefore, it is premature to discount low maternal vitamin D as a possible factor in autism and more research is warranted.

Vitamin D deficiency during pregnancy has yet to be proven to be causative of ASD in the developing fetus. Yet deficiency is associated with pregnancy complications like preterm delivery, preeclampsia (chapter 3H), which apparently increase the risk of autism.

The American College of Obstetrics and Gynecology (ACOG) recommends vitamin D measurements and supplementation if a deficiency is revealed for individuals in high risk groups. It is logical to screen mothers at high risk for autism (which have already one child with ASD) for vitamin D levels during subsequent pregnancies (23). Although this assumption is logical its efficiency in reducing rates of ASD requires further research and support.

Conclusions

Although many of the epidemiological studies examining the association between vitamin D and autism do not show significant causality, the research investigating the role of vitamin D in embryological development and neurogenesis does suggest there is an association between vitamin D and normal development of the nervous system. Additionally, there has been new research suggesting a connection between serum levels of insulin-like growth factor (IGF) and autism (23) (chapter 6D). None of the hypotheses or mechanisms appear to work in isolation and they all may have a role in the development of ASD.

There appears to be some type of correlation between vitamin D autism. However, it is unclear at this time how the two interact and whether they are linked directly or indirectly. Therefore, further research on this association is needed. Furthermore, all of the factors (genetic and environmental) of ASD need to be accounted for collectively and simultaneously, rather than separately, as was done in the past. There need to be studies comparing and contrasting the differences when the vitamin D deficiency specifically occurs, and if it stops, when it does. In other words, there should be studies that examine developmental vitamin D deficiency prenatally, postnatally, and throughout childhood, in order to specify exactly when and if vitamin D deficiency may be detrimental and when there is a point at which the vitamin D deficiency may cause irreversible damage.

It was disturbing to realize how many neuropsychiatric disorders are now being loosely associated with hypo-vitaminosis D. Most of the literature related to this topic has been cross-sectional; more longitudinal observational studies are warranted before any advice regarding vitamin D supplementation can be offered to any population. Additionally, there are insufficient data on the "normal" levels of vitamin D for anyone, especially pregnant women with regard to the development of ASD. However, the ACOG recommends vitamin D levels be above 32 ng/ml. Therefore, more research examining healthy plasma levels of vitamin D are necessary prior to establishing the association between vitamin D and any of the neuropsychological disorders, and more specifically, ASD.

Vitamin D has many effects on normal physiology. Therefore, a deficiency in it may exert a stress that indirectly affects brain development. Given the high prevalence of vitamin D deficient pregnant women, the apparent rise of ASD, and the accessible nature of vitamin D, further investigations are indicated. It is not clear when a developmental vitamin D deficiency is pathological for a child. For example, comparing the outcomes of low vitamin D in patients who were deficient *in utero* or in infancy should be studied in sufficient numbers to be statistically powerful. Only after examining these different situations and identifying a healthy serum level of vitamin D, with regard to autism, may we begin to draw further conclusions.

It is a public health necessity to try to reduce the incidence and prevalence of ASDs, and as such, we are obligated to complete further research to help draw definite conclusions about the association between vitamin D and ASD. Currently, there appears to be a relationship between vitamin D and ASD. However, the mechanisms and extent of this relationship remain unclear.

Chapter 5D – Mercury (fish)

Section I: Minamata source

Nimrah Ahmed, Julia Brothers

[Because of neurologic harm found with ingestion of mercury-laced fish, concern has been raised about its possible association with autism. The relationship between the amount and type of fish consumed, and the resultant exposure to mercury is discussed – Ed.]

Introduction
In the years following the end of World War II, Japan entered an era of rapid industrialization and modernization, in order to recover from its devastating loss. This period of increased productivity led to the growth of both new and old corporations. Factories arose within rural towns, providing a new industrial identity as well as a source of jobs and income for the families that resided there. Minamata, Japan was originally a quiet fishing village on the coast of the Japanese island of Kyushu, which relied heavily on its namesake bay for vitality before the establishment of the Chisso Corporation factory between the Minamata Bay and River.

Opening into the Shiranui Sea, the Bay provided the townspeople with a wide variety of fresh seafood – the primary foundation of their diet and livelihood. Although it began as an electric power company in 1906, the Chisso Corporation adapted to the changing times and switched from providing hydroelectric power and chemical fertilizers to mass producing acetaldehyde in the 1930s, which was used in manufacturing plastics and other industrial products (1). Inorganic mercury was necessary as a chemical catalyst to increase the rate of production; however, toxic methylmercury was a byproduct of the synthesis and was continuously dumped into the bay up until the late 1960s. The pollution of Minamata Bay would later become known as the Minamata Disaster (2). Because of its neurotoxicity, the question arose if mercury caused autism, in particular.

Observations

The first signs of the impending catastrophe in the fishing community were in 1953, when the villagers of Minamata noticed that fish were found belly-up near the waste pipes of the Chisso factory. Cats that were fed fish from the bay developed strange "dancing" behaviors and convulsions (3). The first human victim was reported in 1956. Data collected by doctors and scientists found that most of the significant pathological changes were in the central nervous system (4). Notable symptoms included sensory disturbances such as visual field constriction, hearing impairment, ataxia (uncoordinated movement), speech disturbance and disequilibrium (5). Methylmercury poisoning was shown to affect the brain unevenly, with most damage shown in the cerebral and cerebellar regions. (In the initial stages of evaluation, autism in particular was not singled out as one of the possible consequences of mercury pollution.)

In addition to the neurological symptoms, patients also displayed facial nerve palsy, dysarthria (speech muscle impairment), limitation of neck movement, muscle atrophy, weakness and abnormal muscle tone. Other signs of disturbance were noted in other organ systems, including erosive inflammation in the digestive tract, hypoplasia of the bone marrow (leading to anemia), atrophy of lymph nodes, fatty degeneration of the liver and kidney, and the alteration of pancreatic islet cells (6). Due to its origin within the town of Minamata, the affliction was dubbed "Minamata Disease."

In the preliminary stages of the epidemic, it was unknown how it was contracted or if it were contagious. Therefore, patients exhibiting the visibly disturbing symptoms were hidden away from society in isolated hospital beds and psychiatric wards. The cause of Minamata disease did not remain a mystery for long, however. In 1959, animal experiments done by researchers at Kumamoto University proved that the Chisso factory had been the source of the mercury food poisoning. In spite of overwhelming evidence, the Chisso Corporation denied the link to the contamination and the issue was dropped. Silence would not only benefit the country socially, but also economically. The Chisso Corporation was at the head of the new industrial age and to challenge them would undoubtedly stunt the country's growth. In addition, the fishermen of Minamata preferred to keep the matter private, in order to keep the fishing community free of stigma.

Following the initial outbreak of Minamata disease, doctors reported increasing incidence of cerebral palsy and other congenital disorders among local children, whose mothers were asymptomatic. In 1961, scientists began to investigate these reports, and found symptoms of acute mercury poisoning among children born after the initial crisis who had never been fed contaminated fish. They were found to exhibit severe musculoskeletal deformity, spasticity, seizures, deafness, severely impaired cognition and other developmental delays. Researchers concluded that these children were suffering from a congenital form of Minamata disease, which ultimately led to a rethinking of the role of the placenta in protecting the fetus. Prior scientific opinion had held that the placenta protected the fetus from heavy metal toxicity. In the case of mercury, however, it was determined that the placenta in fact filters methylmercury from maternal blood and concentrates it in the fetus (7).

In 1965, a similar tragedy took place in Niigata, Japan. Contamination was traced to a factory that had been using a mercury catalyst in a process similar to the Chisso Corporation's industrial process in Minamata (8). Based on the similarity of symptoms and the discovery of mercury pollution, scientists concluded that Niigata patients were suffering from the same disease seen in Minamata. Unlike in Minamata, victims of the Niigata contamination lived a considerable distance from the factory and did not have connections to the company. As a result, the community was more supportive of victims' pursuit of legal action, and a lawsuit was filed in 1968. The reaction to the Niigata outbreak prompted a more sympathetic response to the initial outbreak in Minamata. The Citizens' Council for Minamata Disease Countermeasures was established to provide support for victims and their families, and in 1969 a lawsuit was filed against the Chisso Corporation. The silence was finally broken. The Japanese government ruled that mercury poisoning was the probable cause in both incidents. While families took action against the Showa Denko Company in Niigata, Chisso Corporation preemptively stopped dumping mercury into the bay – thirty-five years after it began.

These incidents in Japan merited enough global recognition that, in 1970, a California State Task Force on mercury and health officially recommended the public to limit consumption of "sport fish" – specifically, striped bass, catfish, and sturgeon (10). Pregnant women, in particular, were warned not to eat any sport fish at all, and in 1971, this warning was extended to any woman who had a chance of becoming pregnant (9). The task force based its recommendation on Swedish research which estimated a lethal dose as 60-70 ppm (parts per million) and set the upper limit of safety to 50 ppm, based on casualties from the Niigata disaster. American researchers had become aware that high mercury levels in pregnant women could cause neurological damage to their children.

Minamata disease symptoms bore enough similarity to other neuropsychiatric disorders that, over the ensuing decades, Japanese health experts took an aggressive stance on diagnosis and screening of various known neuropsychiatric disorders among children. In the decades following the outbreaks of disease in Minamata and Niigata, diagnosis of autism became more prevalent. Scientists worldwide began to examine prenatal exposures in their broad search for a cause. Incidence of autism was comparatively high in Japan, prompting an examination of the association of mercury exposure and autism (10). Researchers ultimately concluded, however, that Japan's autism prevalence had been higher in early decades as well, likely due to broader diagnostic criteria, and had not significantly increased among generations affected by mercury contamination (11).

As further evidence against the autism-mercury association, scientists have pointed out that symptoms of mercury poisoning bear little similarity to those of autism. The characteristic motor findings in mercury toxicity are ataxia and dysarthria, tremor, muscle pains, weakness, and spasticity. In patients with autism, however, the only common motor manifestation is repetitive behavior – such as flapping, circling, and rocking, in addition to hypotonia and "clumsiness" (10). Mercury poisoning can cause bilateral constriction of the visual fields, compromised contrast sensitivity, paresthesias, and peripheral neuropathy. In contrast, autistic patients sometimes show decreased responsiveness to pain, as well as increased sensitivity to other sensory stimuli, including hyperacusis (abnormally acute hearing). Hypertension, skin eruptions, and thrombocytopenia are sometimes seen in mercury poisoning, but are seldom seen in autism. Congenital and early postnatal mercury poisoning leads to reduced head circumference and microcephaly, whereas autism is associated with increased head circumference. The clinical signs of mercury toxicity, therefore, do not appear to be similar to the typical clinical signs of autism (11).

The Minamata tragedy made a lasting impression upon the American public consciousness through the work of photographer W. Eugene Smith, in a photo essay published in the June 1972 issue of *Life* magazine (12). A striking photograph from the essay, "Tomoko Uemura in Her Bath," of a severely deformed child held naked in her mother's arms, turned heads around the world toward Minamata disease. Its caption narrated the heart-wrenching story of how Tomoko soaked up mercury from her mother's blood, as a fetus, and paved the way for healthy birth of all her siblings. This emotional introduction was not without its consequences. Parents began to fear seafood entirely, but the American scientific community did respond. In the early 1970s American research journals began to discuss neurotoxicity induced by marine pollution (13).

Public interest drove funding for research in the area of mercury pollution. The existence of two types of organic mercury – ethyl- and methylmercury – caused confusion in regards to which derivative was linked to birth defects, autism, and even Minamata disease. The structures of the compounds differ by one methylated sidechain, but the names of the two chemicals were often used interchangeably by the press.

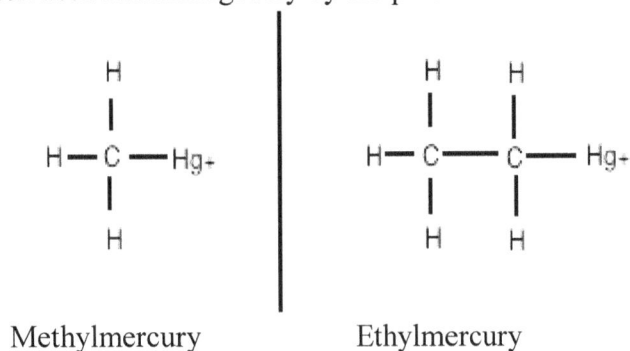

Methylmercury   Ethylmercury

Methylmercury is an organomercury formed by marine bacteria that scavenge inorganic metal molecules. After small fish consume the low levels of methylmercury in bacteria, larger fish eat the small fish. With no way to excrete the ingested mercury, they accumulate it in their tissues. When sharks and other predatory animals consume the larger fish, their levels of methylmercury become even higher. Thus, once methylmercury enters the marine ecosystem, it tends to accumulate in predatory fish, in a process known as bioaccumulation.

Ethylmercury, by contrast, is a biological metabolite of thimerosal (chapter 7B). Ethylmercury does not bioaccumulate and is excreted from the body faster than methylmercury (14). While methylmercury has been shown to cause pathogenesis (disease), ethylmercury was found to be safe at pharmacological concentrations, and has been used in thimerosal as an antimicrobial agent in vaccines for nearly a number of decades. The implication of methylmercury in Minamata disease and other environmental disasters, however, ignited concerns about the use of ethylmercury in thimerosal, which continues to linger to this day, despite scientists finding no evidence of harm with either pre- or postnatal exposure (12).

Just as American journals began discussing mercury poisoning in earnest, a second deadly disaster broke in Iraq in 1971, where over six thousand farm families were hospitalized for methylmercury poisoning due to its presence in an agricultural pesticide. Although the incident in Iraq was not related to seafood, it helped the FDA (US Food and Drug Administration) determine preliminary safety values for mercury exposure in adults. The next step was determining safe intrauterine and postnatal levels, but this presented a new and complicated challenge (12). All fish contain some level of mercury, but at what threshold does consumption become unsafe?

The Seychelles Child Development Study was a landmark in this search. The Republic of Seychelles is an archipelago comprising 115 islands off the coast of Zanzibar. Eighty-five percent of its population eat fish daily (14). Their fish contains mercury levels comparable to that of fish in the US market, making Seychelles an appropriate place to study the effects of a diet high in fish on health. A longitudinal study was designed, where 771 mother-child pairs were tracked over years for mercury level (measured in hair and nails) and performance on neurodevelopment tasks. Though Seychellois children had ten to twenty times higher methylmercury levels than American children, there was no evidence of developmental delays in any of the children. In fact, in the early years, postnatal consumption of fish, which caused a higher concentration of mercury in hair and nails, actually showed positive developmental effects, with children scoring higher on the neurodevelopmental tasks (15). The researchers theorized that consumption of good nutrients — such as the omega-3 fatty acids in fish and the beneficial molecules in breast milk (chapter 9A) — could be more important than the detrimental effects of mercury (16).

A similar study in the Faroe Islands of Denmark also found positive effects on neurodevelopment in toddlers that correlated with low postnatal exposure through mercury in breast milk. However, at around seven years of age, it was apparent that children with higher prenatal exposure had worse developmental outcomes - with deficits in attention, language, verbal memory, motor speed and visual-spatial function (17,18). One important difference between the populations of Seychelles and the Faroe islands is the source of their methylmercury: people in the Faroe islands consumed pilot whale meat and whale blubber, which contains over five times higher level of methylmercury, than the fish consumed either in Seychelles or the US. These larger doses taken in by the mother might be more difficult for the fetus to detoxify before the brain sustains damage. Additionally, several other pollutants, such as polychlorinated biphenyls (PCBs), tended to concentrate in whale blubber (17). This finding has led, recently, to recommendations against inclusion of pilot whale in the Faroe diet, due to modern pollution levels (18).

The average methylmercury concentration in hair of the US population is 1 ppm or less. The severe, debilitating doses of mercury in Iraq (see above) during the agricultural disaster ranged up to 674 ppm of mercury in hair, a concentration which caused the type of horrifying symptoms that characterized Tomoko Uemura in her tragic photograph: microcephaly (small heads), seizures, mental retardation, and cerebral palsy (recall that the maximum "safe" dose determined by Swedish researchers was 50 ppm). In Iraq, developmental delays were found in cases where maternal methylmercury levels were estimated to have been as low as 10 ppm (15). In Seychelles, where no adverse effects on development were noted, concentrations ranged up to 29 ppm. In the Faroe Islands, neurological deficits were found at a median concentration of 24.2 ppm.

In 1990, to determine the safe limit of exposure for neonates, the World Health Organization (WHO) divided the maximum adult dose by a factor of ten, and adopted 5 ppm as the international standard for tolerable level of mercury in hair (15). Drawing on new data from the same studies, in 2013, the WHO established a Provisional Tolerable Weekly Intake (PTWI) of 1.6 micrograms per kilogram body weight per day, considering this PTWI "sufficient to protect developing fetuses, the most sensitive subgroup of the population," while emphasizing the importance of fish to a balanced, healthy diet (19).

Although it is generally neurotoxic, it is now doubted that mercury toxicity can be a direct causative agent for autism. This is apparent from the failure of the rate of autism to decrease once mercury was removed from the thimersol additive of vaccines (chapter 7B).

Conclusions

In summary, the industrial waste disaster at Minamata – repeated at Niigata, Japan – introduced the world to the neurotoxic and neurodevelopmental dangers of organomercury pollution. These dangers include both cognitive and motor deficits, but autism was not identified as one of the many consequences – at any level of exposure. The agricultural disaster in Iraq provided an early opportunity for determination of fatal organomercury exposure levels, after which large-scale cohort studies were performed on the seafood-dependent populations of Seychelles and Faroe Islands to determine safe exposure levels for fetuses and infants. Although the unique diet of the Faroe population introduced challenges to the comparison, the WHO came to the conclusion that 5 ppm is the maximal tolerable exposure and that dietary limitations on fish intake should be balanced with the potential health benefits from its consumption.

Chapter 5D, Section II: Molecular mechanism

Andrew Ross

[The localized inflammatory effect may explain the harmful effects of mercury on nervous tissue in general and autism in particular. – Ed.]

Introduction

Numerous studies have examined the potential association between maternal mercury exposure and the fetal development of autism. Animal and neural cell models have demonstrated that high levels of laboratory mercury exposure can create phenotypes analogous to those observed in autism spectrum disorder (ASD). However, it remains to be determined if consumption of mercury from contaminated fish is responsible for the phenotypes observed in humans with ASD. It has been reported that mercury can depress insulin-like growth factor-1 (IGF-1) (chapter 6D), create a proinflammatory state via cytokine modulation (chapter 6C), decrease myelination (chapter 6A) and alter typical brain connectivity, and propagate a hyperoxidative state causing endothelial stress and decreased cerebral blood flow (chapters 8B,8C). Intriguingly, all of these molecular abnormalities are also observed in cases of ASD andthe potential mechanistic link between mercury and ASD will beexplored in further detail in this section.

Observations

Uterine transfer of mercury

To consider the mercury-autism link, uterine transfer of mercury from mother to fetus first warrants examination. In contrast to other heavy metals, including zinc, copper, cadmium, and lead, methymercury (MeHg) crosses the placenta into cord blood with relative ease (chapter 4B). The ability of MeHg to pass to fetal tissue suggests that the toxicity of fetal mercury exposure may be enhanced compared to other common heavy metals. An examination of 48 mother-fetus pairs found that lead, zinc, cadmium, selenium, and copper were all found at higher concentrations in placental tissue compared to umbilical cord tissue. Conversely, MeHg levels were reported to be 1.6 times greater in cord blood than placental blood (1). Consistent with this finding, an analysis of 649 mother-child pairs documented an increase in both fetal mercury levels during pregnancy and infant mercury levels in the hair during breastfeeding while maternal mercury concentrations decreased (2). In addition, kinetic analysis demonstrates a half-life for MeHg in human blood of 50 days (3). Thus, the relatively poor ability to detoxify and excrete mercury, coupled with the ease of its transfer from maternal to fetal blood, highlights the concern that mercury exposure may be a potential contributor to the symptoms observed in children with ASD.

Insulin-like growth factor-1 (IGF-1)

Of the data suggesting a mercury-autism association, the capacity for mercury to alter levels of IGF-1 in particular was investigated (4). IGF-1 is a relatively small protein with structural similarities to insulin. Functions include growth regulation, neurogenesis, and cortical organization (chapter 6D).It has been shown that a loss of IGF-1 function can cause abnormalities in the development of neurons in animal models (5,6). Similar neuronal abnormalities have been observed in children with autism, and a decreased fetal concentration of IGF-1 has been associated with other neurological diseases as well (4).

Supporting these findings, rescue studies in animal models indicate that IGF-1 supplementation is able to ameliorate neuronal phenotypes similar to ASD (7). Furthermore, it is known that brain tissues of children with autism display a decrease in neuron myelination, a decrease in oligodendrocytes, and an increase in astrocytes (4). Mirroring these findings, a decrease in IGF-1 during development creates a parallel set of conditions (8).

With a clear understanding of the crucial role of IGF-1 for neuronal development, the molecular interaction of IGF-1 and mercury can be investigated. There is evidence that ionic mercury can inhibit IGF-1 activity in human neuroblastoma cells in a dose-dependent manner (9). Additionally, MeHg has been shown to decrease the motility of migrating neurons in the CNS with full motility restoration achieved by exogenous IGF-1 injection (10). If MeHg can inhibit both neuronal IGF-1 activity and motility with inhibition ameliorated by exogenous IGF-1 supplementation, this suggests the mechanism of mercury toxicity in neural development may involve IGF-1 signaling. If mercury is capable of inhibiting IGF-1 signaling within the developing nervous system, mercury exposure via maternal fish consumption could potentially be associated with the deficits observed in ASD.

Neuronal organization and myelination

In addition to a decrease in IGF-1, a defining characteristic of autism includes altered neuronal organization and myelination (chapter 6A,9A). Neurons in the prefrontal cortex of children with ASD show decreased myelination, a decrease in axon connectivity between brain regions, and an increase in short-spanning axon proliferation (11,12). Myelination of cortical axons is crucial for brain function and deviation from typical myelination patterns could be a contributing factor in autism (13). This decrease in long-distance connectivity is often coupled with growth of axons within designated regions of the brain (14). The proliferation of local dendrites may be a compensatory mechanism to offset the disruption of long-distant axon growth, but this remains to be proven. Of note, mercury also causes a decrease in myelination and neuron growth (15). Offering further support for this mechanism, oligodendrocytes, the cells responsible for myelinating neurons, display receptors for IGF-1. Additionally, mercury disrupts larger axons that travel greater distances in the brain with a higher specificity than smaller, local axons (16). Exposure to mercury could be a contributing cause of local axon proliferation and a decrease in neural connectivity across regions of the brain seen in patients with ASD (15, 16).

Hyperinflammatory state

In conjunction with neural architecture defects, it has become increasingly evident that inflammatory cytokines are elevated in ASD (chapters 6B,6C). Many of the major pro-inflammatory cytokines, including TNFα, IFNγ, MCP, and IL-6, are upregulated in ASD and contribute to a hyperinflammatory state (17,18). Intriguingly, mercury exposure has been correlated with an increased expression of TNFα, and IFNγ *in vivo* and is also able to stimulate pro-inflammatory cytokine release in isolated peripheral-blood mononuclear cells (19, 20).

Mercury can also activate microglia and astrocytes, which function as modulators of inflammation in the central nervous system (21). The over-activation of these cells leads to atypical inflammation and immune responses. Consistent with these observations, microglia and astrocyte activity is increased in patients with ASD (17). It may be hypothesized that atypical activity of these defense cells in the central nervous system is inducing an inflammatory state that acts in tandem with the altered brain connectivity seen in autism. Similar aspects of inflammation occurring in both mercury exposure and ASD exposure suggest a potential mechanistic association, or at least a co-morbidity.

Cerebral blood flow

Providing an additional association, cerebral blood flow is decreased in cases of mercury exposure and in autism. Following the Minamata disaster (Section I), it was shown that cerebellar blood flow was decreased in those exposed to high levels of mercury (22). Interestingly, blood flow was only reduced to the cerebrum, the area of the brain altered in ASD, and not the cerebellum. Despite an increase in the head circumference of children with autism compared to age-matched controls, cerebral blood flow is decreased, similar to what is observed with mercury poisoning (23). This hypoperfusion could potentially contribute to the altered function in the prefrontal cortex observed in ASD.

Mercury has additionally been shown to activate vascular endothelial cells, leading to an increase in phospholipase D and phospholipase A2 (24). In a similar manner, vascular endothelial markers are increased in children with autism (25). The hypoperfusive state and vascular endothelial cell activation observed in both ASD and mercury exposure provides another mechanistic similarity between the two conditions.

Conclusions

Despite the evidence indicating an apparent molecular and mechanistic connection between autism and mercury, additional research needs to be conducted to clarify this view. One of the most promising areas of investigation concerns the parallel molecular deficits related to IGF-1 signaling observed in both ASD and mercury toxicity. This neuropeptide has a wide range of actions encompassing many of the observed defects seen in autism and mercury exposure. Importantly, mercury has been shown to directly inhibit IGF-1, and IGF-1 receptors appear on cell types instrumental in maintaining cerebral architecture.

Mercury is able to accumulate in fetal tissues as a result of maternal exposure at high levels compared to similar toxins. This suggests that a critical amount of mercury obtained from fish consumption might lead to significant fetal deficits. While there is a well-documented set of similar phenotypes and molecular mechanisms in mercury exposure and autism, there is not enough evidence to warrant a conclusion of definitive causation. It is possible, for instance, that mercury toxicity provides an instructive experimental model of ASD, while the actual etiological factors in autism have not yet been identified. It may be that neonates with a propensity for autism are affected by precarious levels of mercury acting as an environmental trigger.

Chapter 5D, Section III: Mercury versus Omega-3 Fats

Tatiana Carillo, Dimple Chhatlani, Cynthia Clarke, Susan Ko, Victoria Pham

[In defining the recommended levels of fish consumption by pregnant women, a balance needs to be reached between the potentially harmful effects of mercury contamination on neural tissue and the nutritional value of omega-3 fats for the growing fetus. – Ed.]

Hypothesis

Fish are an important source of nutrients for proper neurological development in humans. Although fish consumption provides essential omega-3 fatty acids that promote fetal brain development, recent studies have emphasized the apparent correspondence between high fish consumption and autism spectrum disorders. The Seychelles Child Development Study (SCDS) evaluated prenatal methylmercury exposure from fish consumption over the course of 5 years (Section I). Although brain development is most crucial during fetal development, it continues for years postnatal; hence, continued exposure of methylmercury may have prolonged adverse effects. The SCDS main cohort collected data from postnatal exposure at different time points to establish causal relationship with methylmercury exposure and child neurological development (1). The study found associations with methylmercury biomarkers and child development, but no definite direct relationship.

Observations

The concern about women consuming fish during pregnancy is related to the potential for mercury poisoning. In the body, mercury is converted to methylmercury which binds to red blood cells and easily passes through the placenta to the developing fetus (mechanism – Section II). Potentially adverse effects of mercury poisoning include neurodevelopmental deficits which may increase the risk for autism in the newborn.

One of the main ways mercury enters human bodies is via consumption of fish that have retained mercury content. Similarly, fish accumulate mercury as they eat other fish containing the heavy metal. In this way, larger and/or older fish at the upper end of the food chain are known to have higher mercury content (2). Accordingly, dietary recommendations for pregnant women call for limiting fish consumption overall, and specifically for avoiding shark, swordfish, king mackerel, and tilefish. In response to these recommendations, many pregnant women simply avoid eating fish altogether. However, because fish are also a good dietary source of lean protein and omega-3 fatty acids which are essential nutrients for a developing fetus, eliminating an entire category of nutritious food is not desirable. To encourage pregnant women to consume appropriate amounts and types of fish, the Food and Drug Administration (FDA) teamed up with the Environmental Protection Agency (EPA) to enhance existing nutrition recommendations (see below).

Biological gradient effect of methylmercury ingestion

The purpose of the 2004 FDA/EPA Consumer Advisory was to emphasize the positive benefits of eating fish while minimizing exposure to mercury. The Advisory recommended that women who may become pregnant, pregnant women, and nursing mothers consume as much as 12 ounces (two average servings) per week of fish that are typically low in mercury (specifically mentioning the most commonly consumed lower mercury fish/shellfish, including shrimp, canned light tuna, salmon, pollock and catfish). The Advisory also explained that albacore ("white") tuna usually has more mercury than canned light tuna, so only one of the two average servings of fish allowed per week (or up to 6 ounces per week) should be albacore/white tuna.

Although most fish contain trace amounts of mercury, consumption of certain species should be avoided to prevent reaching potentially harmful levels. The species targeted were those that accumulated the highest levels of mercury, measured over a two decade time-span. This information is of value to the public and should be disseminated to provide guidance on acceptable levels of fish consumption before it poses a health threat.

Tilefish, swordfish, and shark ranked at the top of the list, with salmon at the bottom. When comparing mercury levels in commercially available and commonly eaten fish species, it can be observed in Table 1 that tilefish has the highest level at 1.45 ppm and salmon has the lowest level at 0.01 ppm (parts per million) (3).

Table 1: Examples of total mercury levels (ppm) in some commercially available fish species (n = sample size. FDA, 1990-2010) (3).

Species	Mean Mercury Concentration	n
Tilefish (Gulf of Mexico)	1.45 ppm	32
Swordfish	0.99	636
Shark	0.98	356
Mackerel King	0.73	213
Grouper (All Species)	0.45	53
Tuna (Fresh/Frozen, Albacore)	0.36	43
Tuna (Canned, Albacore)	0.35	451
Salmon (Canned)	0.01	34

Bluefish with different lengths were collected from the New Jersey Atlantic coast in 2011. Tissue dissections of the brain, kidney, liver, skin and scales, and red and white muscle were conducted. It was determined that mercury levels generally increased with fish size. Furthermore, results showed that liver tissue had the highest concentration of total mercury, while the skin or scales has the lowest amount compared to other tissue of bluefish (4). According to the United States Environmental Protection Agency (EPA) the reference dose of methylmercury to protect the nervous system was calculated to be 0.1 µg/kg body weight per day. These guidelines can be utilized during pregnancy to help determine a low toxicity diet (5).

Table 2: Total mercury (ppm, wet weight; µg/g) in bluefish collected from New Jersey using Kruskal–Wallis Chi-square. (sample size: n = 40; *skin/scale n = 15) (4).

Tissue	Mercury (mean ± SE)
White Muscle	0.32 ± 0.02 ppm
Red Muscle	0.37 ± 0.09
Brain	0.09 ± 0.01
Kidney	0.57 ± 0.09
Liver	0.38 ± 0.06
*Skin/Scales	0.05 ± 0.01

Additional research has been conducted on the link between fish consumption, blood mercury content, and the apparent risk for autism in the newborn. The Centers for Disease Control and Prevention conducts a series of surveys each year, known as the National Health and Nutrition Examination Survey (NHANES), collecting epidemiological data for the purpose of developing sound public health policy (6). A survey on the trends in blood mercury content and fish consumption among U.S. women of childbearing age found that the blood methylmercury level in women who consumed fish six or more times per month was well below the toxic level of 5.8 micrograms per liter (7). Also, the Seychelles Child Development Study, a large longitudinal cohort study, assessed the prevalence of autism-like behaviors in children born to mothers who consumed large amounts of ocean fish. No consistent association between prenatal mercury exposure and autism behaviors in the children was found among the 1784 Seychellois women participants with prenatal methylmercury levels 10-20 times higher than mothers in the United States (8) (Section II).

Wild vs. farmed fish

When pregnant women consider eating fish, they are often wary of high mercury levels in some fish. It is known that fish types have variable mercury content. For example, tuna contains more mercury than salmon. However, what about wild fish vs. farmed fish? Farmed fish are typically considered safer, especially during pregnancy, because they are raised in a controlled environment with known feedings.

According to a study in *Environmental Toxicology and Chemistry,* accumulation of mercury depends on various factors such as fish growth cycle, age, and trophic position (9). Trophic position is defined as the fish's position in the food chain - what the fish eats and who eats the fish. Therefore, it was observed that some of the larger fish generally have higher concentrations of mercury. Kelly et al. studied the levels of mercury in farmed and wild salmon from British Columbia, Canada due to the large amount of farmed salmon imported from there to the United States. They examined various species of salmon and reported higher concentrations of mercury in wild salmon compared to farmed salmon.

Another study conducted by Hites et al. assessed organic contaminants in farmed salmon. They performed a preliminary study which did not show a difference in levels of mercury between wild and farmed salmon (10). A third study conducted by Yamashita et al. found higher levels of mercury in farmed blue-fin tuna compared to the wild fish. Overall, the results are inconclusive and more studies should be conducted to increase the validity and reliability of any findings.

Cooked vs. uncooked fish

When a toxin is ingested, one must take into consideration the biological processing and breakdown it undergoes in the body. Although not much research exists on this matter, a study from the University of Montreal sought to elucidate the effects of cooked fish on the bioaccessibility of mercury (Hg). Bioaccessibility or availability is the dosage of any compound that reaches the systemic circulation after *in vitro* digestion. Spurred by previous studies that mercury consumption models vastly overestimated actual mercury levels in specific fish-eating populations, Ouedraogo et al. studied three fish species (tuna, mackerel and shark) prepared in three different ways (raw, boiled, and fried) and measured the mercury levels in dry weight. The results showed a slightly greater amount of methylmercury (dry weight) in boiled fish compared to fried and raw fish. However, they also reported that the bioaccessibility of mercury levels was higher in raw fish compared to boiled or fried fish (both had decreased bioaccessibility of Hg by 40% and 60%, respectively). Black/green tea and coffee were found to synergistically reduce the bioavailability of mercury during co-digestion. More studies will be needed to improve the reliability and validity of the findings; however, the nascent ideas of decreasing bioaccessibility of Hg through differing culinary preparations are promising, and warrant further consideration (11).

Omega-3 fatty acids

Fish consumption during pregnancy provides nutrients essential for proper fetal neurologic and cognitive development (chapter 6D). Cold water fatty fish such as salmon and tuna provide high levels of docosahexaenoic acid (DHA), an omega-3 fatty acid essential to proper brain development prenatally and even after childbirth (12). Inadequate intake of omega-3 fatty acids decreases DHA and increases omega-6 fatty acids in the brain. This leads to decrease in neurogenesis, neurotransmitter metabolism, and retarded cognitive abilities. Adequate maternal intake of nutrients rich in omega-3 fatty acids, such as fish and plant oils, is essential for fetal brain development.

Ingested omega-3 fatty acids are transferred to the developing fetus via the placenta. Restriction of omega-3 fatty acids in the maternal diet have been linked to decrease in neuronal body size, impaired mitotic cell migration, and decreased embryonic brain development (12). In spite of the beneficial nutrients found in fish, consumption during pregnancy has been restricted to limit methylmercury exposure to the fetus. Current FDA consumption guidelines limit the amount of fish intake to no more than 6 oz. per week during pregnancy as mercury poisoning prevention.

Mercury exposure during pregnancy has been associated with the onset of neuropathologic disorders in the offspring (13). One of the major factors contributing to methylmercury toxicity is its ability to accumulate in biological organisms, especially in aquatic animals such as fish. Swordfish, a top predator, occurs worldwide in temperate and tropic climates, predominantly the Gulf of Mexico and Pacific Ocean. They prey on king mackerel, herring, barracudinas, and crustaceans. The accumulation of methylmercury in swordfish is due to the ecological effect of biomagnifications: large predator fish consume smaller organisms rich in Methylmercury, thereby increasing their mercury levels exponentially (10). Swordfish have been shown to contain 0.5 parts per million of mercury, this level of mercury can lead to mental retardation, cerebral palsy, deafness and blindness.

Table 3. Typical omega-3 fatty acid level in various fish species.

Species	Source	Total Omega-3 Fatty Acid content* (μg/g)
King Mackerel	Marine	2.2
Salmon	Marine	1.9
Herring	Marine	1.8
Bluefin Tuna	Marine	1.6
Lake Trout	Freshwater	4.6
Canned Sardines	Marine	1.4
Red Snapper	Marine	0.2
Striped Bass	Freshwater	0.8
Pollock	Marine	0.5

*1)Wang, YJ, Miller LA, Ferren M, Addis PB (1990) Omega-3 fatty acid in Lake Superior fish, Journal of Food Service 1990; 55(1):71-3;

2) Exler J. (1987) Composition of foods: Finfish and Shellfish Products. Agriculture handbook No.8-15. Washington, DC. USDA.

Conclusions

Fish consumption in general has not been found to be linked with increased risk for autism in the newborn. However, moderation of fish consumption and the avoidance of certain fish for pregnant women may still be warranted due to other possible adverse effects of mercury on the fetus such as cognitive and motor deficits. For pregnant women who choose to limit their intake of fish, other dietary sources of omega-3 fatty acids (an important nutrient for fetal brain development) include walnuts, chia seeds, flax seeds, canola oil, soybean oil, and omega-3 fortified eggs.

[Note of caution: While this chapter has presented a review of published data on the subjects of mercury and omega-3 fatty acids in fish, it is essential that pregnant women or women anticipating a pregnancy in the near future should consult with their physician specialist on this subject before modifying their diets. – Ed.]

MATERNAL INFECTION; NEUROGENIC DISORDERS

Chapter 6A - Myelination

Katherine Redford

[Axonal myelin sheathing is fundamental for effective functioning of nerves, especially in the bran. Deficiencies of this insulating material is commonly found in brain biopsies of autistic children – Ed.]

Hypothesis

The cause for disruption of neuronal communication in the autistic brain is not yet completely understood. A current hypothesis is that myelin, the insulating structure in the human nervous system, undergoes departures from normal in individuals with autism. A number of studies have been conducted examining the brain of the autistic individual on a macroscopic level (1-3), in addition to looking at densely myelinated pathways (4,5) and microscopic changes in myelin in the post-mortem autistic brain (6). Significant changes to myelin integrity in the such brains have been observed, but the cause for these changes is not certain. Multiple theories have been suggested. These will be reviewed in this and other chapters of this book.

In order to understand these changes, their potential causes, and what they mean for the function of the nervous system in the autistic individual, we must first explore the role of myelin in some detail.

Observations

Myelin structure and function

Myelin is a substance found in the white matter of the nervous system (7). White matter refers to the parts of the central nervous system in the brain and the spinal cord that appear to be shiny and light in color (as opposed to gray matter, which is darker). The concentration of myelin is responsible for this color difference. Functionally, neurons serve as conductors of the electrical impulses acting as the messages of the central nervous system. Myelin sheathes increase the speed and accuracy of the information being sent.

Composed of both protein (mostly myelin basic protein and proteolipid protein) and lipid (primarily cerebroside, cholesterol, and phospholipids), myelin surrounds nerve axons as they travel from one part of the nervous system to the next. Oligodendrocytes (in the central nervous system) and Schwann cells (in the peripheral nerves) produce myelin using their cell membranes. The membrane coils around the axon in a spiral fashion and segmentally produces periodic interruptions, the nodes of Ranvier.

In unmyelinated fibers, surface conduction at the nerve surface is very high and depolarization happens steadily along the cell membrane, causing the transmission of the impulse to be very slow. Fibers that are myelinated, on the other hand, will only depolarize at the nodes of Ranvier. This allows the impulse to "jump" from node to node, resulting in rapid message transmission by saltatory conduction. This more efficient method of depolarization saves space, time, and energy when the nervous system communicates. While the reason is unclear, this increased conduction results in improved information processing in the human brain (8). Tracts are bundles of neuronal axons forming nerves with the brain. The velocity of impulse conduction is 50-100 times faster in myelinated nerve axons than in nonmyelinated ones. The adult human brain contains 100 billion neurons.

Development of myelin in the human brain

Myelin begins to develop in humans in the first and second trimesters of pregnancy, reaches a maximum rate within the first year of extrauterine life, and continues until the second or third decade. Myelination of axons in the central nervous system (CNS) is almost complete by the end of the second postnatal year. The brain is not myelinated all at once, but rather in stages which generally occur from deep to superficial, and posterior to anterior (8). As noted, most myelination occurs in the first post-natal year; the corpus collosum and the internal capsule are rapidly myelinated during this time (1). These two structures connect the two hemispheres of the brain, and the brain to the spinal cord, respectively. They are highly myelinated and are vital in the decision-making and reasoning processes of the CNS. One of the last portions of the brain to undergo myelination is the cerebral cortex, the outer portion of the front of the human brain, responsible for many higher level functions including perceptual awareness and thought (1) (chapters 3B-3F).

MYELINATION CONTROL

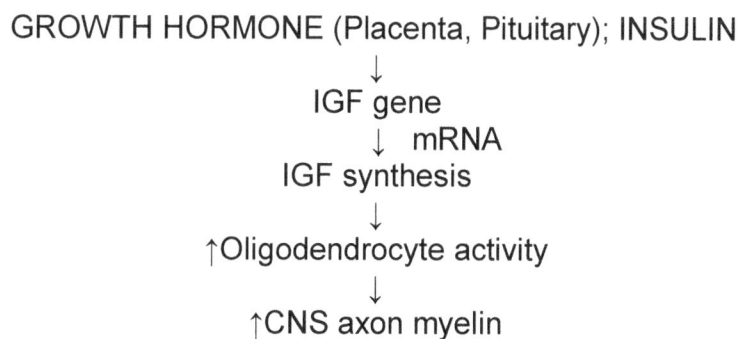

GROWTH HORMONE (Placenta, Pituitary); INSULIN
↓
IGF gene
↓ mRNA
IGF synthesis
↓
↑Oligodendrocyte activity
↓
↑CNS axon myelin

Role of myelin in autism

There are many studies investigating the structure of the central nervous system and of its myelin, specifically in autistic individuals. While information is constantly being updated and improved, a general trend has revealed itself. First, on a gross scale, the brain of an autistic child does not develop at the same rate as in a child without neurologic pathology (2). Second, certain parts of the brain have demonstrated decreased connectivity mainly due to decreased or disrupted myelination of white matter (4). Generally, connections in the autistic brain appear to be hindered or reduced over long pathways, and inefficient between adjacent parts of the brain, when compared to a control group (5).

MRI-based studies on autistic children have demonstrated that there is increased brain volume by the age of two to five years. Interestingly, this same study showed that older children with autism do not possess the enlarged volumes that younger subjects demonstrate, suggesting that there is abnormal regulation of brain growth in children with autism (2). Other studies had similar age-dependent findings (3) (chapter 6D). This may be due to defective patches in the cortex (see below).

Multiple studies have used diffusion tensor imaging studies to compare white matter in subjects with autism to a control group, with varying results (chapter 3A). These studies measure fractional anisotropy, the degree of density and directionality, and mean diffusivity (a value reflecting the displacement of molecules). Such measurements assess the integrity of myelin in a pathway; a high fractional anisotropy and a low mean diffusivity indicate normal white matter structure. A recently published meta-analysis of twenty-five such studies demonstrated significant reductions in the fractional anisotropy in the corpus callosum, left uncinate fasiculus, and left superior longitudinal fasiculus, as well as increased mean diffusivity in the corpus callosum and the superior longitudinal fasiculus bilaterally (4). These studies were performed after the diagnosis of autism and were compared to an undiagnosed control group; the patients were between the ages of 3 and 30 years.

Changes in these parts of the central nervous system correspond to the symptoms and classical presentation of autistic individuals (chapter 3C). The corpus callosum is the main connection between the two hemispheres and has the largest concentration of white matter in the brain. Connectivity disruption at the corpus callosum can cause impairments in social and emotional functioning as well as cognitive functioning performed by the cerebral hemispheres they connect (9). The superior longitudinal fasiculus connects the frontal to the occipital lobe, and is thought to play an important role in language processing (10), often deficient in individuals with ASD.

Moving to an even more microscopic level, a study performed at Harvard investigated changes in prefrontal axons in post-mortem brains of individuals diagnosed with autism. The investigation focused on regions of the brain that are responsible for social interaction and emotion. Overall, since these brains were from older adults, white matter density was overall similar in autistic individuals and unaffected controls, consistent with previous MRI findings (2,3). However, the investigation demonstrated that the number of white matter myelinated fibers meant to travel long distances were significantly fewer in the autistic individual, specifically in the area below the anterior cingulate cortex. Also in this region, autistic individuals have increased concentration of short fibers traveling to adjacent regions. Another part of the brain, the orbitofrontal cortex exhibited decreased myelin thickness under light and electron microscopes. Overall, these findings suggest inefficiency in pathways that affect emotion (6). As previously noted, myelin is vital for the efficient relay of neuronal conduction, and these regions of the brain are the areas where social interactions and emotions are processed. When there is hindered connectivity, an individual may present with difficulty in social interactions and emotion handling.

In looking at the complexity of the CNS and its development in the autistic patient, it seems that changes are notable in the brain as a whole, as well as in specific tracts composed of large amounts of white matter. In contrast, it is unclear to date what is occurring to cause these changes in myelination. Many theories have been suggested, each requiring further investigation.

Situations affecting structure, function, and concentration of myelin.

The reports in the research literature have identified many different changes that happen in the brain of the autistic individual throughout development and into adulthood. A common finding is the disruption of normal myelin structure and function, especially in parts of the brain that control the processing of emotion and decision making (2-4,6,9). Currently, there is no consensus as to what causes these changes but many investigations have suggested possibilities. Below are some of these hypotheses. Many of these topics are discussed in greater detail in other chapters of this book as well.

Autoimmunity

Myelin-associated glycoprotein is a molecule that makes up part of the structure of the oligodendrocyte's processes that surrounds axons. It appears to play an important role in the transmission of a nerve impulse and in the regeneration of young neurons. One study investigated the levels of anti-myelin associated glycoprotein antibodies in the blood of thirty-two autistic children, compared to thirty-two age-matched control unaffected children (11). Autistic children were found to have a significantly higher level of these antibodies in their serum, and their concentrations correlated with the severity of their autism (chapter 6E). Also, the autistic patients reported a higher rate of auto-immune diseases in their family history, suggesting that this may play an important role in the development of autism in some people.

Another study undertook the task of assessing the levels of neuron-specific antigens in the serum of children with autism. Included among these antigens were myelin basic protein (MBP), myelin-associated glycoprotein (MAG) and myelin oligodendrocyte glycoprotein (MOG). All were found to be elevated in patients with autism (12). Additionally, these children had elevated levels of cross-reactive proteins from milk, Chlamydia pneumoniae, and Streptococcus Group A, suggesting that these cross-reactive proteins and infectious agents may be affecting neuronal tissues negatively.

Hyperserotonemia

Serotonin plays an important role in neurological development before it takes on a neurotransmitter role in the mature brain. In the early human brain, there is a refining process where vital connections are retained and unnecessary ones are eliminated. Serotonin and its receptors play a part in this process (13). Additionally, myelin basic protein (MBP) is involved in the process of myelination in the developing brain. Auto-antibodies to MBP and the neurotransmitter, serotonin, have been found to be simultaneously elevated in many individuals with autism (chapter 6D). One study addressed the obvious and important question: Are these two findings related? Is serotonin contributing to the autoimmunity to MBP? A study of fifty children with autism found levels of both to be high, but concluded there was no significant correlation between serotonin levels, anti-MBP antibodies, and the severity of autism in these patients (14).

IGF-1

Insulin-like growth factor 1 (IGF-1) plays a vital function in normal myelination as the central nervous system develops. A number of studies have correlated decreased levels of IGF-1 in the autistic individual's serum and myelination activity. An investigation recently published suggested following infants from birth for changes in serum IGF-1 concentration and determining if those with abnormal low levels developed autism later in life (15). Such a prospective study might define a measure of causality as a potential mechanism for the etiology of autism. It has been proposed that neonatal measurement of umbilical cord levels of IGF, anti-MBP, and serotonin may serve as a biomarker (the "Autism Index") for the potential of future development of autism (16) (chapter 6D).

A recent investigation reported "focal disruption of cortical laminar architecture" in the brains of autistic children (17). This could be consistent with dysmelination in such individuals. Of particular interest is the observation that newborn females reach a peak myelination rate earlier than males (18). Such a phenomenon may explain why autism is four times more common in boys than girls (chapter 1C).

Conclusions

The reports in the literature have demonstrated that disruption of myelin structure and function are commonly seen in individuals with autism. However, there is little consistent evidence identifying what causes this. Most of the investigations to date have used small patient cohorts and have linked autism with increased levels of antibodies against neurological antigens without demonstrating the mechanism by which these entities cause symptoms.

Such research may well be a stepping stone to delving deeper into the understanding of what causes autism, but there is much to be elucidated and documented. Many studies have demonstrated high correlations, but none to date have convincingly demonstrated causality. With multiple investigations identifying dysmyelination in autistic individuals, there needs to be further investigation into a potential mechanism for this change. Large cohorts of infants should be followed prospectively from birth until the time when psychogenic symptoms present themselves in order to relate them to cause. It is impossible to rule out any possibilities yet without such a comprehensive investigation.

Despite the uncertainty surrounding these myelination changes, there is hope that a focus can be placed on finding a solution to the challenges facing the increasing number of families facing the diagnosis of autism.

Chapter 6B – Infection

Bina Kviatkovsky, Gabrielle Rozenberg, Cindy Agu

[The occurrence of infections during pregnancy in the gravida can initiate and stimulate Maternal Inflammatory Activation leading to an increased incidence of autism in the infant-. – Ed.]

Hypothesis

If given the opportunity, would you receive a flu vaccination?

Should I get a flu vaccination while I'm pregnant?

How does the flu vaccine affect my unborn baby?

If I get sick, does the baby get sick too?

These are many of the questions expecting mothers ask doctors when it comes to the administration of vaccines while pregnant. In April, 2013, the Centers for Disease and Prevention (CDC) conducted a survey on 1,702 self-selected pregnant women asking whether or not they had received the flu vaccination while pregnant. According to the survey 50.5% of women reported receiving the vaccine before or during their pregnancy. However, what about the other 49.5% of pregnant women? Why are pregnant women deciding not to receive the vaccination? According to the survey conducted by the CDC, one of the reasons why women did not receive the vaccine is because they were concerned about the possibility of actually getting the flu after receiving the vaccination. This is an interesting finding because research is now looking into the possibility of maternal immune activation caused by viral, bacterial and fungal infection as the possible cause of autism.

Observations
Maternal Infections

Recent research has focused on the connection between maternal infection while pregnant and childhood autism. Expecting mothers are generally informed about the precautions that are needed to be taken in order to prevent infection. These bacterial, viral and parasitic agents, which have the ability to enter the fetal bloodstream, are known as the TORCH infections. The TORCH group of infections includes toxoplasma, rubella, cytomegalovirus, herpes simplex virus and a group designated as other. This group consists of such infectious agents as syphilis, varicella-zoster virus, measles, mumps, parvovirus, adenovirus, HIV and influenza. These organisms are currently known to cause a variety of complications, including spontaneous abortion, intrauterine growth restriction, prematurity and postnatal infection. With this knowledge researchers have proposed that prenatal or early infantile viral infections maybe a factor in the genesis of autism.

The placenta houses the growing fetus and allows for gas exchange, the elimination of waste, and the delivery of nutrients. This process occurs by the delivery of maternal blood to the chorionic villi of the placenta. The maternal blood bathes the villi allowing for the exchange to occur. If the mother has parasitic, viral or bacterial infection depending on the makeup of the invading organism, this could lead to the possible infection of the fetus. An infection that is the result of a bacterium will trigger the production of cytokines from placental tissue itself, triggering adverse reactions [1]. Infection of the mother will also cause for an increase in her own cytokines, which may also have the ability to cross the placenta leading to central nervous system developmental defects.

The central nervous system of the developing fetus is highly susceptibility to damage [2]. Researchers have studied the effects that the TORCH organisms have on the developing central nervous system (CNS). Toxoplasma, rubella, cytomegalovirus (CMV) and herpes simplex virus (HSV) are all known to cause CNS damage. Toxoplasma specifically leads to altered human behavior, while rubella, cytomegalovirus and HSV cause a various range of CNS abnormalities for instance encephalitis and mental retardation [3]. Studies have also suggested that prenatal exposure to rubella virus CMV increases the risk of Autism Spectrum Disorder (ASD) in children [3].

These finding lead to studies that focused on the effects of viral infection on the developing fetus [4]. The response to pathogen exposure depends on a range of factors, which include maternal immune status, the infecting pathogen, the strain of virus, the developmental stage of the fetus, and the pathogen concentration infecting the fetus [2]. When a woman becomes pregnant her immune system weakens causing an increase in susceptibility to infections. Intrauterine infection and inflammation may lead to fetal CNS injury by cellular injury or due to such insults as hypoxia [1].

A fairly recent study that took place in Denmark further investigated the possibility of autism being caused by prenatal viral infections. Atldortir, the principal investigator, began his research with insight on the fact that infectious disease was a common path to maternal immune activation during pregnancy. The goal was to determine the occurrence of common infections, febrile episodes and use of antibiotics reported by the mother during pregnancy and the risk for autism spectrum disorder in offspring [5]. Research was conducted on a population based cohort which consisted of over 96,000 children aged 8-14 and born in Denmark from the years 1997-2003. Information on infections, febrile episodes and the use of antibiotics was self-reported through telephone interviews during pregnancy and early postpartum.

Atladottir's data suggested that there was inadequate evidence in support of his original hypothesis, which stated that mild common infectious diseases or febrile episodes during pregnancy were directly associated with an increased risk of childhood autism [5]. However, he did note that maternal viral infection during the first three months of pregnancy and maternal bacterial infection during the third through sixth months of pregnancy were found to be associated with a diagnosis of ASD. His research also suggested that maternal influenza infections were associated with a "twofold increase in the risk of infantile autism" and babies whose mothers had fever that lasted for a long period of time while pregnant were three times more likely to become autistic [6]. It was also reported that viral infections that occurred specifically during the third trimester of pregnancy lead to a greater risk of developing autism [5].

A focused examination was conducted by Libbey et al. in 2005. This study suggested that chronic prenatal infection could lead to high levels of cytokines such as interleukins 1, 2, and 6. These cytokines could either be produced in the developing fetal brain or could be produced in the mother and then cross the under developed fetal blood brain barrier and potentially cause abnormal central nervous system development. Animal models have been used to test the effects of cytokines produced by the maternal immune response and the later development of autism in children. The models focused on the actual or artificial infection of pregnant mice or rats. The simulated response involved the activation of the maternal immune response devoid of the actual pathogen. This was done by injecting synthetic double-stranded polyribonucleotide [poly (I:C)] into the expecting mother, triggering an antiviral immune response. They also did the same with the injection of lipopolysaccharides (LPS) to trigger the antibacterial immune response. One infectious agent of interest was the human influenza virus. It is believed that an influenza infection at early to mid-gestation triggers behavioral abnormalities, believed to indicate that maternal antiviral immune response has an effect on fetal brain development.

Researchers further investigated the effects of the antiviral response by injecting Lewis rats with Bornea disease virus and observing its affects. They noted that rats born to these mothers demonstrated autistic behavior. These experiments among others give light to the fact that the antiviral immune response could in fact disrupt normal fetal brain development leading to autism like developmental abnormalities [2].

Maternal Immune Activation (MIA)

Related research suggested that there may be a link between maternal infection and ASD due to maternal immune activation (MIA). MIA includes the response to any infection in the mother during pregnancy that sets off an immune response. MIA has been linked to developmental defects such as ASD in the fetus (using rat models) in the first two trimesters, especially the middle to late first trimester [7].

Findings have supported the postulated MIA association in the first trimester with the development of ASD by statistically analyzing and evaluating 10,000 ASD cases as well as a smaller but still significant risk in the second trimester, with bacterial infections [8].

In order to understand the possible link between ASD and MIA, it is pertinent to appreciate the mechanism behind MIA. When an infection occurs in the mother, her internal immune response includes an increase in molecules called chemokines. Chemokines are molecules that regulate the immune system by directing lymphocyte development (B cells and T cells) and control immune cell migration to sites of inflammation [9]. However, inflammation may also result in a response to the infection, which may alter the fetal environment, leading to possible cellular and tissue damage. Inflammation in the mother has also been associated with central nervous system defects in the fetus [10]. Additionally, once exposed to MIA, the child may be subjected to altered cytokine and chemokine levels from the mother, which could lead to long lasting detrimental developmental effects throughout child's life.

There is strong evidence that points to the maternal cytokine response as a vital component in maternal immune activation and endocrine changes within the placenta, which then leads to changes in fetal neural development [7]. Several cytokines have been noted to play a key role in MIA, including interleukin 6 (IL-6), tissue necrosis factor alpha (TNF-α), IL-12, and IL-1. Special significance exists with IL-6 and the MIA process in particular. As will be discussed later in this chapter, MIA up-regulates pro-inflammatory cytokines, such as IL-6, in the brain and blood of the fetus.

Different models have been used to test this MIA response. In various studies, both bacterial and viral stimuli were implanted in pregnant non-primate animal models, and the resulting chemokine and cytokine levels as well as the effects of these on the behavior of the offspring were measured. The stimuli used in these models included influenza virus, synthetic double stranded RNA (which mimics influenza virus), and bacterial lipopolysaccharide (LPS; found on the surface of gram negative bacteria). Mouse models tested for autistic-like behavior (defined as elevated anxiety, latent inhibition, and working memory) [7]. These behavioral patterns are exhibited from infancy through adulthood.

Two hypotheses have been proposed to determine how the MIA leads to pathological and behavioral changes. The first hypothesis involves the contribution of maternal cytokines to altering the fetal brain [7]. The second comprises placental inflammation, causing a disruption in the transfer of oxygen and nutrients to the fetus, which can subsequently lead to hypoxia and cellular stress (see chapter 3G) [10].

Current data suggest that maternal cytokines play a key role in normal brain development and function, as indicated by cytokine receptors found on neuronal and glial cells [7,11]. Cytokines function to mediate many aspects of the central nervous system development [11]. They possess the innate ability to regulate gene expression by activating signal transduction pathways that regulate transcription factors. Additionally, normal physiologic levels required by the cytokines vary only slightly compared those which pathologic changes in the host. Thus, homeostasis exists to keep these levels in balance. If the levels are disrupted by MIA, pathologic changes can result [7].

Induction of maternal cytokines alters their expression in the fetal brain including, but not limited to the following molecules: IL-6, IL-1b, IL-17, IL-13, monocyte chemotactic protein 1 (MCP-1) and macrophage inflammatory protein (MIP1a). In one study, 23 cytokines were measured in the blood and three different brain regions (frontal cortex, cingulate cortex and hippocampus) control (saline-injected) and ASD offspring. In both groups, the cytokines were found to be present throughout their lifespan and modulated in an age and region specific manner. Notably, in the MIA/ASD group, the frontal and cingulate cortices showed elevated pro- and anti-inflammatory cytokines and chemokines early on in the post-natal life, followed by a decrease from the normal levels in the adolescent years (see chapter 6D). This was then followed by a steady rise of cytokines compared to normal adulthood levels [7].

More data which report that cytokines play a critical role during the formation of synapses (neuronal connections) and plasticity (learning), a decrease in cytokine levels relative to the controls, have demonstrated altered brain connectivity in individuals with ASD. The varying levels of cytokines throughout the lifespan of individuals with ASD suggest that MIA leads to chronic changes in the fetal brain cytokine levels, which then mediate alterations in the central nervous system (brain and spinal cord), and influence and alter the behaviors of the affected child [7].

While MIA leads to changes in the levels of pro-inflammatory cytokines (such as IL-6, and tumor necrosis factor alpha; TNF-α), this phenomena also changes the levels of anti-inflammatory cytokines and chemokines in the blood and brain of affected offspring. This indicates that it may be the disruption of the balance between the many pro- and anti-inflammatory molecules that leads ultimately to autistic behavior, as opposed to changes in a solitary chemokine [7].

Based on the mechanism by which inflammatory cytokines may affect fetal development, one way to explore the effects that these molecules have on the placenta and the fetal environment. The developing fetus relies on the mother to supply oxygen, and vital nutrients such as glucose, which are transferred through the placenta into the fetal circulation. During the MIA process, inflammation may alter the placental tissue and consequently disrupt the transfer of these critical supplements to the fetus. This is thought to lead to the induction of a number of genes associated with hypoxia (chapter 3G), oxidative cellular stress and cellular death (apoptosis) (see chapter 4B). As a consequence, cellular stress and hypoxia in the fetal brain are likely to result [10].

There are several gene families that are regulated during the hypoxic conditions in the fetal environment. The most commonly altered gene family is BH3, which is a family of pro-cellular death genes. The second most altered protein is alpha hemoglobin stabilizing gene, otherwise known as erythroid associated factor or, *eraf*. The main task of eraf is to remove reactive oxygen species (ROS) created by an excess of alpha-hemoglobin, which can be damaging to cells. Once these genes are turned off, tissue damage most likely ensues. In most cases, this leads to permanent damage to the developing fetus [10].

Hypoxic stress can also affect the neurons in the developing CNS. The fetal cerebral cortex is primarily composed of two main types of neurons: Glutamergic pyramidal projections and GABAergic (γ-aminobutyric acid) interneurons (see chapters 3B-3F). The loss of the latter due to hypoxic stress is responsible for the excitatory neuronal firing that may cause seizure-like activity. The cognitive deficits seen in autism are in part due to excitatory/inhibitory imbalance caused by the loss of GABAergic interneurons. Improper cortical interneuron development and function may play a role in maladaptive social behaviors associated with autism [10].

As previously noted, the placenta acts as the selective barrier between the maternal and the fetal circulation. Many nutrients and immunoglobulins (IgG) can cross the placenta; cytokines diffuse through as well and can be protective to the growing fetus or cause harmful outcomes. The key cytokine causing the latter effect is interleukin-6 (IL-6) [8]. Elevated maternal IL-6 can cross the placenta after MIA and activate the immune cells in the decidua (uterine lining in pregnancy which forms the maternal part of the placenta). This then activates the Janus Kinase (JAK) signal transducer and activator of transcription 3 (STAT3) pathway (shown in figure 1), resulting in activation and elevation of more pro-inflammatory cytokines [8]. The IL-6 induction of JAK/STAT leads to an increase of acute phase proteins (synthesized from the mother's liver), which also contributes to an inflammatory response. While these inflammation stimulating proteins (e.g.SOCS3; suppressor of cytokine 3) are activated, placental growth hormone is down regulated. This down regulation leads to a reduction of insulin like growth factor binding protein 3 (IGFBP3), and insulin like growth factor 1 (IGF1). All of the above changes in endocrine factors may ultimately lead to placental pathophysiology. These changes have also been associated with long term behavioral deficits linked to autism (see chapter 3C) [8].

Although there is much work to be done to move forward in our understanding of this autism spectrum disorder, recent studies show promising methods to combat the negative effects of MIA on the fetus. Numerous therapeutic approaches both during pregnancy and postnatally, have shown encouraging results in attenuating autistic behaviors in the MIA offspring. For example, researchers have developed antibodies against IL-6, which have been shown to be effective in combating the inflammatory JAK2/STAT3 pathway [8]. The anti-inflammatory cytokine, IL-10, intrinsically blocks the inflammatory effects of MIA. However, if IL-10 is increased in the absence of MIA, this can also lead to behavioral abnormalities. This emphasizes the delicate balance between pro and anti-inflammatory cytokines in maintaining normal development.

An example of a compound that attenuates the adverse outcome of MIA is N-acetyl-cysteine. Pregnant mice were infected with lipopolysaccharide (found in the outer membrane of gram negative bacteria and elicits a strong immune response) and pre-treated with N-acetyl-cysteine in an experiment to determine the benefits of the substance [12]. Normally, N-acetyl-cysteine binds to glutamate receptors in the fetus, which leads to an increased calcium influx. In this study, this influx of calcium suppressed the fetal inflammatory response to LPS and prevented many of the behavioral effects of maternal LPS infection [8,12].

Another example of a class of compounds that weaken the MIA signal is the bioflavonoids. These are compounds found in plants products. They have a protective role in MIA offspring by dampening the signal responsible for the pathological increase in cytokine expression (such as IL-6 and TNF-α), as well as the attenuation of the JAK2/STAT3 pathway which has been implicated in ASD. This was supported by the LPS microglial model [11, 13]and mouse models [14]. Two particular bioflavonoids have specific importance to MIA are diosmin, a structural analog of luteolin, and luteolin. Diosmin was studied *in-vivo* in conjunction with IL-6 injection in pregnant mice. The data showed a decrease in pro-inflammatory cytokine levels such as IL-1β and TNF-α in the fetal rat brain by almost 50 %, as well as an attenuation of the IL-6 (invoking the abnormal behavior observed in MIA/adult offspring). IL-6 has been discussed as being crucial to the development of ASD; therefore, the attenuation of its levels was demonstrated to lessen the behavioral changes observed in ASD offspring. The other bioflavonoid, luteolin was studied *in-vitro* and similar results to diosmin (as discussed above) were observed. It is important to note that luteolin inhibited JAK2 and STAT3 phosphorylation by almost 50 % [13,14]. This study evaluated the protective doses in mice using FDA guidelines and applying comparable values to humans.

Conclusions

MIA is a complex process that results in detrimental changes to the developing fetus, specifically to the CNS. There are many mechanisms that seem to work synchronously, such as the imbalance of cytokine levels during the critical milestones in the CNS development in combination with the hypoxic environment (generated by the infection) that result in the observed ASD behaviors.

With the continuation of research in this area, new diagnostic and treatment options are developing and show great promise for the future of ASD intervention. If we look back at the classical TORCH infections, we see that there are a number of viral infections included in the group. As discussed in this section, research has focused primarily on infections such as influenza and how these can lead to maternal infection which may progress to devastating outcomes (i.e. learning, behavioral and developmental delay) on the evolving fetus. Potentially preventative measures may be taken by the pregnant mother to substantially decrease the risk of ASD development by getting an annual flu vaccine early in gestation. According to the Center for Disease Control and Prevention (CDC), pregnant women are significantly susceptible to influenza infections compared to non-pregnant women and recommend that pregnant women get their influenza vaccine at any period prior or during their pregnancy to avoid potential harm to the woman and/or the developing fetus. Although the development of autism has not been attributed to one single cause or factor, arming a prospective mother with the knowledge of how to reduce the developing fetus' risk of developing ASD is paramount.

Chapter 6C – Inflammation

Mina Mosaad, Maryan Nasralah, Thomas Quinn, James Yu

[The apparent deleterious effect of inflammatory processes on fetal and neonatal brain development may be the result of excess circulatory interleukins. – Ed.]

Hypothesis

The nature of autism spectrum disorder (ASD) truly is a spectrum not only in phenotype, but in pathogenic mechanisms too. Various factors are associated with the pathogenesis of autism, and in many cases, there is more than one single mechanism that can account for the etiology of each specific aberration. Considering the multifactorial nature of ASD, a thorough study on the intricacies pertaining to the numerous implicated mechanisms is a necessity for developing an understanding how and why autism manifests as it does.

This chapter will investigate the role of inflammation in the pathogenesis of ASD. The chapter will first examine the implications of systemic inflammation mediated by mast cell activation, discuss the inflammatory role of microglia in neuroinflammatidiscern the transient and long-term effects of inflammation on neuronal function and development, study the various inflammatory mediators and signaling cascades implicated in autism, and conclude with an exploration on potential anti-inflammatory therapeutic modalities for ASD using the lessons learned.

Observations

Mast cell activation in utero and autism susceptibility

A fetus's condition in utero has always been a main concern in prenatal care. With more research in ASD, it is becoming more evident how factors like stress and the environment an expecting mother is exposed to may affect her fetus. With the apparent growing incidence of autism, research has begun to show a correlation with mast cell activation.

Mast cells contain heparin and histamine, which are substances with the capacity to cause inflammation and potential injury to body tissues. Mast cells have a variety of activators, but their activation in utero has now been linked to inflammation in the brain of the fetus. According to TC Theohardies; "In utero inflammation can lead to preterm labor and has itself been strongly associated with adverse neurodevelopmental outcomes. Premature babies have about four times higher risk of developing ASD and are also more vulnerable to infections…" (1). Later in the chapter we will explore how mast cell activation can lead to neurological damage and potential development of autism. The resulting in utero inflammation can also cause preterm labor, increasing the risk even more for the development of ASD, rendering a vicious cycle.

Evidence of mast cell's link to autism can be seen in the prevalence of "allergic-like" symptoms in children with ASD (1). Mast cells are critical in the manifestations of allergies. In a case control study references by Theoharides et. al., allergic problems like asthma, atopic dermatitis and high serum IgE were present in 70% of Asperger patients, while food allergies were noted more in autistic children than in the healthy control group (1). Another study showed that 30% of autistic children had a family member with a history of allergies (2). Additionally, a report specified that the prevalence of ASD is 10 times greater in mastocytosis patients, patients that have mast cell activation in the skin, urticarial pigmentosa for example (1).

Environmental factors triggering the activation of mast cells

There are specific factors triggering the activation of mast cells in the brain of an individual with ASD. Environmental and neuropeptide triggers are important factors that trigger this cascade. Two related factors are; mammalian target of rapamycin (mTOR) and neurotensin. Both of are crucial components that work hand in hand to stimulate mast cells. Mammalian target of rapamycin (mTOR) is a kinase that is a component of the phosphoinositide 3-kinase (PI3K) pathway that mediates the regulation of growth and cell survival signaling. (2)

On the other hand, neurotensin is a neuropeptide (3). Neurotensin is released along with corticotropin releasing hormone under times of stress stimulating the brain's mast cells. Interestingly, neurotensin levels are increased in the serum of children with ASD, a role of stimulating mast cell secretion of mitochondrial adenosine triphosphate and DNA. Corticotropin-releasing hormone, neurotensin, and environmental toxins could further trigger the already activated mTOR, leading to stimulation of the brain's mast cells in those areas responsible for ASD symptoms (4).

Along with these intrinsic factors, there are important extrinsic environmental stress factors that target mast cell activation. Prenatal stress releases excessive amounts of corticotropin-releasing hormone (CRH) from the hypothalamus, which has pro-inflammatory effects via mast cell activation (1). CRH can cross the placenta and can even be produced by the placenta when responding to external stressors.

Increased CRH serum levels are seen in mothers who delivered preterm babies. It is becoming more evident that preterm babies have a strong correlation with autism. In a retrospective study it was seen that children born <33 weeks gestation had a two-fold increase in the risk for autism, 21% of those born <28 weeks gestation were diagnosed with autism, and 26% of those cases with a birth weight less than 1500 g tested positive for autism (1).

One of the most alarming effects of elevated CRH is its ability to disrupt the blood brain barrier (BBB) through mast cell activation. The disruption of the BBB leads to serum auto-antibodies against brain proteins, thus causing inflammation (an important factor of the pathogenesis of ASD). Indeed, serum of mothers and children with autism have shown auto-antibodies against brain proteins, especially against the cerebellum, that have cross-reacted with encephalitogenic proteins from milk, Chlamydia pneumonia and group A Streptococcus (1).

Another potential environmental trigger neurotoxicity is mercury (II) chloride (chap. 4C, 4D, 5D). According to a study done to find the effects of mercury on mast cell activation, mercury (II) chloride triggers the release of VEGF and IL-6 .VEGF is an inducer of inflammation and IL-6 is a cytokines that aids in maturation of mast cells. The BBB acts as a gatekeeper that keeps away not only pathogens, but also components that could harm the brain (5).

According to the study, there is a positive correlation between high levels of IL-6, VEGF, and high mercury(II) chloride. Data support the hypothesis that the inflammatory cytokines which induce inflammation and maturation of mast cells are increased in cases of exposure to mercury(II) chloride, and therefore can be a co-factor leading to ASD. (5)

Another report, which looked at children of nurses who were exposed to certain heavy metal pollutants in their area of residency during the mother's pregnancy and birth, shows a correlation of heavy metal toxicity to the incidence of ASD. The study showed that mothers who were exposed to high levels of lead, manganese, methylene chloride, mercury, and nickel had a higher risk of conceiving children with autism, there were 279 males affected as opposed to 46 females. The figure below shows the correlation of heavy metal exposure to diseased children; it is important to note that exposure to mercury resulted in one of the highest odds ratio of developing ASD. This fact correlates to the previous study, of exposure to mercury (II) chloride, in that high mercury levels can lead to increased VEGF and IL-6 and therefore induce inflammation and maturation of mast cells (3)

Microglial model of autism pathogenesis

A mounting body of literature suggests that the progression of (ASD) may be influenced by immune mediators during early development of the brain. Many of these theories revolve around abnormal activity of microglia, the resident macrophages of the central nervous system (7). Under normal conditions, microglia exhibit sentinel-like activity, responding to infection and monitoring and maintaining neuronal function within a localized region of the brain. Following an insult to the central nervous system, microglia produce a host of cytokines that mediate neuroinflammation. Microglia are also responsible for synaptic stripping, a process that is characterized by the pruning of diseased or dysfunctional neurons, promoting a remapping of neural circuitry. This phenomenon has been suggested to be active during pre- and post-natal brain development and may have considerable implications in the pathogenesis of autism through altered or augmented microglial activity during early development (8).

Aberrant microglial activity has been suggested to persist into adulthood based on recent studies that demonstrate excessive microglial activation in the brains of autism. These studies examine this hypothesis from a pathological, molecular, and clinical perspective. The symptoms of increased microglial activation correlate with deficiencies in language and cognitive and motor function, as seen in ASD (7).

The ongoing neuroinflammation caused by microglia has been examined from multiple perspectives. Several studies have revealed activated microglia in post-mortem brain tissue of autistic subjects, indicating the presence of chronic inflammation that is thought to persist from childhood to adulthood. A study by Tetreaul et al, compared the densities of microglia in different parts of ASD brains (9). Microglia were found in increased densities in two areas of the cerebral cortex that are functionally and anatomically different. Therefore, the authors concluded that microglia are likely denser throughout the cerebral cortex in autistic brains (7,9).

Another experiment investigated Rett syndrome, a neurodevelopmental disorder in which patients exhibit autism-like behavior. This disorder is characterized by language, motor, and cognitive defects due to synaptogenesis impairment. A mouse model of this impairment causes changes in the brain such as decreased neuron size and decreased dendritic branching. Rett Syndrome has been linked to a gene, methyl CpG binding protein 2 (MECP2) which represses transcription. It is thought to be expressed in all cell types of the brain. A mouse model of Rett syndrome was used and phagocytic activity was shown to be strongly reduced. Mice with a missing MECP2 gene have poor locomotor function and shorter life spans. It was shown that when the MECP2 gene was reintroduced to the mice missing the MECP2 gene, these symptoms partially improved. The results of this experiment suggest that microglial function, particularly phagocytic activity, is essential for the maintenance of neuronal activity (8).

Studies done on samples of cerebrospinal fluid taken from living ASD patients revealed increased levels of proinflammatory cytokines, such as tumor necrosis factor-α (TNF-α), interleukin (IL)-6, and chemokine (IL-8) (7). These results further support the hypothesis that increased neuroinflammation plays an important role in ASD.

The chronic neuroinflammation noted in autism has been suggested to be attributed toward abnormal expression of nuclear factor kappa-light-chain enhancer of activated B cells (NF-$_\kappa$B), which can result in chronic and excessive inflammation. A study of human post-mortem brain tissue of the orbitofrontal cortex revealed increased expression levels of NF-$_\kappa$B in neurons, astrocytes, and microglia compared to controls. It was concluded that NF-$_\kappa$B is aberrantly expressed in ASD subjects in the orbitofrontal cortex as part of the molecular cascade resulting in neuroinflammation. Another study of autistic children's blood samples also yielded similar results, demonstrating a significant increase of NF-$_\kappa$B as compared to controls (7).

Glutathione (GSH) is also thought to play a role, as it mediates microglial activation. Astrocytes supply GSH to microglia and neurons. However, when reduced glutathione is depleted, microglia and astrocytes are activated and release proinflammatory cytokines such as TNF-α and IL-6. In addition, the depletion of glutathione may render neurons sensitive to cell death due to oxidative stress. Studies have demonstrated that autistic subjects have inadequate GSH production, due to abnormalities in the transulfuration pathway, where GSH is made. Another study demonstrated low plasma GSH levels in ASD, which would provide a possible explanation for the increased microglial activation seen in ASD patients. However, oxidative stress due to microglial activation can also deplete GSH levels, resulting in a cascade of events that further induces GSH depletion. Lastly, there has been evidence suggesting that depletion of neuronal GSH results in increased production of cytotoxic nitric oxide (NO) (7).

When microglia are activated, they release large amounts of NO (nitric oxide) and superoxide as an attack mechanism. NO metabolites are derived from the cytotoxic effector enzymes such as neuronal nitric oxide synthase (nNOS), endothelial-NOS (eNOS), constitutive-NOS (cNOS), and inducible-NOS (iNOS), the latter of which is activated by IFN-γ, the bacterial products lipopolysaccharide (LPS), and to a lesser extent TNF-α and IL-1β (10). Elevated plasma levels of NO have been seen in autistic children (11). High concentrations of NO damage cells by oxidizing surrounding nucleic acids, proteins, and lipids, resulting in neuronal cell death, and may disrupt normal brain synaptic connections and neurodevelopment in ASD (12).

Many studies indicate that ASD symptoms result from disrupted connectivity between the different regions of the brain and appear to be most severe in the later-developing regions of the cortex (chap. 3B-3F). A study using fMRI showed decreased functional connectivity in the brains of those with ASD compared with control subjects, including regions involved in sensory and emotional processing (13) (chapter 3C). Similar connectivity abnormalities have been noted in studies of both children and adults. It has also been found that greater underconnectivity abnormalities are correlated with more severe ASD symptoms.

The hypothesis that excessive microglial activation plays a role in ASD is very interesting. The role of microglia warrants further investigation to more clearly delineate its role in this complex disorder. There are studies which suggest a role for excessive microglial activation in the development of ASD.

Neuroinflammation in ASD and an established framework for comparison

The central nervous system (CNS) is usually considered immune privileged, with limited access for leukocytes due to the BBB. Increased levels of inflammatory mediators, either originating from a peripheral inflammatory response or an underlying neurodegenerative process, can increase BBB permeability, subsequently contributing to the initiation or progression of focal neuroinflammation within the CNS (14). ASD is associated with immune dysfunction in the brain, periphery, and gastrointestinal tract (chap. 5B), as well as antibodies against the fetal brain, suggesting a disruption in the BBB (15,16).

Although a disruption in BBB permeability is implicated in the pathogenesis of ASD, earlier neuroinflammation can also cause BBB disruption. Therefore, BBB disruption may either initiate neuroinflammation, or be an exacerbating consequence of earlier neuroinflammation. It is still up for debate whether BBB disruption is primarily via assault from peripheral inflammatory mechanisms such as mast cell activation or auto-immune induction, or is actually a secondary consequence of earlier neuroinflammatory processes such as microglial activation originating from BBB-permeable cytokines (15,17). Although the precise etiology of neuroinflammation in ASD is unknown, the pathogenic consequences are significant.

Hypotheses for neuroinflammation's effect on the developing brain include immediate cell death, and long-term alterations in the vasculature and function of the BBB, leading to increased susceptibility to toxins, drugs, and peripheral inflammatory mediators. Models of neuroinflammation on developing brains have shown changes in cortical and subcortical white matter, cortical neuron density, and cerebellar grey and white matter (18). The functional and histopathological defects in ASD are likely manifestations of neuroinflammation. They include impaired perinatal and postnatal neurological development, increased BBB permeability, gliosis, and synaptic stripping (2,7,19).

Animal models of disease have proven useful as a means to study the relationships between inflammation, demyelination, and neurodegeneration. An animal model of multiple sclerosis (MS) called experimental autoimmune encephalomyelitis (EAE) has been particularly valuable in MS research (20). Although EAE and MS are phenotypically disparate from ASD, EAE has utility in a pathophysiological discussion of ASD as it has both the benefit of being very well characterized, and shares several pathological features with ASD, including inflammation, increased BBB permeability, gliosis, synaptic damage, and demyelination (20,21).

By considering the shared inflammatory mediators, and clinical and histopathological manifestations of neuroinflammation seen in EAE, we can demonstrate the importance of minimizing the severity of damaging inflammatory reactions, thereby preserving CNS structure and functionality. In addition, EAE provides a framework for testing various neuroprotective therapies that could potentially be useful for ASD.

EAE: A speculative neuroinflammatory framework for ASD pathogenesis

EAE is a CD4+ T-cell-mediated autoimmune disease, with activated Th1 and Th17 cells thought to be the major immunological culprits in pathogenesis (20). Th1 cells release IFN-γ which has the ability to activate CNS-resident microglia and astrocytes. Th17 cell differentiation is induced by IL-6 and TGF-β1, the former via the signal transducer and activator of transcription 3 (STAT3) signal transduction pathway (22). The disease is characterized by the breakdown of the BBB and lesions disseminated throughout the central nervous system, namely the brain, spinal cord, and optic nerves, consisting of demyelination, axonal loss, and glial scaring (21). These inflammatory, demyelinated lesions show accumulations of hypertrophic, glial fibrillary acid protein (GFAP) and vimentin immunoreactive astrocytes within and at the margins of the lesion. GFAP and vimentin are markers associated with the proliferation of immature astrocytes, indicating reactive astrogliosis. Oligodendrocytes are depleted within these lesions. This possibly indicates that migration into the lesion by oligodendrocyte progenitors, which could potentially remyelinate the damaged tissue, is physically blocked due to intense gliosis (23).

A plethora of aberrations associated with neuroinflammation are implicated in the progression of EAE, including, but are not limited to: NFκB-induced activation of endogenous microglia and infiltrating macrophages, TNF-α induced aminomethylphosphonic acid (AMPA) receptor upregulation, N-nitrosodimethylamine (NMDA) and AMPA associated glutamate excitotoxicity, mitochondrial stress and reactive oxygen species (ROS), antibodies-mediated complement fixation, antibody-dependent cytotoxicity by Fc-receptors, oligodendrocyte apoptosis, phagocytosis of myelin, secretion of proteases, and interrupted axonal transport (24-27).

The temporal and mechanistic relationships between neuroinflammation, demyelination, and neurodegeneration vary between EAE models, highlighting the overtly multifactorial nature of the disease (20). Wide heterogeneity in histopathological findings, MRI morphological alterations, and clinical presentations is a feature shared by EAE, MS and ASD. It is unclear what precisely causes the different courses for any of these diseases. Such wide diversity may indicate that EAE, MS, or ASD may individually actually be a collection of unique diseases with distinct etiological causes that have been phenotypically lumped together. Another possible explanation arises from the observed dependence that genetics and immunizing antigen plays on the disease phenotype in EAE (28). Genetic differences may translate to the CNS having variable levels of vulnerability to inflammation or reduced ability to repair damage (27). Keeping these possibilities in mind is vital during discussions on ASD.

Variable findings are commonly seen in ASD studies and seem to have a dependence on region of interest, age, and severity of disease (29). For example, both increases and decreases in glutamate have been seen in ASD patients (30-33). Although glutamate is generally promising, due to variability between studies no biomarkers have yet been unequivocally elucidated as the definitive biomarker characteristic of ASD (34). The phenotypic and mechanistic variability that EAE and ASD exhibit presents challenges when trying to understand their etiology and pathogenesis. The details surrounding their most common factor, neuroinflammation, are also difficult to elucidate. Some models of EAE show a clear link of neuroinflammation being the root cause of neurodegeneration and demyelination. Meanwhile, other models suggest inflammation is just a secondary response to independent neurodegenerative processes. Even others show neurodegenerative processes are able to occur in the absence of neuroinflammation (28). Although there are diverse pathogenic mechanisms underlying the variations in EAE, and possibly ASD, a neuroinflammatory component is involved in the majority and is worth exploring.

EAE's clinical correlates with ASD

We can appreciate the significance that an acute bout of neuroinflammation can have on normal neurological function in general by examining the clinical time-course of either relapse-remitting EAE (RR-EAE) or relapse-remitting MS (RR-MS). In RR-EAE and RR-MS, we tend to see neurological function decline during acute inflammatory attacks called relapses. Visual, motor, sensory, coordination, balance, cognitive, and various other functions are negatively affected during bouts of acute inflammation (27). These relapses are followed by periods of remission as inflammation diminishes in intensity along with the severity of the symptoms. The resolution of symptoms during seen in RR-EAE highlights the devastatingly harmful effects of acute neuroinflammation on nervous system function (28). Based on this relationship, corticosteroids are occasionally used in MS to relieve symptoms of acute inflammation (35).

Unfortunately, the story does not end as inflammation subsides in EAE and the animals go into remission. Although corticosteroids have utility in the short term treatment of symptoms arising from active inflammation, there are long-term consequences to each inflammatory relapse that corticosteroids do not seem to prevent (35). Long-term damage following even a single inflammatory attack has been described in the CNS. Significant anatomical and functional defects are seen in the retina, an outpouching of the brain embryonically derived from the diencephalon, following a single bout of optic neuritis (ON). ON is inflammation of the optic nerve, and is one of the first clinical presentations seen in many MS patients (36). Highly significant reductions in retinal nerve fiber layer (RNFL) thickness and macular volume have been seen following a single bout of ON (37).

The previously described RNFL loss is a form of neurodegeneration, and is a sign that other relatively permanent degenerative processes can occur in other locations within the CNS following a single inflammatory episode. The potential for permanent damage from neuroinflammation has implications for ASD. Considering the permanence and severity that a single episode of neuroinflammation can have in adults, the potential consequences of perinatal inflammation are profound. Inflammatory assault while the brain is still in the earliest stages of development can lead to lasting damage; with the severity of the disorder being dependent upon the intensity and duration of inflammation. Indeed, ASD shows abnormal regional and global elevations in white matter tissue water content via T2 MRI, and abnormal cortical connectivity in both white and grey matter (38,39). To make matters more complicated, there is evidence that ASD-associated neuroinflammation is not only restricted to the perinatal time period, but may also consist of chronic inflammation throughout adulthood too (19).

Considering the chronic inflammatory aspect of ASD, it is imperative to examine the long-lasting effects of chronic neuroinflammation beyond just the scope of potential developmental aberrations. Relapse-remitting and chronic progressive EAE models show repeated relapses and chronic inflammation can lead to the accumulation of various types of neurological damage over time. A quantitative decrease in the number of neurons due to neurodegeneration will result in the disruption of normal neurological function and is closely associated to the progression of long-term disability. Delayed impulse conduction speed and neuronal misfiring are consequences of demyelination. Considering the complexity of the interconnections between neurons in the CNS and the distances they have to transverse to communicate throughout the body, faulty neuronal conduction will severely disrupt cognitive, neuromuscular, and end-organ function. In addition, sub-lethal apoptosis without neuronal cell death can occur in synapses resulting in dendritic spine loss (25). This synaptic stripping has been shown to occur early in the disease course, is independent of demyelination, and is strongly associated with massive release of TNF-α from activated microglia. As practically no new neurons can be generated during adulthood, any neurons lost in ASD due to any of these injurious mechanisms will lead to permanent impaired brain function (40).

Relevant immunological mediators in the pathogenesis of ASD

Given the vast breadth and depth of complexity governing the inter-relationships between proinflammatory signal cascades, their upstream and downstream mediators, and the extensive cross-talk among them, an exhaustive exposition is beyond the scope of this book. Nevertheless, considering the inflammatory mediators implicated in ASD, and their multifaceted interactions and effects is vital for understanding the pathogenesis. Mothers with elevated serum levels of IFN-γ, IL-4 and IL-5 has been associated with an increased risk for ASD, while increased concentrations of IL-2, IL-4, and IL-6 were associated with an increased risk of developmental disorder without autism. Although the placenta forms a barrier between maternal and fetal circulation, some immune factors, such as IgG and IL-6, have the ability to cross the placenta (41). Meanwhile, some other inflammatory mediators that are unable to cross, like IFN- γ, are still able to respond to receptors on the maternal-fetal interface and alter the fetal compartment. The cumulative effect may alter aspects of neurogenesis, neuronal migration and synaptic plasticity. This fetal immunological link is demonstrated in a prenatal mouse model of autism, which showed injected IL-2 crossed the placenta and entered the fetus. Lymphocytes from IL-2 pups showed accelerated T cell development and TH1 differentiation, suggesting that maternal levels of certain cytokines during pregnancy can induce in their offspring an increased long-lasting vulnerability to neurobehavioral abnormalities (42).

The specific T-cell response seen in ASD varies from study to study. One study examining cytokines in ASD brain tissue found proinflammatory cytokines (TNF- α, IL-6 and granulocyte-macrophage colony-stimulating factor [GM-CSF]), Th1 cytokine (IFN- γ) and chemokine (IL-8) increased compared to controls. Th2 cytokines (IL-4, IL-5 and IL-10) showed no difference. Therefore, the Th1/Th2 ratio was found to be significantly increased in ASD brain tissue, indicating an increased innate and adaptive immune response via the Th1 pathway (34). Other studies examining cytokine levels in children with ASD show variable findings (43). Increased plasma levels of the Th1 cytokines IL-12 and IFN- γ, and increases IFN- γ in the supernatant of whole blood cultures have both been found (43-45). In contrast, the use of monoclonal antibodies has shown increased proportions of IL-4 containing $CD4^+$ and $CD8^+$ T cells, and decreased proportions of IFN- γ^+CD4^+, $IL-2^+CD4^+$, IFN- γ^+CD8^+, and $IL-2^+CD8^+$ T cell subsets (43,46).

With evidence that Th1 autoimmune disorders and Th2 allergic diseases are positively associated, and share similar risk factors that cause the generation of both responses, it has been considered that the usual Th1 vs Th2 paradigm, where the predominance of one stifles the other, may be an oversimplification. One study showed increased activation of both Th1 and Th2 responses in children with ASD. Increased IL-2, IFN- γ, IL-4, IL-13, IL-5 and IL-10 in peripheral blood mononuclear cells were seen, with Th2 predominance (43). Other studies showed elevated levels of serum IgE and IgG are also associated with ASD, acting as further evidence of an allergic response and autoimmune response, respectively (43,47-48). In addition to the possibility of concomitant Th1/Th2 responses, elevated serum levels of IL-17A have also been seen in children with ASD and are correlated significantly with the severity of autism, suggesting a Th17 role (49). Interestingly, EAE showed IL-17 production only during the acute phase. Partial clinical recovery observed during chronic EAE was associated with the absence of IL-17 (20). Further research is needed to investigate if increased serum IL-17 is pathogenic in autism.

Several mediators of inflammation, including IL-6, IL-1α, IL-1β, and TNF-α are able to cross the BBB (50). Their permeability opens up the possibility that these interleukins, after arising from a peripheral inflammatory response, may become early mediators of initiating neuroinflammation in ASD. The initial increase in BBB could potentially arise from early neuroinflammation via the activation of microglia. Activated microglia are a major source of TNF-α in the CNS. TNF-α, IL-1β, and IL-17A all increase BBB permeability (51). The case can be made for the origin of BBB permeability to potentially be secondary to TNF-α originating from activated microglia. Activated microglia are thus also implicated in the potential initiation and progression of neuroinflammation in ASD, EAE, and MS (52). With increased BBB permeability, the potential for further neuroinflammatory damage occurs since peripheral mediators and lymphocytes are able to enter the CNS. Autoantibodies play a pathological role in both EAE and ASD, and are able to either cross over into or be generated within the CNS once the BBB breaks down. Autoantibodies against neuronal progenitor cells have been shown in the sera of ASD children, suggesting that autoimmunity may affect postnatal neuronal plasticity (53).

The cortex and cerebellum of ASD patients have shown increased astro- and microgliosis, along with increased levels of IL-6, TNF-α, monocyte chemotactic protein-1 (MCP-1), TGF-β1, IFN-γ, and IL-8 gene expression, among others (19). Th1-mediated activation of microglia and macrophages results in the release of oxygen radicals and proinflammatory cytokines (25,54). It is interesting to note that in a chronic progressive model of EAE, the highest increase of cell number and morphological change in microglia coincided with the peak of clinical disease (55). As mentioned earlier, astrogliosis may prevent remyelination by acting as a physical barrier for oligodendrocyte progenitors. Although the exact signaling pathways mediating astrogliosis has not been precisely elucidated in EAE, other mouse models implicate Janus Kinase 2 (JAK2)/STAT3 activation (56) (chapter 6B). Additionally, IL-6 plays a role as it is upregulated in reactive astrocytes. Blockade of IL-6 has been shown to reduce astrogliosis in a traumatic spinal cord injury murine model (57,58).

Among the proinflammatory cytokines released by microglia is TNF-α. Overexpression of TNF leads to demyelinative damage in EAE via multiple downstream mechanisms (59). An early pregnancy mouse model of maternal immune activation (MIA) with subclinical immune activation by LPS showed that TNF receptor 1 (TNFR1) signaling is required for LPS to affect the placenta. It is striking that very small doses of LPS from subclinical infection early in pregnancy were enough to cause transient placental vasodilation and hemorrhage that ultimately resulted in small tracts of necrosis and permanent tissue injury to the placenta. The lesions were then accompanied by impaired fetal perfusion and hypoxia in the fetal brain (60). Another likely TNF-α inflammatory mechanism involved in ASD is TNF-α induced AMPA receptor upregulation. Neutralization of TNF with anti-TNF antibodies and pharmacological blockade of AMPA receptors have been shown to be protective in EAE, and decrease synaptic degeneration and dendritic spine loss (25,59).

There is evidence that ASD patients have a spectrum of mitochondrial dysfunction of differing severity, with about 79% not associated with any genetic abnormalities, likely signifying secondary mitochondrial dysfunction (61). Mitochondrial dysfunction, activated microglia, infiltrating macrophages, and several other mechanisms are all capable of producing reactive oxygen species (ROS), which are chemically reactive and can cause damage (chapters 8B,8C). ROS has been suggested to play a role in myelin and axonal impairments in MS and EAE (62). In addition, decreased brain-derived neurotrophic factor (BDNF) seen in ASD brains results in the downregulation of both the expression and activation of a serine/threonine-specific protein kinase called Akt. Decreased Akt activity leads to decreased regulator Bcl-2 proteins in the mitochondrial membrane, rendering the neurons more susceptible to apoptotic signaling. This pro-apoptotic state is exacerbated by the observation that p53 expression is increased in ASD brains (63).

Excitotoxicity, oxidative stress, and mitochondrial dysfunction have complex interrelationships, with each able to cause or appear as a result from the others. In addition, mitochondrial dysfunction can result in neurodegeneration, while neurodegeneration can contribute to mitochondrial dysfunction in nearby cells. These interrelationships continue as neurodegeneration, BBB dysfunction, and neuroinflammation are also able to cause or appear as a result from the others. Thus, all of these seemingly disparate pathogenic mechanisms are linked in a complex positive feedback loop (40). This obviously complicates research attempting to ascertain the pathogenesis of ASD. See the chapter on thimerosal for a more comprehensive discussion on glutathione excitotoxicity, reactive oxidative species, and mitochondrial dysfunction (chapterr 7C).

Faulty cholinergic neurotransmitter activity is likely present in ASD as parietal cortex M1 (muscarinic) receptor binding is up to 30% lower than normal and nicotinic receptor binding is 65%-73% lower in autistic parietal and frontal cortices (64). Acetylcholine (Ach) has potent anti-inflammatory actions and suppresses the production of IL-6, TNF-α, high-mobility group box-1 (HMGB1), IL-1, and migration inhibitor factor (MIF) through the efferent vagus nerve. Ach's anti-inflammatory effects seem to be dependent upon the α7 nicotinic acetylcholine receptor (α7 nAChR) subunit (65). Microdeletions of the chromosome 15q13.3, which is the location of the CHRNA7 gene that encodes α7 nAChR, is associated with ASD. The subsequent loss of Ach's anti-inflammatory effects and a lack of inhibitory tone on GABA receptors may play an etiological role in ASD (66). Interestingly, polyunsaturated fatty acids (PUFAs), which will be discussed more in depth later in this chapter, and cholinergic agonists such as nicotine have similar anti-inflammatory benefits to Ach (65). Specifically, PUFAs function to augment levels of BDNF in the brain, augment a type of NO synthesis, and inhibit the production of TNF-α, IL-1, and IL-6 (63).

A closer look into IL-6 signaling and STAT activation

Consideration of pro-inflammatory signal transduction pathways conventionally regarded as unrelated to ASD is merited in light of the recent neurodevelopmental associations ASD has with MIA and IL-6. The aim of this section is to aid in potential future research efforts into the pathogenesis of ASD by discussing various important aspects of IL-6 signaling and STAT activation, and exploring potential inflammatory and neurodevelopmental connections with ASD which may not have been previously considered.

Increased serum IL-6 has been linked to the expression of an autistic phenotype in mice, and may possibly be due to its effects on promoting Th17 differentiation, suppressing CD4[+] Foxp3[+] T regulatory cells which normally function to prevent excessive immune reactions, and STAT3 activation (15,67). Monocytes and macrophages are the main producers of IL-6 in acute inflammation after activation of Toll-like receptors (TLR), which are receptors that recognize structurally conserved motifs commonly found on bacteria or viruses, and T cells appear to also be a source of IL-6 during chronic inflammation (67,68). In C6 glioma cells, TNF-α induces IL-6 synthesis through the JAK/STAT3 pathway in addition to the phosphorylation of NFκB, p38 mitogen-activated protein (MAP) kinase and stress-activated protein kinase (SAPK)/c-Jun N-terminal kinase (JNK) (69). This is interesting, as normally IL-6 activates JAK/STAT (chap. 6C). IL-1β also activates STAT3 in C6 cells (69). The precise role of JAK/STAT in glial cells remains to be elucidated.

IL-6 signal transduction involves the activation of JAK tyrosine kinases, leading to the activation of transcription factors of the STAT family. Another major signaling pathway for IL-6-type cytokines is the mitogen-activated protein kinase (MAPK) cascade, which contains the Ras/Raf intermediary signaling proteins, mitogen-activated protein kinase kinase (MEK or MAP2K or MAPKK), and extracellular signal-regulated kinases (ERK) (70,71). Although there is significant crosstalk between the STAT/JAK and MAPK cascades, IL-6-induced STAT3 activation is MAPK independent, but sensitive to serine/threonine kinase inhibitor H7 (70). IL-6 also activates the PI3K–AKT pathway (67). IL-6 induces gp130-dependent signaling via two modes, either by binding the cognate gp80 IL-6 receptor, which activates Erk1/2, JNK1/2, p38-MAPK and PI3K, but not the JAK/STAT pathway, or via trans-signaling which utilizes soluble IL-6 receptor (sIL-6r), which is involved in JAK/STAT activation (72). IL-6 binding to sIL-6r also results in ERK-MAPK signaling in chondrocytes, and most likely other cell lineages (73).

STAT3 activation is not only mediated by IL-6-type cytokines, but can be mediated by all other cytokine signaling associated with gp130 and JAK1/2, including IL-10, IFNs, TNF-α, IL-21, and IL-23, and various growth factors (74,75). Crosstalk between several related pathways may also lead to STAT3 activation, as Src-transformed fibroblasts, which are fibroblasts expressing the proto-oncogene c-Src, showed that inhibition of p38 and JNK suppresses a type of STAT3 activation, and glioma cells showed protein kinase C epsilon type (PKC-ε) has been shown to mediate activation of a specific STAT3 isoform through integration with the MAPK cascade (RAF-1, MEK1/2, and ERK1/2) (76). It should be noted that the various mechanisms of STAT activation likely result in a divergence of effector functions, as the activators may phosphorylate different regions of STAT or completely different STAT proteins. Cell lineage also likely plays a role. Suppressors of cytokine signaling (SOCS), also known as the signal transducer and activator of transcription (STAT)-induced STAT inhibitor (SSI) or the cytokine-inducible src homology (SH), are negative feedback regulators of the JAK/STAT pathway that are upregulated via STAT activation (77). Nevertheless, inhibition of STAT3 activation by SOCS can potentially be overcome by overexpression of native JAK1 and JAK2 (78).

SOCS have also been shown to negatively regulate insulin-like growth factor-1 receptor (IGF1R) mediated signaling in myoblasts (77,79). This implies that IL-6, which is upstream of SOCS, may decrease serum IGF via the JAK/STAT pathway (77). It has also been reported that IFN-γ activates STAT1 which in turn suppresses IGF1R promoter activity in a human osteosarcoma cell model (77,80). If this finding were to hold true in vivo for humans, STAT1 upregulation could potentially hinder IGF-1 signaling. Meanwhile, it has been shown that in mice, STAT5 is essential for GH-stimulated gene expression and subsequent IGF-1 production in various human cell lineages (77).

The relationship between the activation of the IGF1R downstream signaling pathway and the abundance of STAT was studied in an animal model of periconceptional maternal dietary restriction and/or obesity, which are maternal stressors that results in an increased stress responsiveness of the hypothalamo-pituitary-adrenal axis in offspring. Periconceptional dietary restriction of both normal weight and obese ewes showed upregulation of the JAK/STAT pathway, an increase in STAT1 upregulation, abundance of phospho-STAT1 and phosphor-STAT3, and a downregulation of STAT5, adrenal IGF1R, downstream Akt, and activated phospho-Akt (Ser473) in both male and female lambs and mTOR in female lambs. The exact differences varied between groups. Surprisingly, these periconceptional dietary changes were independent of SOCS1/SOCS3 changes (77). The various aforementioned studies imply that IL-6 induced Jak/STAT activation, and possibly even STAT1 or STAT3 activation, SOCS upregulation, or STAT5 inactivation via different upstream pathways, are associated with decreased serum IGF-1 levels.

Implications of JAK/STAT activation in ASD

Several cytokine signaling pathways, such as NF-κB and JAK/STAT, are involved with the modulation of cell proliferation, differentiation, and migration during prenatal brain development (71). During embryonic development of the CNS, the JAK/STAT3 pathway maintains homeostasis between neuro- and gliogenesis (81). Forced activation of JAK/STAT signaling has been shown to lead to precocious astrogliogenesis (82).

MIA, which is an environmental risk factor of ASD, can initiate IL-6 induced JAK/STAT activation (16) (chapter 6B). LPS or synthetic, double-stranded RNA polyriboinosinic–polyribocytidilic acid (polyI:C) can be administered to pregnant dams to mimic the immunestimulating actions of live bacterial or viral infections, respectively (83). These viral and bacterial MIA mouse models result in offspring with behavioral, social, and neuropathological symptoms of autism (16,83). A poly(I:C) MIA model showed increased IL-6 mRNA as well as maternally-derived IL-6 in the placenta, which mediated activation of the JAK/STAT3 pathway in the spongiotrophoblast layer of the placenta. IL-6 dependent disruption of the GH-IGF axis, characterized by decreased GH, IGF1 and IGFBP3, and IL-6 dependent altered expression of placental lactogen (PL) and pro-lactin-like proteins (PLP) were also observed (84). The pathogenic implications of decreased IGF-1 following IL-6 induced JAK/STAT3 activation in ASD will be discussed in more depth later (chapter 6D).

Protein expression in the prefrontal cortex and striatum of poly(I:C) offspring showed modifications in intracellular signal transduction networks downstream of JAK/STAT, including the MAPK cascade, which includes Ras/Raf, MEK, and ERK, and various other oxidation and auto-immune targets (71). Poly(I:C) offspring are partly immunologically characterized by a systemic deficit in $CD4^+$ $Foxp3^+$ T-regulatory cells, and increased IL-6 and IL-17 production by $CD4^+$ T-helper cells. These permanently hyperresponsive $CD4^+$ T-helper cells, as well as decreased immunosuppressive T regulatory cells, suggest MIA causes a chronic, proinflammatory phenotype in offspring (16). It is interesting to note that STAT3 is proposed to be the main regulator of myeloid derived suppressor cell function and is indispensable for Th17 differentiation, supporting the assertion that STAT3 is a clinically significant downstream consequence of MIA (75).

A mouse model of LPS inflammation, an inducer of MIA, in non-pregnant mice showed that LPS-induced blood macrophage NO synthesis and iNOS expression worked through activation of the ribosomal protein S6 kinase beta-1 (S6K1)-p42/44 MAPK pathway, and is regulated downstream by STAT3 phosphorylation and subsequent STAT3 transcriptional activation. Nicotine inhibits this LPS-induced NO synthesis through suppression of S6K1-p42/44 MAPK and STAT3 phosphorylation (85). This highlights an important mechanistic link between the faulty cholinergic activity seen in ASD and the inflammatory effects of LPS-induced STAT3 activation. It remains to be seen whether the relationship in ASD is due to:

1) faulty cholinergic activity preceding MIA; resulting in a loss of anti-inflammatory cholinergic protection that predisposes individuals to MIA by otherwise innocuous stimuli, or

2) MIA preceding faulty aberrant cholinergic activity; with inflammatory mediators from an initial MIA somehow disabling Ach's potent anti-inflammatory actions and predisposing individuals, or

3) is dependent upon the individual and potentially multifactorial.

Although the precise function of the JAK/STAT pathway in glial cells is unknown, STAT1 and STAT3 are known to play important functions in post-ischemic brain damage (69). In addition to the aforementioned pro-inflammatory associations of the IL-6/JAK/STAT pathway, there is evidence that IL-6 induced STAT3 activation was actually neuroprotective in a mouse model of cerebral ischemia (86). Indeed, TNF-α had a similar result, as pre-treatment of hippocampal cells in culture with TNF-α prior to ischemia was protective against neuronal death. The ultimate fate of cells following activation of STAT, TNF-α, and other inflammatory pathways is likely dependent upon an aggregation of the cellular microenvironment, cytokine co-stimulation, and the concentration and timing of activation. As a simplified example of in vitro glial cells, anti-inflammatory cytokines such as IL-10 prompted STAT3 activation, but not STAT1 activation, while pro-inflammatory signals such as IFN-γ prompted STAT1 activation, but not STAT3 activation, and both STAT1 and STAT3 were activated by IL-6 (87).

STAT3 also plays a role in vascular diseases, as it is activated in response to hypoxia, oxidative stress or ROS, growth factors, and cytokines. It induces vascular smooth muscle cell (VSMC) proliferation, which is a key event involved in neo-intimal growth during post-hypoxic arteriogenesis. Stimulation of VSMC proliferation is also mediated by the MAPK-ERK$_{1/2}$, PI3K/Akt, and p38 MAP kinase pathways (88). Whether pathological vascular remodeling plays a role in ASD is unclear. A viral MIA model with exposure of C57BL/6J pregnant mice to poly(I:C) at gestational age 16 days not only induced significant increases in IL-1β, IL-13, and MCP-1, but also vascular endothelial growth factor (VEGF) in the cerebrospinal fluid of the fetal brain. Besides its roles in vasculogenesis and angiogenesis, VEGF also contributes to various mechanisms of CNS development including neuronal migration, differentiation, axonal growth, and path-finding, indicating that deregulation of VEGF expression during critical periods of brain development may be pathogenic (89). Elucidating potential STAT3 involvement in subsequent vascular disorders following fetal hypoxia and placental lesions is thus far an untapped area of research.

Considerations for targeting inflammation as a potential therapeutic modality

This chapter has discussed how neuroinflammation and systemic inflammation are associated with the pathogenesis of the developmental and functional deficits observed in ASD. The association with neuroinflammation makes it an excellent target for study in elucidating the precise etiology and pathogenesis, with the long-term goal of preventing the onset or severity of autism. Although no curative therapies currently exist, the potential for utilizing anti-inflammatory diets and supplements for the prophylactic and therapeutic treatment of ASD is discussed in this section.

Ketogenic diets

Evidence supporting the therapeutic effects of ketogenic diets (KD) for ASD patients exists. KD's have been shown to suppress the expression of inflammatory cytokines and chemokines, as well as the production of ROS in an EAE model. By attenuating the inflammatory response and oxidative stress, the KD had a protective effect on spatial learning and memory functioning in this model (90). The BTBR mouse model of autism, which is characterized by impaired reciprocal social interaction, impairments in communication, and repetitive behaviors, showed behavioral improvements from a KD (91,92). KD-fed BTBR mice showed decreased self-directed repetitive behavior, improved social communication of a food preference, and increased sociability in a three-chamber test (91). The three-chamber test assesses these via two scenarios. The mice are first given a choice of exploring a new chamber vs. an identical novel chamber with an unfamiliar mouse. Time spent in each chamber and number of entries into each chamber was scored. The second scenario gives the mice a choice between exploring a chamber with the now-familiar stranger mouse vs. a new stranger (93). KD-fed mice showed improved chamber time in the first scenario. Although KD mice did not exhibit preference for social novelty in the second scenario, the time spent in frontal contact with the mouse-containing cages or stranger mice themselves significantly improved (91).

There is also a case report of a 12 year old child with regressive autism who, once placed on a gluten-free, casein-free KD high in medium-chain triglycerides, showed marked improvement of autistic and medical symptoms (94) (chapter 5B). Seizures were significantly improved clinically within several weeks of achieving ketosis. In addition, the patient's morbid obesity was resolved with 60 pounds of weight loss, improved cognitive and language function, marked improvement in social skills, increased calmness, and complete resolution of stereotypies, which is a term that encompasses the restricted, repetitive, and stereotyped behavior seen in autism (94,95).

As a relatively high proportion of ASD patients have associated non-mutation mitochondrial dysfunctions, causing increased oxidative stress and associated glutathione depletion, the KD is thought to ameliorate these conditions (94, chap. 4B). Since some ASD patients have concomitant cerebral folate deficiency with autoantibodies against their folate receptors (FR), a casein-free KD has an additional advantage in ASD (96, chap. 5A). A milk-free diet has been shown to downregulate these autoantibodies since milk contains substantial amounts of FR, and seems to present the triggering antigen for the autoantibody response (96).

Unfortunately, a mouse model has shown prenatal and early postnatal exposure to a KD consisting of primarily 58.6% (by weight) hydrogenated vegetable shortening (e.g.,Crisco®), 17.3% casein, 8.7% cellulose, and 8.6% corn oil to have deleterious effects on neonatal brain structure and results in retarded physiological growth. Specifically, KD brains were shown to have bilateral decreases in the cortex, hippocampus, corpus callosum, fimbria, and lateral ventricles, and increases in the hypothalamus and medulla (97). Whether this finding holds true for all KDs or in humans remains uncertain as there is a paucity of research studying the effects of KDs on human pregnancy, perinatal development, and childhood neuronal development. In addition, a pediatric epilepsy clinic in Korea utilizing a calorie restricted "classic KD" with 90% of calories from unspecified long-chain fatty acids, 6% calories from proteins, and 4% calories from carbohydrates has associated their diet with early and late onset complications such as GI disturbances, hypertriglyceridemia, hyperuricemia, osteopenia, renal stones, cardiomyopathy, and others. Most findings were transient and were successfully managed by careful follow-up and conservative strategies (98). Height and weight growth impairment was also seen in children from this clinic following the long-term administration of the "classic KD," and was more severe and permanent if the KD was started prior to the age of 3 years old (99). Despite the apparent growth retardation seen in KDs started prior to 3 years old, there is also the possibility of a bias, as children that young would not normally be placed on a KD that young unless their epilepsy was poorly controlled and particularly severe.

The specific composition of KDs plays a very important role in both the safety and efficacy. A modified "Atkins" diet, low-gylcemic index diet, or diet rich in polyunsaturated fatty acids may confer many of the same benefits with a more tolerable safety profile than the aforementioned "classic KD" used in the Korean epilepsy clinic (98). KDs have also shown to be beneficial and relatively safe in mice and case studies of children suffering from epilepsy, including those with pre-diet hyperlipidemia given diets high in mono- and poly-unsaturated fats, and even type-1 diabetes despite the generally assumed increase risk of developing diabetic ketoacidosis and nephropathy (100,101).

More ASD specific research would elucidate whether the anti-inflammatory benefits supersede any growth risks in early KDs, however care must be taken to conduct such research ethically and safely. Also, any potential research on the effects of human dietary modifications on MIA should be cautious, as maternal dietary restriction and weight loss in ewes during the periconceptional period was shown to increase in adrenal growth and in the cortisol strength response in offspring, and a decrease in adrenal IGF1R (77). This may be due to an interplay of cortisol and insulin on the GH/IGF axis. However, the exact relationship is likely complex and multifactorial. Overall, more mature, adult ASD patients seem to currently be the safest population to test the anti-inflammatory KD treatment until more research is conducted on the safety of a modified, less severe KD in young children and pregnancy.

Omega-3 polyunsaturated fatty acids

Marine omega-3 PUFAs (n-3 PUFAs), specifically eicosapentaenoic (EPA) and docosahexaenoic acids (DHA) but colloquially known as fish oil, have various anti-inflammatory properties that may prove useful in the treatment and prevention of ASD (102) (chapter 5D). In general, PUFAs have also been shown to augment memory and cognitive function, as well as enhance NO formation, especially from eNOS and cNOS. Although NO is normally considered pro-inflammatory, NO, BDNF, PUFAs, and Ach interact with each other to regulate neuronal activity and synaptic function, and have a modulatory influence on immune responses and inflammation (63). See chapter 5D for a more thorough discussion on the risks vs. benefits of fish consumption and methylmercury (MeHg) poisoning. This section will focus on the anti-inflammatory considerations of n-3 PUFAs, with a reliance on knowledge of the inflammatory mediators we have discussed earlier as they relate to autism.

Pregnant rats fed a diet with 5% total fat intake consisting of either a standard diet of 0.8% of total fatty acids as n-3 PUFAs (<0.02% total fatty acids as EPA and <0.02% DHA), or a high omega-3 (Hn3) diet with 33.2% of fatty acids as n-3 PUFAs (5.4% EPA and 23.8% DHA), showed that the Hn3 diet increases protectin and resolvin levels in the placental labyrinth zone which is the site of maternal-fetal exchange (102). Protectins and resolvins are two families of pro-resolving lipid mediators that promote the resolution of acute inflammation by a wide variety of mechanisms, thereby preventing the onset of chronic inflammation. While enzymatic oxygenation of arachidonic acid (AA), an n-6 PUFA, generates both pro-inflammatory and pro-resolving lipid mediators, analogous pathways for EPA and DHA primarily lead to the formation anti-inflammatory, pro-resolving and cytoprotective lipid mediators such as protectins and resolvins (103). The ability of DHA and EPA metabolism to circumvent the initial inflammatory prostaglandin and leukotriene increases associated with AA oxygenation and instead primarily increase levels of the aforementioned pro-resolving lipid mediators has been shown to be protective in many autoimmune, traumatic, infective, ischemic, and inflammatory disease models (104).

N-3 PUFAs seem to exert a protective effect against neuroinflammation. In a spinal mouse model of carrageenan-induced neuroinflammation, dose-dependent spinal injection of DHA reduced carrageenan-induced microglial activation, p38 MAPK phosphorylation which mediates microglial activation, and the production of the proinflammatory cytokines TNF-α and IL-1β. In addition, in vitro results from the same study also showed that DHA blocked LPS-induced p38 activation and the subsequent expression of other inflammatory mediators including IL-6 and the chemokines CCL2, CCL3, and CXCL10 that are chemoattractant for various immune cells (105). Another study showed that when RR-MS patients treated with interferon beta-1b were given 4 g/day of fish oil for 12 months, there were significant decreases in serum levels of TNFα, IL-1β, IL-6, and nitric oxide metabolites. However, no differences in serum lipoperoxide, which is a free radical, or clinical disease severity were seen after 12 months of supplementation (106).

One study demonstrated that DHA and EPA inhibit IL-6-induced STAT3 phosphorylation and C-reactive protein expression in an IL-6-treated human liver carcinoma cell line (107). The study also showed that DHA and EPA do not suppress the activity of ERK1/2, which is unfortunate considering ERK1/2 is also downstream of IL-6 activation, and that Raf/ERK upregulation can alter cortical cell migration, neurogenesis and maturation, as well as impair the development of excitatory synapses and dendritic spines (72,108). These findings, as well as the observation that Ras/Raf/ERK1/2 signaling is enhanced in the frontal cortex of autistic individuals and BTBR mice, supports the hypothesis for the Raf/ERK pathway as one of the many signaling pathways implicated in the pathogenesis of ASD (108). Despite the evidence against the ability of DHA and EPA to suppress the activity of ERK1/2, the finding that they inhibit IL-6 induced STAT3 phosphorylation in human liver cancer cells is still interesting. Further investigation on whether DHA and EPA inhibits placental JAK/STAT3 activation in MIA models is warranted due to ASD's association with MIA-induced, IL-6 mediated activation of the JAK/STAT3 pathway (chapter 6B).

Although the effect of n-3 PUFAs on MIA models is a necessary future step, another study fortunately showed that 2.5g/day n-3 PUFA supplementation (2085 mg EPA and 348 mg DHA) in medical students resulted in decreased TNF-α and IL-6 production by peripheral blood mononucleated cells, which include lymphocytes and monocytes, as well as a modest decrease in serum TNF-α. Considering their average dietary n-6:n-3 ratio was already 10.82 at baseline compared to the typical ratios of 15:1 to 17:1 seen in North Americans, the results are encouraging in that the anti-inflammatory effects of n-3 PUFA supplementation may be even more significant in the general population (109). It is interesting to note that that early human hunter-gather diets had an estimated n-6:n-3 intake of 2:1 or 3:1 (110).

There are several practical aspects to n-3 PUFA supplementation that must be considered in a discussion on the safety and efficacy of therapeutic supplementation for ASD. It has not yet been ascertained whether the observed anti-inflammatory effects are a direct result of increased n-3 PUFA consumption, a decrease in the high dietary n-6:n-3 PUFA ratio that is prevalent in modern North American diet, or a combination. In any case, it should be noted that AA is still vital in human metabolism, and its metabolites prostaglandin E2 (PGE2) and lipoxin A$_4$ (LXA$_4$) facilitate the synthesis of BDNF, which is deficient in ASD, even better than DHA and EPA derived resolvins and protectins. Interestingly, very high unbalanced levels of either n-6 or n-3 PUFAs adversely affect development and have been associated with ASD-like symptoms. Appropriate amounts of both n-3 and n-6 PUFAs are necessary in balance for proper neuronal development and synapse formation (63). Also, the dietary source of n-3 PUFA matters as dietary conversion of alpha-linolenic acid (ALA), which is found in plant sources such as flaxseed, canola and soybean oil, to DHA and EPA is inefficient in humans, and may thus be inferior to marine n3 PUFA's in reducing markers of systemic inflammation (111). The optimal dosing is also unknown with one study showing more efficient incorporation of EPA into the plasma and mononuclear cell phospholipids of older males (53-70 years old) than younger males (18-42 years old) (112). The innate immune responses of young males were not affected by an EPA intake of < or =4.05g/day, which is over the 3g/day upper limit of marine n-3 PUFAs intake that the Food and Drug Administration (FDA) has ruled as "Generally Recognized as Safe (109,112)." The study asserted that an EPA + DHA intake of 1.65 g/d is below the threshold required to exert anti-inflammatory effects in healthy men (112).

The matter is complicated by the risk of mercury poisoning from fish consumption and the effects on pregnancy and child development (chapter 5D) for a more in-depth discussion). It is important to note that while refined and concentrated n-3 PUFA products contain virtually no methylmercury and are very low in organochloride contaminants, less controlled preparations may contain appreciable amounts (113). The consumption of krill oil may potentially be a viable, safe alternative as a source of n-3 PUFA for a few reasons. N-3 PUFAs in fish oil are stored as triglycerides whereas 30% to 65% of fatty acids are incorporated into phospholipids in krill oil. These differences may affect bioavailability, with evidence supporting both krill and fish oils as comparable sources of n-3 PUFAs despite krill oil EPA and DHA doses being 62.8% of that found in fish oil (114). In addition, marine sources of n-3 PUFAs that are not predatory, shorter-lived, or smaller species, such as krill and algal oil, have lower levels of MeHg (115). A study comparing 6 weeks of fish oil and krill oil consumption in a mouse model with persistent low-grade exposure of human TNF-α showed that fish oil and krill oil were comparable dietary sources of n-3 PUFAs. Interestingly, fish oil was shown to significantly increase IL-17 in the liver compared to controls, whereas krill oil diet tended to decrease MCP-1, which regulates migration and infiltration of monocytes, in mesenteric adipose tissue. Although differences in IL-6 detected in mesenteric adipose tissue were not significant, krill oil tended to have the lowest concentrations (116).

At the time of the 2011 Cochrane meta-analysis examining the efficacy of n-3 PUFAs for improving the core features and symptoms of ASD, only two randomized controlled studies investigating the efficacy of n-3 PUFA supplementation in a total of 40 ASD children were available. Doses ranged from 1.3 g/day (700 mg of EPA and 460 mg of DHA) to 1.5 g/day (840 mg EPA and 700 mg DHA). The duration of supplementation ranged from 6 to 12 weeks (117). A 2009 systematic review and the aforementioned 2011 Cochrane meta-analysis are in agreement that thus far, there is no high quality evidence that n-3 PUFA supplementation is effective for improving core and associated symptoms of ASD (117.118). The meta-analysis called for a large well-conducted randomized controlled trial is needed that examines both high and low functioning individuals with ASD, with longer follow-up periods (117).

The lack of efficacy for n-3PUFAs seen thus far in randomized controlled studies in improving the core and associated symptoms does not necessarily preclude potential clinical benefits for ASD. A discussion on or investigation into the potential benefits of maternal n-3 PUFA supplementation were not included in either analysis. Also, as mentioned prior, there is evidence that EPA incorporation into plasma and mononuclear cell phospholipids is negatively correlated with younger age in males, that innate immune responses of young men were not affected by an EPA intake of $\leq$ 4.05g/day, and that EPA + DHA intake of 1.65 g/d is below the threshold required to exert anti-inflammatory effects in healthy men (112). The studies included in the meta-analysis were below this supposed minimum therapeutic threshold. Any future randomized controlled trials on the efficacy of n-3 PUFAs in ASD may need to investigate larger doses than conventionally used.

Other various anti-inflammatory strategies

Vitamin D supplementation is discussed in more detail in chap. 5C - Vitamin D. A quick discussion on the inflammatory pathways it may affect is warranted. Vitamin D has significant immunomodulatory effects, and has been shown to inhibit Th17 cytokine production, enhance Treg activity, induce natural killer T cell functions, suppress Th1, and promote Th2 cytokine production, skewing T cells toward Th2 polarization (119). Vitamin D has also been shown to downregulate monocyte toll-like receptor 2 (TLR2) and TRL4 expression, thereby causing monocytes to be less responsive to activation by LPS. Upon TLR-ligand engagement addition, impaired NF-kappaB/RelA translocation and reduced p38 and p42/44 MAPK phosphorylation was observed (120). Interestingly, knockdown of TLR2 in gingival fibroblasts showed decreased IL-6 and IL-8 in response to LPS (121). In addition, administration of vitamin D upregulates the expression of MAPK phosphatase-1 (MKP-1) in human monocytes and murine bone marrow-derived macrophages (BMM). Indeed, at physiological concentrations, two forms of vitamin D, the active form $1,25(OH)_2D_3$ called calcitriol and the stored form $25(OH)D_3$ called calcifediol, dose dependently inhibited LPS-induced p38 phosphorylation, IL-6 and TNF-α production by human monocytes via the upregulation of MKP-1 (122).

EAE models have supported the role of resveratrol as potential neuroprotective agent. Resveratrol is thought to be neuroprotective due to its intrinsic radical scavenger properties, and upregulation of sirtuin 1 (SIRT1) and nuclear factor erythroid 2-related factor 2 (Nrf2), and inhibition of NF-κB and AP-1 (123). In particular, SIRT1 has been shown to inhibit IFN-γ-induced JAK-2 activation in mouse blood macrophages, and thus the JAK/STAT1 pathway (124). Although resveratrol did not reduce the occurrence or severity of active neuroinflammation in some models of EAE, it as effective in preventing some of the long-term consequences of neuroinflammation, including demyelination and neurodegeneration. This lead to a decrease in neuronal death and lasting functional deficits observed during periods of inflammatory remission in EAE (65,125). Another EAE model showed resveratrol was associated with rises in IL-17[+]/IL-10[+] T cells and CD4 IFN-γ[+] cells, and with repressed macrophage IL-6 and IL-12/23 p40 expression (126).

Resveratrol's ability to reduce demyelination and neurodegenerative damage following neuroinflammation may give it some utility in ASD. Unfortunately, another study has shown resveratrol to exacerbate demyelination and inflammation without neuroprotection in the CNS in both autoimmune and viral EAE models (127). In addition, the question remains whether SIRT-1 activators would be efficacious in preventing the neurological remodeling that neuroinflammation may cause, since some studies that showed resveratrol to be neuroprotective observed that resveratrol did not prevent or alter CNS neuroinflammation (65,125). There is a chance that even without long-term pathological changes like demyelination or neurodegeneration, inflammation itself can still cause detrimental neurological remodeling in-utero. This would make a therapeutic agent that is more effective in preventing neuroinflammation from occurring in the first place, more ideal.

An herbal compound plumbagin (PL) has been shown to be immunosuppressive to encephalitogenic T cell responses in EAE through down-regulation of the JAK-STAT pathway. PL selectively inhibited IFN-γ and IL-17 production by CD4+ T-cells. PL also suppressed pro-inflammatory molecules such as iNOS, IFN-γ and IL-6, accompanied by inhibition of IκB degradation as well as NF-κB phosphorylation. Given ASD's pathogenic association with these inflammatory mediators and the JAK-STAT pathway, PL or similar compounds may have utility in ASD (128). Unfortunately, PL has been shown to have anti-fertility, abortifacient, and anti-estrogenic effects in female Wistar rats (129). This disqualifies PL from potential maternal supplementation. Futures studies would most likely focus on functionality improvements in adolescent or adult animal models of ASD. As with every potential treatment modality, care must be taken in determining efficacy and safety.

Prenatal prophylactic flavonoids are another potential therapeutic strategy against autism for its anti-inflammatory effects (81). In vivo treatment of quercetin, a flavonoid, has been shown to ameliorate EAE by inhibiting IL-12 production and neural antigen-specific Th1 differentiation. In vitro treatment indicated blocked IL-12 induced JAK2, STAT3, and STAT4 activation (130). Other studies have shown that multiple bioflavonoids can be used to inhibit IFN-γ induced STAT1 activation and attenuate production of pro-inflammatory cytokines in microglial cells. Importantly for ASD, the flavonoid diosmin has a protective effect against IL-6/MIA mediated pathological and behavioral effects. A MIA model showed adult offspring of pregnant mice co-treated with IL-6, in order to induce JAK2/STAT3 activation, and diosmin have attenuated behavioral deficits and pathological outcomes such as increased inflammation (81).

Conclusions

These potential therapeutic strategies barely scratch the surface of possibility. By studying the pathogenic mechanisms of and risk factors contributing to ASD, we can identify new potential targets for treatment. Investigating the unique benefits and limitations of both recognized and hypothetical therapeutic strategies then enables us to better understand ASD. We hope to apply our ever increasing knowledge to ameliorate and hopefully even one day prevent autism.

Chapter 6D - Insulin-like Growth Factor
Gary Steinman

[Several conditions which have been observed to increase the chance of a child developing autism are based, in part, on reduced production of insulin-like growth factor. Measuring this biochemical, which affects the degree of myelination of developing nerves, may provide a biomarker for anticipating the subsequent appearance of this condition. – Ed.]

Hypothesis

As of now, no proposed origin of autism has been clearly and convincingly supported with laboratory and clinical data. Essentially all of the hypotheses that have been advanced have either been disproven with subsequent observations or remain to be investigated thoroughly. Many hypotheses endeavor to explain the cause of autism, but none has produced sufficient supportive data to substantiate any of them. Without a general mechanism to define the genesis of this disorder, the search for one must continue to facilitate treatment and/or prevention. Insulin-like growth factor-1 (IGF), the subject of the present chapter, is one such example.

It appears to be the consensus of the majority of researchers now examining the etiology of autism that the origin of this malady rests with two essential, interconnected factors:

1) Genomic aberrations set the stage for the expression of this propensity into the classical neurologic characteristics of the disorder.

2) Any one of a number of prenatal environmental triggers (e.g., hypoxia, inflammation, viral infection, oxidative stress, or teratogens) promotes this neuropathologic tendency to be overtly translated into classical autism. It is interesting to note that each of these conditions can have a controlling effect on the level of IGF.

As one of the newest hypotheses, it is proposed that levels of IGF in the fetus and newborn correlate with the potential of autistic characteristics appearing in the first two or three years of life (1). As discussed in the Conclusions and Prospectus section of this book, such a model should account for the dominance of male-over-female occurrence (chapter 1C), the relationship to maternal antepartum infection (chapter 6B), and the potential benefit of breastfeeding in preventing or reducing the manifestations of autism (chapter 9A).

Observations
Recent findings

If one sibling has been diagnosed with autism, the chance of his/her parents later conceiving a second affected child increases to 1-in-5, about 10-20 times the rate in the general population (2). It is twice as common in siblings as half-siblings. This suggests that this condition might occur as an autosomal recessive trait or a dominant trait with partial penetrance, where one or both parents could bear the modified gene without exhibiting the trait themselves. Furthermore, some sets of monozygotic (genetically "identical") twins have one affected and one normal member (chapters 1C,8A). This would intimate that autism involves both an environmental trigger and an inherited genetic tendency.

Autism is apparently the result of a continuum of defective neural development in the fetus, neonate, and young child. The behavioral characteristics of this disorder are usually not evident until early childhood. It is commonly diagnosed at age 1-3 years through special neurologic/psychological testing when the child does not meet expected development milestones such as speaking and social interaction (chapter 1D). These examinations entail subjective impressions derived by the testing professionals; hence, a difference of opinion of the true diagnosis between examiners may result. It is desirable to develop a quantitative, objective approach to the diagnostic process.

Insulin-like growth factor (IGF) is a single-chain, small protein containing 70 amino acids (3). The primary antepartum source of IGF is the placenta, and, postpartum, the liver. IGF influences numerous functions in the body, most of which are anabolic in nature. For example, it was previously reported that the rate of multiple ovulations resulting in twinning is influenced by the level of IGF (4).

Recent related findings help to develop a general theory that may ultimately formulate an all-encompassing explanation for the origin of autism:

1) Fetal hyperglycemia in cases of poorly controlled maternal diabetes and obesity has been correlated with epigenetic effects on the IGF gene (chapters 3H,3I). In early pregnancy, the primary modulator of circulating fetal IGF-1 appears to be insulin, rather than growth hormone (5);

2) Birth hypoxia (chapter 3G) and oxidative stress (chapters 8B,8C), experienced by children who subsequently developed autism, can be considered correlative or co-morbid factors in this setting. Cell membrane receptors mediate the translation of message-bearing agents, such as IGF, to interpret their signal into cell functions. IGF receptor has been shown to regulate resistance to oxidative stress (1).

3) Women affected by viral illnesses (chapter 6B) or exposure to pesticides (chapter 4E) in the first trimester of pregnancy express an increased incidence of giving birth to children who subsequently exhibit autistic behavior. Such an occurrence may be related to the presence of increased levels of inflammatory cytokines (chapters 6C) which decrease the production of placental IGF.

4) Gene polymorphisms (chapter 8A) can down-regulate the production of IGF (1). It has been proposed that carriers of pairs of such gene variants would more likely exhibit autistic behavior. Similarly, several polymorphisms found in some autistic children can alter their capacity to deal with oxidative stress (chapters 8B,8C).

Myelination

Many autism hypotheses are based on findings in affected children discovered only once abnormal behavior is detected. Thus, it is often not possible to ascertain if such factors are fundamental causes of the disorder or are co-morbid products of abnormal functions at the molecular or tissue levels. For example, 60% of autistic youngsters have decreased plasma glutathione in the reduced state. This leaves the issue of oxidative stress (chapters 4A,8B) open to question since no rationalization is readily given for the other 40%.

The most meaningful study would be a prospective investigation where specific parameters and biomarkers in randomly selected children are followed from birth until such time as autism can be ruled in or out by conventional psychological testing. Ongoing inquiries have collected umbilical cord blood samples for quantitation of IGF. Possible correlations of neonatal blood findings are then being compared with neurologic observations in the children later in life (Steinman, Mankuta, unpublished results).

For lack of sufficient experimental data, it is premature to conclude that IGF by itself is at the heart of the genesis of autism. However, that some phenomena such as oxidative stress (chapters 8B,8C) and maternal viral illnesses (chapters 6B,6C) may exert their influence through IGF-related basic pathways tends to support a general mechanism for the genesis of this disease (see below). This appears to be based on this growth factor's effect on neural myelination in the fetus and newborn (chapter 6A):

a) Defective myelination (dysmyelination) leads to inadequate shielding of nerve cell axons in the central nervous system.

b) Under-activity of the oligodendrocytes in the brain, which perform the myelination process, may be due to IGF deficiency or oxidative stress.

Pertinent observations concerning the role of this growth factor in neural myelination in autism before and after birth include the following:

1) At 28 weeks of pregnancy, a higher level of placental growth hormone (GH) has been found in the sera of women carrying female fetuses (6). GH is the primary controlling factor in determining the level of IGF in the second half of pregnancy. On average, four times as many males display autistic behavior as females (2) (chapter 1C). This would support the contention that defective neurogenesis actually starts prior to delivery.

2) A series of lumbar punctures performed on autistic children (for other medical indications) displayed lower levels of IGF in the cerebrospinal fluid surrounding the brain and the spinal cord up to the age of four years than in normal children (7). Above four, the concentration rises, possibly explaining the phenomenon of megalocephaly found in some autistic children.

3) Neonates born very-small-for-gestational-age (VSGA) have lower levels of IGF in their umbilical cord blood than normal-sized babies (8). Such under-sized children also have a higher incidence of autism.

4) IGF stimulates gene expression in the oligodendrocytes in the brain of the fetus and neonate to myelinate (insulate) portions of the nerve components being developed (9). This process begins in the late second trimester of pregnancy and reaches its peak growth by one year post-delivery. Biopsies of the brains of deceased autistic children reveal hypomyelinated neurons, whereas neurologically unaffected children display

normal nerve insulation (10,11). Hypomyelinated nerves are more susceptible to injury under oxidative stress because of reduced function of oligodendrocytes (12). The deficiency of myelin shielding in the nerves of the central nervous system (mainly the brain) can be detected by magnetic resonance imaging (MRI) as early as 6 months post-delivery as well (chapter 3A).

5) IGF genetic polymorphism may account for the depressed levels of the growth factor in neonates destined to eventually develop overt autism (13) (see below).

6) Maternal infection-related fever in the first trimester of pregnancy (e.g., with influenza) increases the chance of autism appearing in the offspring (chapter 6B). This has been related to the ability of the cytokine, interleukin-6 (IL6), released in such inflammatory situations to reduce the production of IGF by the placenta before birth.

7) Fetal IGF-1 is also sensitive to maternal nutrition (5). Maternal under-nutrition leads to decreased fetal IGF-1 and decreased fetal growth.

8) The longer children are breast-fed, the lower is the likelihood of their developing autism (14). Breast milk contains a higher level of IGF than bovine milk or formula (chapter 9A). This might also point to an appropriate preventative to reduce or eliminate the subsequent manifestations of autism. Another means for elevating blood IGF in the newborn is massage therapy (chapter 2D).

9) Antepartum chorioamnionitis (placental membrane inflammation) or peripartum hypoxia can be accompanied by reduced IGF in the newborn and autism, subsequently (chapter 3H,6C).

10) A primary result of axonal myelination is the increased velocity of nerve conduction (15). Impulse velocity is much lower in uninsulated axons than in myelinated ones. Myelination allows impulses to move 100 times faster along nerve conduits and serves to fix such pathways for efficient function. Myelin is a neuronal insulating material composed of several layers of glial membranes. Unmyelinated axons display conduction velocities up to 10 m/sec, whereas myelinated fibers have speeds as much as 150 m/sec (16,17). This enhancement depends on restriction of action potential generation only at spaces between myelin patches (i.e., nodes of Ranvier).

11) Using magnetoencephalography (chapter 3A), autistic children have been found to have latency delays in their right-hemisphere cortical functioning, compared to neurologically normal children (16). This is consistent with auditory and speech deficits typically noted in such youngsters. Thus, delayed auditory evoked responses might serve as imaging biomarkers for autism.

These and other findings suggest that depressed serum IGF levels at birth can forecast deficient CNS myelination later, and, ultimately, the appearance of pervasive developmental disorders from defective neural development such as autism. The random movements of the newborn represent trial-and-error experimentation, testing which neuromuscular processes are most productive. Once such a pathway is ascertained, it is finalized by myelination of the axons to improve impulse velocity and reproducibility. Insufficient myelination would result in neural dysfunction. Since autism is apparently the result of a process initiated before birth, it is important to detect such a deficiency of IGF at birth, so that enhanced supply and replacement can begin immediately, whether by breastfeeding, massage, injection of the growth factor, or other means.

As noted earlier in this chapter, the recurrence of autism in families with at least one affected child is 1-in-5 (2). These statistics suggest an underlying autosomal recessive genetic trait that may possibly be detectable in the parents prior to conception. Alternatively, preimplantation genetic testing could select out the unaffected embryo conceived by *in vitro* fertilization. This finding becomes especially important where close relatives marry and procreate together, since by the Founder Effect, the incidence of the disorder would be enhanced further.

Decreased myelination can be observed by brain imaging in some cases several months following birth (chapters 3A,6A). Recently reported studies point to the prospect that stimulated stem cells collected from the umbilical cord at birth may enhance nerve myelination (19) (chapter 9B). This remains to be examined in greater detail. If successful, compatible matching would be more likely since the stem cell donor and the recipient would be the same individual.

As noted above, one cause of decreased serum IGF is gene polymorphism. For example, such nuclear variation of the IGF-I gene influences the age-related decline in circulating total IGF-I levels. These modified genomes are typically found in children born small for gestational age. If such genetic alterations are found in both children with autism and their parents, it is plausible that pre-conception gene testing can identify couples with an increased probability of conceiving autistic children later.

Early neurogenesis

Embryonic stem cells (chapter 9B) can be stimulated to differentiate by:
a) introduction into mature, living tissue under the influence of local molecular signals, or
b) exposure to appropriate molecular "instructions" *in vitro* (17).

In vivo signal production is controlled by specific genes. Tyrosine kinase receptors transduce the molecular signals locally. Most directing molecules in neurogenesis are peptide hormones such as fibroblast growth factors (FGF), a central player in this scenario. Neuronal cell migration in the fetal/neonatal nervous system promotes spatial relationships with the increasingly active organs and tissues under development. Movement of neural crest cells is guided by locally released signal molecules (17).

The axon growth cone extends from the cell body to its ultimate pre-synaptic terminus under the control of nerve growth factor (NGF) and brain-derived neurotrophic factor (BDNF), for example. The preferred target of nerve outgrowth is an active site (e.g., a contractile element), whereas less demanding neural pathways are reduced by apoptosis. The more correlated and repeatedly active a particular synapse is with parallel pathways, the more persistent is that overall pattern of nerve function (17). This may explain the apparently random motions of infants, who seem to be maximizing the functionality of the motor components of their nervous systems by trial-and-error.

Glial cells follow existing axon pathways as migratory guides, thereby directing the finalization of each circuit by myelination. CNS neural synaptic density and myelination both reach a maximum around 10-12 months of neonatal age. Genetic mutations affecting the release of growth factors (e.g., IGF) can disrupt the ability of glial cells to migrate and properly function in axonal myelination, thereby disrupting neural connectivity (chapters 3A,3B). This may be at the heart of the pathogenesis of such maladies as schizophrenia and autism (17).

Supportive evidence

IGF gene polymorphism (chapter 8A), especially involving the promoter region of the gene, can be the basis for reduced production of this growth factor by the baby (18). However, a definite cause-and-effect relationship of this genetic variation and autism remains to be demonstrated. If such a trigger is substantiated, routine testing of all neonates for IGF deficiency, with and without known prenatal inflammation or toxin exposure, would allow early detection of autistic tendencies and the potential benefit of IGF supplement in such children.

Two additional serum biomarkers often increased in cases of autism are serotonin and anti-myelin basic protein (MBP) (19) (chapter 6B). Combining these two values with the level of IGF in the umbilical cord makes possible the calculation of an Autism Index (**AI**). Such a value could quantitate the likelihood of a newborn later developing overt manifestations of autism. Thus, the AI in a hypothetical example of an (impending) autistic newborn would be >0.00, and in a perfectly normal newborn would be ~0.00. The magnitude of AI may also correlate with the subsequent psychological results (i.e., the severity of the condition in an individual child on the autism spectrum), but this remains to be investigated.

Pertinent correlative examples supporting such an etiologic pathway would be:

1) IGF inhibits oxidative stress-induced apoptosis in stem cells (20).
2) IGF-1 receptor regulates resistance to oxidative stress (21).
3) Levels of serum IGF-1 can be decreased antepartum by pesticides (22).
4) Hypoxia can down-regulate IGF-1 and IGF-1 receptor gene expression (23).
5) By inhibiting the pathway to IGF production, mercury can decrease myelination (24).
6) Folic acid is able to modulate IGF-1 receptor gene expression (25).
7) Maternal inflammation decreases placental IGF production (chapter 6D).
8) Reduced expression of mRNA for IGF-1 has been found in diabetics with peripheral neuropathy (26).
9) That IGF is involved with brain development was noted when the IQs of young children were found to be directly correlated with their IGF levels (27)
10) Although some investigators have suggested that children conceived by *in vitro* fertilization are at greater risk for autism, possibly related to depressed IGF levels (1), recent studies report no association found (28).

11) Inflammation may influence the level of IGF through increased capillary permeability. In such a setting, circulating protease inhibitors could gain greate access to extravascular IGF binding proteins, thereby releasing decreased amounts of free IGF to cell surface receptors (29).

12) IGF-1 is multifunctional in the nervous system by stimulating myelination, among its many roles (30).

13) Transgenic mice which lack the ability to produce IGF have reduced axonal diameters and decreased nerve conduction velocities (31).

14) In the absence of myelin sheaths, there is less brain white matter (32), and nerves exhibit impaired function (33).

15) Brain IGF mRNA is highly expressed during fetal life, reaching a peak in the early postnatal weeks. IGF receptor is found in abundance in the growth cones of early neurites and actively promotes neuronal motility and outsprouting (34). Reduced IGF accelerates neuron apoptosis.

16) In unmyelinated axons of diameter α, nerve impulses travel at a velocity of about $1.8(\alpha)^{1/2}$ meters/second, whereas with myelination of thickness β, the conduction speed is about $12(\alpha+\beta)$ m/s (chapter 6A) (35).

17) Milk is a good source of IGF which survives digestion. Neonates breastfed up to one year of age subsequently develop autism less often than those who are not (36).

Conclusions

It is here hypothesized that reduced neonatal IGF concentration may forecast increased risk of subsequently developing autism. If proven correct, it would be rational to utilize this concept to quantitatively predict in the newborn the risk of infantile autism than waiting for later subjective psycho-neurologic signs alone.

The concept presented here is that determination of the level of IGF at birth may help uncover the odds that a particular neonate may subsequently exhibit autism. More than being just a coincidental biomarker, this parameter may also point to the advisability of supplementing IGF in the newborn (e.g., with prolonged breastfeeding) to enhance neuronal myelination in the central nervous system. In this way, the "mis-wiring" of neural pathways characteristic of autism might be reduced.

Taken as a whole, the findings reviewed in this chapter would support the contention that almost anything which acts to reduce the level of IGF in the fetus and/or neonate would disrupt the myelination process or hinder synaptic maturation, triggering the appearance of the typical hallmarks of autism and it special behavioral characteristics.

As Hertz-Picciotto summarized (37): "Interactions of environmental, modifiable factors with common gene polymorphisms or possible sequence variants may be involved in the vast majority of autism cases, dictating that large sample sizes are needed to unravel these causes."

Glossary

AI: autism index

CARS: childhood rating scale

IGF: insulin-like growth factor

MBP: myelin basic protein

M-CHAT: modified checklist for autism in toddlers

MEG: magnetoencephalography

INOCULATION

Chapter 7A: Vaccination/MMR

Bethlehem Kassaye, Nicole McGill, Renata Segal, Araj Sidki, Nathaniel Strock, Kseniya Svyatets

[The saga which has had the greatest (negative) effect on researching the cause of autism thusfar relates to the fear of a connection between childhood vaccination and the occurrence of this disorder. Even though several studies invalidated this pronouncement, unfounded concern remains in the general public. – Ed.]

Hypothesis

The controversy linking vaccines to autism has had some of the most dangerous effects in medical history. A 1998 publication by Andrew Wakefield and 12 of his colleagues attempted to link children with intestinal abnormalities who began to show developmental delays after vaccination with the measles, mumps, and rubella vaccine (MMR vaccine). The paper itself did not prove conclusively that there is an association between the MMR vaccine and children with autism or developmental disabilities (1). However, the damage had been done; the number of unvaccinated individuals had begun to rise, as did outbreaks of diseases that vaccines were made to prevent.

Observations

Vaccines are biologically created substances that incorporate weakened or dead parts of microbes that can be injected into the human body. Once a vaccine is introduced into the human body, the immune system develops antibodies specific to the microbe. These antibodies protect the person from the illness if the person ever comes in contact with the live form of the virus (2,3).

MMR is a vaccine that at one time was thought to be linked to inflammatory bowel disease (IBD) and autism (4). The MMR controversy has induced a perpetual fear in many parents, who now refuse to vaccinate their children, which has compromised the herd immunity for the general population. Herd immunity is the idea that vaccination of the majority is protective to the minority population that cannot get inoculated (e.g.,immuno-compromised individuals). When the majority of people (the herd) are immune to a certain disease, it serves to shield the unvaccinated from contracting disease. If contraction of a disease in a population is decreased then transmission to those that are not immune is also decreased. Although the theory of association between MMR and autism was proposed and dismissed more than ten years ago, parents still continue to worry about adverse effects of the inoculations. As a result, this has led to new problems, such as recent outbreaks of these currently rare diseases that were mostly eradicated before the MMR/autism controversy (5).

MMR is a trivalent vaccine given to young children to provide immunity against measles, mumps, and rubella in a single shot. Besides being extremely infectious and contagious, each of these diseases can have severe life-threatening complications. For example, the measles virus (MV) is an infection that presents with the triad of cough, coryza and conjunctivitis, as well as photophobia in the early stages. However, a rare complication of MV is progression to subacute sclerosing panencephalitis (SSPE), in which the virus persists in the brain. It functions as a slow-acting virus, resulting in behavioral and intellectual changes, and, more importantly, chronic central nervous degeneration. The majority of SSPE cases are fatal (6).

In appraising the severity of this disease, prior to the availability of the MMR vaccine, approximately three to four million people contracted measles every year (7). Between 1964-1965, 12.5 million people in America were infected with rubella. 2,000 babies died due to rubella complications, and 11,000 rubella related miscarriages occurred (8). In addition, the World Health Organization estimated measles cases in 1998 to be 30 million worldwide, which led to 888,000 measles-related deaths, as well as contributing to an astounding 10% of deaths in children less than 5 years old in developing countries (9).

The inoculations for the measles, mumps, and rubella were combined into one injection in 1971 (10). The vaccine was so successful at reducing the prevalence of these diseases that by the end of the 1970s-early 1980s, the Centers for Disease Control and Prevention (CDC) declared their goal in eliminating measles from the United States by the year 2000. During 1989-1990, the United States saw a major resurgence of the measles in unvaccinated individuals. The CDC then recommended a second dose of the MMR vaccine to children of elementary school age. After this change, from 1992-1993 the number of reported cases of measles decreased from 2,237 to 312. There was hope of eradicating measles in the Americas by the year 2000 (11).

Like the United States, Great Britain (particularly England and Wales) followed suit with the same immunization schedule. Both countries had a more gradual decline in measles cases after the vaccine was introduced. Following the introduction of the booster shot for the MMR vaccine to children, reported cases of measles in England and Wales dropped from 26, 222 in 1989 to 9,680 in 1991. Also, like the US, England, and Wales had a measles outbreak in 1994 due to an increased number of unvaccinated individuals. Reported cases of measles rose to 16,375 (12). Since 1995, there has been a relatively steady decline in reported measles cases. However, it was not until 1998 that number of parental consents to administer the MMR vaccine to one's child in both the United States and the United Kingdom began to decline. Several reasons may have caused this decline; there could have been speculation as to the safety of these injections, creating doubts in the public's mind about whether or not to have each child vaccinated.

The MMR hypothesis grew out of a case study that was conducted by a research group in the UK in 1998. Andrew Wakefield, a gastroenterologist, was the lead author of the 1998 article published by *The Lancet*, a prestigious medical journal in Great Britain, titled "Ileal-lymphoid-nodular hyperplasia, non-specific colitis, and pervasive developmental disorder in children".

Prior to his work on autism, Wakefield's research interest was in finding a link between persistent MV infection (via monovalent vaccine or wild-type) and IBD (inflammatory bowel disease) (13). IBD is a group of diseases that includes ulcerative colitis and Crohn's disease. Wakefield and his team believed that the development of Crohn's disease might be the result of chronic MV infection at a critical time during early childhood and that an increased risk may be associated with giving the live attenuated vaccine at that time (14).

When approached in 1996 by a mother concerned that her child with gastrointestinal (GI) problems had developmentally regressed shortly after receiving MMR, Wakefield shifted his research focus onto this possible phenomenon that could have a tremendous effect on his prior research. The original study in 1998 consisted of 12 children (with a mean age of 6 years), who had begun to experience diminished developmental skills, such as language, along with diarrhea and abdominal pain, who were referred to a pediatric gastroenterologist (4).

The goal of the report was to find out if there was some kind of link between children who had (IBD), regressive developmental disabilities (autism spectrum disorder), and the MMR vaccine. The children involved in this study were put under a variety of assessments to examine and evaluate their conditions. The numerous tests conducted involved neurological, developmental, and GI studies via colonoscopy and biopsy sampling. These tests demonstrated that each of the 12 children exhibited an "intestinal abnormality" ranging from lymphoid nodular hyperplasia to aphthoid ulceration (4). Other endoscopic findings indicated that the children suffered from other colonic and rectal abnormalities as well. Interestingly, four of the 12 cases demonstrated a "'red halo sign' around the swollen cecal lymphoid follicles, which is an early endoscopic feature of Crohn's disease" (15).

Wakefield and colleagues then collected detailed histories, paying particular attention to the temporal relationship between vaccinations and dates of infections. When the children's parents and physicians were both asked for detailed histories, it was only the parent's observations that indicated eight out of the twelve children had begun exhibiting developmental delays which the parentsthought were linked to MMR (4). There was a 63-day average interval from exposure to the onset of the first signs of behavioral delay. Although the article ultimately concluded there is inadequate evidence of a link between the vaccine and any of the health issues of the children involved (4), once the media had become aware of this study, they quickly began to publicize these results, which caused a massive increase of concerned parents worldwide because of the suggested link between MMR, IBD, and regressive type of autism (15). Since Wakefield was the lead author of the article and had continued to endorse the theory, he has been primarily associated with the controversy.

After the news had spread, journalists began to interview numerous parents. Many of these parents shared their personal experiences of how they felt the vaccine had adversely affected their child's development. Although there was no scientific proof of this correlation, they continued to endorse the belief that MMR had induced adverse effects (15). A simple headline saying a doctor believes there is a link between vaccines and autism was enough to create doubts in the public mind. For an individual who does not know how to differentiate between credible versus unreliable resources, the vast amount of information available to a lay person can be overwhelming. Thus, the controversy created a health scare and caused many parents not to vaccinate their children in the UK. Furthermore, several parents worldwide began to boycott the MMR vaccine in a protective attempt to keep their child safe.

Signs and symptoms of autism usually appear in the second year of life, a time that happens to coincide with administration of MMR. Whereas MMR is first given at 12-15 months, the first signs of autism appear at 15-18 months. However, an efficient diagnosis of autism is made around 24 months or later (16). This gave credence to the possibility that there might be a connection between MMR and autism. However, Wakefield's study states, "We did not prove an association between measles, mumps, and rubella vaccine, and the syndrome described [autism]" (1). What the authors did was identify the possibility of a link, stating that, "Further investigations are needed to examine this syndrome and its possible relation to this vaccine." Unfortunately, once any relative connection is made to developmental disorders, parents are rightly hesitant to give their children the vaccine. Furthermore, other data demonstrated that there had been a general increase in the number of autistic diagnoses since the MMR vaccine was introduced in 1988 in the UK; this only led to further concerns (17). As a result, only two months after the article was published in London, doctors and other health care providers were receiving a variety of questions regarding the vaccine and its possible neurologic side effects (18).

Another particular concern about Wakefield was that the combination of three live viruses into one vaccine could cause vulnerability in particular children (14). An interview was conducted in 2000 with Barbara Loe Fischer, the president of the National Vaccine Information Center and leading advocate for parental informed consent in regard to childhood vaccines, during which she discussed Wakefield's findings. Wakefield had been concerned that the live trivalent vaccine was causing some "genetically vulnerable children" to develop an MV infection in the intestines that was negatively impacting their immune and nervous system. In addition, she referred to his recommendation for children to obtain the three vaccinations at separate times with a span of at least one year between each one. Interestingly, the vaccines are available separately in the United States; however, in countries such as Great Britain, the public health authorities have banned this option (14). As a result, parents are essentially forced to vaccinate their children with the trivalent vaccine or nothing at all. This makes it difficult for informed parents with ongoing anxiety about MMR to choose between the possible risk of autism versus the risk for diseases they had never seen before.

Wakefield's paper originally appeared in *The Lancet* in 1998, creating a worldwide discussion and encouraging a large body of scientific research on the link between the MMR vaccine and autism. Several years after Wakefield's paper was published, reporter Brian Deer came to *The Lancet* with claims that the doctor had been given money by attorneys of parents of the autistic children in Wakefield's study, these parents had financial interest in finding a causation result (19). Accusations were also made that Wakefield falsified medical histories of his subjects (20). These actions could result in a measurement bias with his results. If the information gathered was in fact distorted, the reliability of his outcomes became questionable.

In 2004, *The Lancet* initiated investigations into allegations of misconduct in Wakefield's study. When these investigations started, 10 of the original 13 authors decided to write a retraction of the paper's interpretation, leaving only Wakefield and 2 others as proponents of the MMR hypothesis. During this time, there was also discussion that the doctor may lose the right to practice medicine in the UK based on the proposed misconduct in the research reported in the 1998 article (21). According to the *Independent* newspaper, Wakefield was facing charges for serious professional misconduct by the General Medical Council and "publishing inadequately founded research, failing to obtain ethical committee approval, obtaining funding improperly and subjecting children to unnecessary and invasive investigations." Consequently, the General Medical Council struck Wakefield from the medical registry in the UK in January of 2010 and *The Lancet* formally retracted Wakefield's original paper soon thereafter.

The outcome of the 1998 publication seemed to have struck a personal cord with parents worldwide. At the time of the publication, the criteria for making an autism identification were continuously evolving. Thus, the number of children diagnosed with the disease was on the rise (chapter 1D). Parents were increasingly frustrated because the lack of sufficient therapeutic resources available (22). Wakefield's theory appealed to parents, politicians, and celebrities because it suggested that there was a direct etiology for autism. It offered parents hope of a cure or effective therapy for an increasingly complicated and contested disease (22). In his paper, he stated that eight of his subjects began exhibiting behavioral manifestations of autism in a range of 1-14 days after receiving the MMR vaccine (1). However, he argued that despite this, the history of intestinal pathologies with autism spectrum disorders was enough to suggest a real correlation (1). This made for a convincing argument to concerned parents.

Even though the article on its own was not damaging, the media bombardment that followed proved to be detrimental. A variety of media sources, including the *New York Times, USA today, CNN,* and the *Washington Post* announced that a possible link has been found, causing many parents to panic and stop vaccinating their children (19). In 2009, it was found that 20% of parents in the United States felt that vaccines were responsible for the onset of autism (20). Media reports and even celebrities developed an anti-vaccine campaign. Although his article has since been retracted by Th*e Lancet* along with countless researchers disproving his findings (see below), All over the US and parts of Europe, parents were, and still are, choosing to refuse vaccinations for their children.

Subsequent findings

The research detailed below disproves the MMR hypothesis which is dependent on three conjunctive findings in autistic children after MMR inoculation:
1) persistent MV in the intestinal tissues,
2) development of an inflammatory-type bowel disease
3) regression of development.

A fourth factor that was deemed pertinent when Wakefield started his research on autism, later disregarded due to non-support, was epidemiological evidence that the rising incidence of autism had a positive correlation with the introduction of the MMR vaccination.

The following observations are with respect to the four criteria above, explaining research findings chronologically to arrive at present day conclusions. It is important to refer back to chapter 1A: Scientific Approach in this book when assessing the details of these studies, as well as the observations above detailing inaccuracies and false claims of the Wakefield et al. study in 1998 (1) that marked the beginning of this controversy.

Persistent MV in the intestinal tissues

1) Prior to Wakefield's efforts to relate autism to MMR, he took part in gastrointestinal research searching for a connection between the monovalent measles vaccine and chronic IBD. In one such study unrelated to autism in 1997, Wakefield and other researchers report detecting MV (via TEM - transmission electron microscopy - and immunocytochemistry, a method later found to be unreliable and nonspecific in such cases (23)) in the guts of chronic entercolitis subjects (24). This fact is pertinent because, although the central tenet to the MMR hypothesis is chronic infection by MV in the intestinal tissues, virological studies were not available to support the hypothesis in 1998 (1), although Wakefield already had a method of doing so as detailed in the previous report (24).

2) Kawashima et al. reported virological evidence in a paper in 2000. Peripheral blood samples (PBS) from three of the nine autistic children in the 1998 study were found to have MV RNA of the MMR vaccine strain (via nested reverse transcription PCR with direct sequencing) with MV also found in one of eight patients with Crohn's disease, in one of three with ulcerative colitits and in none of the eight healthy child controls (25). This study was done on PBS, not on the intestinal tissues of the subjects, which were also collected during the 1998 study. The authors acknowledged in the paper that MV may be present in the intestines of these subjects, but did not give further information as to why they did not use GI tissue for MV detection. Since the basis for the MMR hypothesis is chronic inflammation caused by persistent MV, it is of interest that the virological evidence published is from PBS and not GI tissue.

3) In 2000, Afzal et al. analyzed five different detection methods for the presence of MV in the intestinal tissue of children with IBD (4). Since persistent infection with MV is Wakefield's basis of association between MMR and autism, it is necessary to make sure detection methods used to make this correlation are precise, accurate and specific. Afzal et al. chose studies from research facilities that used different methods other than those associated with the 1998 study at RFH (the Royal Free Hospital). Methods from each laboratory are detailed, including the original method from RFH, as well a new method developed at RFH with variation thought to be more sensitive and specific than the first. The authors concluded in the paper that, although it is possible for MV to persist in many different tissues and should be detectable by certain molecular diagnostics, no one has been able to do so in any of these cases.

4) In 2002, Uhlmann et al. reported detection of MV in the ileolymphoid tissue of 75 out of 91 children with autism and five out of 70 in a control group (via reverse transcription TaqMan polymerase chain reaction (PCR) *in situ*). All samples were obtained from RFH (26). Another report in 2002 by Martin et al also announced detection of MV in ileolymphoid tissue of children diagnosed with autism (via the same detection method). This study was with 73 of 77 in the affected population and five of 44 in the control population (27). It is hard to determine if these two studies, with similar authorship (Wakefield named on both), were using similar samples from RFH. There is no detail in the Martin publication of how or where patient samples were obtained. In comparing the two papers, details of test and control populations in each study are remarkably similar. Both papers noted that presence of persistent MV in the general population is unknown and should be subject to greater study (26,27). Although it may be considered quite important, neither paper mentioned MMR vaccination status of the subjects or for what the tissues were tested, specifically, MMR vaccine-strain or wild-type MV (23).

5) In 2006, D'Souza et al. recreated the experimental conditions for MV detection reported in the 2000 Kawashima study and the 2002 Uhlmann study to test the real-time and nested reverse transcriptase polymerase chain reaction (RT-PCR) primers used in those studies (23). (In a real-time RT-PCR test, the detection of the intended section of RNA is made as the process progresses, as opposed to the end of the reaction. In a nested PCR, the initial product is amplified further with a second set of primers to make the detection even more specific to the RNA being sought out.) Peripheral blood samples were used for detection instead of intestinal tissue because in this, as well as many other studies, it is hard to ethically justify performing invasive procedures on young patients to obtain an intestinal sample. While researchers did generate overwhelmingly positive results when using the Uhlmann assays, further investigation, including melting analysis and assessment of amplicon (piece of DNA or RNA generated from the PCR) size via gel electrophoresis, did not yield any positive matches to MV RNA in test or control populations. No positive results were seen when using the Kawashima assays for either population. This study was monumental in that its methods were meticulously reported. Its analysis of the previous research points to where contamination may have occurred and how it was avoided. The authors pointed out that the detection methods used previously with the MV monoclonal antibody were shown by other studies (28) to cross-react with an unidentified human protein and that amplicons used in previous studies (25-27) were actually derived from a human, not a viral gene (23). This is why a reaction occurred in human intestinal tissues providing a false positive result for MV RNA. All of this together solidifies the assertion in this study that the previous PCR data published by those authors is unlikely to be true.

6) In 2008, Hornig and coworkers set out to replicate the 1998 RFH study by testing intestinal tissues of children with GI disturbances and developmental regression for MV (29). Although D'Souza's study was important to discredit the detection methods that had been previously used, it utilized PBS to do so. Hornig wanted to appease the public more by using intestinal tissue for analysis. All subjects are noted having received the MMR vaccine; the test group consisted of 25 children with autism and GI disturbances, and the control group was

children with GI disturbances without a diagnosis Ileal and cecal biopsies were taken from the children via ileocolonoscopy (clinically indicated due to the severity of abdominal pain and GI symptoms). The specimens were sent to three separate labs (including the lab where the original RFH results were obtained) and were blinded to both the labs and researchers. As a result, researchers found no difference in detection of MV RNA in the guts of the autistic children with GI disturbances in comparison to the non-autistic children with GI disturbances. In fact, only two ileal samples, one from the test group and one from the control group, were found to have MV RNA again providing strong evidence against the association of MMR, autism and entercolitis.

Inflammatory-type bowel disease and regression of development

With regard to regression, there are two aspects of note:

1) the loss of developmental skills after MMR vaccination, and

2) an increase in reporting of regressive symptoms after an MMR program was introduced.

Both factors are necessary to distinguish autistic entercolitis as a new phenotype of ASD. Loss of development (such as language) can be arbitrary at ages younger than 2 years old (30). Researchers note that parents are often dismissive of early developmental symptoms because they do not want to believe that their child may have a problem. This leads to symptoms being reported later than they actually start, making parents think that their child has regressed when the problem was there all along.

As mentioned earlier, Wakefield et al. in the 1998 paper linked the MMR vaccine with regressive development solely based on parental memory. Of the twelve children (nine with autism), it was only eight that were associated with autism after receiving MMR (1).

In 2001, Fombonne analyzed factors deemed necessary for autistic entercolitis to be considered a new phenotype of autism caused by MMR (31). Ninety-six child subjects from an epidemiologic study in the UK were assessed for a connection between IBD and regressive development: 76 via pediatrician/parental questionnaires, 20 via pediatrician questionnaire alone. This sample was statistically compared to two controls:

1) 98 autistic children before receiving MMR, and

2) 68 autistic children after receiving MMR.

The authors found no association between regression and GI problems in the test sample and no statistically significant difference from the control samples (31). This, along with finding that regressive rates had actually *decreased* after MMR introduction (attributed to the use of a more stringent definition of regressive development), led the authors to reject the case for autistic entercolitis.

In 2002, a UK population study by Taylor et al. investigated the possibility of autistic entercolitis as a new phenotype of ASD in relation to regression and bowel symptoms (32). The study consisted of 278 children with autism and 195 children with atypical autism (PDD-NOS) born from 1979 to 1998, assessing reports of bowel symptoms lasting more than three months and looking for increased reports of regressive symptoms after the 1988 introduction of the MMR. Of the 473 children, there were 81 who reported bowel symptoms with only two of these having IBD. The study found no significant trend in report of bowel symptoms by birth year, an important observation being that it spanned the period before and after MMR introduction in 1988. The study showed that report rates of regressive autism have not changed proportionately since MMR was introduced to the UK in 1988. Although regression and bowel symptoms seem to be reported together in many neurological developmental disorders, there is no correlation to be drawn with MMR vaccine and the authors reject autistic entercolitis as a new phenotype of autism.

In 2009, Sandhu et al. analyzed bowel patterns (number, color and consistency) of children with ASD compared to those without ASD to determine if a significant difference was present in these two populations (33). Of the 12,984 children in this prospectively conducted study, 78 were eventually diagnosed with ASD and compared with remaining non-ASD children in the group. All data sets used had similar results leading the researchers to conclude that entercolitis is not associated with ASD.

Epidemiological evidence

Wakefield noted in the 1998 case study that if MMR were to have a causal relationship to autism there would be an increased incidence in the population after the introduction of the trivalent vaccination in the UK (1).

In 1999, Taylor et al. evaluated the incidence of autism diagnosis in the UK in eight North Thames health districts before and after the MMR vaccination program started in 1988. Evaluation of 498 cases of autism in children born since 1979 found no change in the trend of incidence of autism diagnoses after the introduction of MMR: a steady rise was noted in the diagnosis of autism year by year, but slope of the graph remained unaffected by the introduction of MMR in 1988 (34).

In 2002, a retrospective cohort study by Madsen et al. reviewed records of children born in Denmark from 1991 to 1998 for significance of MMR vaccination as a cause of autism (35). This is considered a particularly reliable study because in Denmark every child is given an ID number at birth to which the Danish Board of Health thereafter attaches vaccination status. Any medical or psychiatric diagnoses are assigned to this ID number; the latter by the Danish Psychiatric Central Register, which is the reporting body for autistic disorders. After identifying 440,655 children that had received the MMR vaccination during the time period (out of 537,303 born), the study assessed the relative risk of an autism diagnosis. Relative risk assesses the probability of having a disease (autism in this case) in a population of individuals exposed to a certain factor (MMR) versus the probability of disease in those not exposed to that same factor. The relative risk was calculated to be less than one (0.92); including consideration of those diagnosed with an ASD, relative risk with even lower (0.83). These numbers, taken in a 95% confidence interval, provided strong evidence against MMR as the cause of autism, with the risk of autism diagnosis being similar in both vaccinated and unvaccinated children.

Epidemiologic studies coming out of Japan have a unique and valuable element to them: Japan started their MMR program in 1989 only to discontinue it in 1993 due to outbreaks of aseptic meningitis resulting from the Urabe strain of mumps being used in the formulation (36).

This allows Japanese studies to evaluate autism incidence before, during and after MMR. One such study by Honda et al. in 2005 assessed the cumulative incidence of childhood autism and other ASD for children born in Kohoku Ward in Yokohama, Japan from 1988-1996 following them until age seven. The authors note that if MMR were a causative agent of autism, incidence should have decreased significantly in children born after the withdrawal of the MMR program in 1993. Instead, the incidence steadily increased from 1988 with a spike in the trend after the withdrawal in 1993. This is yet another epidemiologic study opposing MMR as a causative agent of autism.

Conclusions

Although we have discussed four factors in order to be thorough, the MMR hypothesis could hinge on one detail: persistent MV in the gut. Regression is hypothesized to result from the chronic inflammation and hyperplasia, which is precipitated by MV in the intestinal tissue. This is why so many researchers have gone to great lengths to show the inability to detect a chronic MV infection (4,29,31), while others have pointed out why earlier detections (25-27) were inaccurate (23,28).

The possible linkage of autism and MMR has been given an enormous amount of undue press, instilling a massive fear within many parents. Parents are still apprehensive about giving their children MMR, although, as shown above, there is a lack of epidemiological evidence to show MMR as being causative of autism. Researchers often look for correlations to point them in a direction to investigate causation. We have all heard the phrase, "correlation does not imply causation," and here is a good place to explain its significance. A correlation, in its simplest sense, is two things occurring together or having an apparent association. These two things can have a relation to one another, but that does not mean that one *causes* the other. If the implementation of MMR had been correlated with an increased incidence of autism, which it has not been, as clearly evidenced above, this would still by no means imply that the administration of MMR *causes* autism (see Prologue for Koch's criteria). All that being said, exposure to MV without prior immunity may cause one to become sick with measles. Since many parents have never seen a child with measles or understand what the disease entirely consists of, it is difficult for them to comprehend the severity and danger of this disease.

The CDC and Public Health England are beginning to push for more legislation requiring vaccinations, because of increasing measles outbreaks in the United States and England in recent years. The number of individuals being vaccinated has increased in 2012, but is still not where it needs to be in order to eradicate the diseases. In the UK, more and more children are receiving the MMR vaccine; however, a slightly smaller number of children are receiving the booster shot now (37). There is no clear indication as to why parents are choosing to not follow through with the vaccination schedule. Without the provided immunity the vaccine offers, children are still at risk of getting the measles, mumps, or rubella.

Because of multiple outbreaks in communities in the United States and United Kingdom, health officials have been administering vaccinations in hospitals and private clinics throughout each respective country. According to recent CDC details for 2012, vaccination rates in the United States reached 90.8%, down from 91.6% in 2011 (38, 39). The United Kingdom also reported increased vaccination rates. As of 2011-2012, they have risen to 91.2%. According to the CDC and Public Health England, the goal is to keep vaccination rates at 90% or higher, with hopes to eventually reach 95% inoculation coverage (37,38).

Whether or not Wakefield expected these kinds of results and consequences to evolve from the original article is hard to say. The main issue at hand is that some parents are still keeping their children from being immunized against harmful diseases because they think it may lead to autism. When otherwise healthy people are not immunized from deadly diseases like measles, they can become infected with these diseases causing prevalence in the population. While these healthy people may or may not suffer serious complications from measles, they are compromising those individuals that are unable to get vaccinated.

The appeal of citing MMR as a possible cause of autism could be because the vaccine is administered shortly before a diagnosis of autism can occur. Other than the coincidental timing of the vaccine and the diagnosis of autism, there is no proven cause or correlation between the two. The MMR vaccine has been shown to provide effective immunity against the measles, mumps, and rubella for over 40 years. With or without the vaccine, the rate of autism diagnosis continues to rise, for reasons yet to be elucidated (chapters 1B,1C,2B). It is important to get the vaccination program back on track so that many fewer children will become unnecessarily infected with life-threatening diseases that should have been eradicated long ago (chapter 1A)0.

Chapter 7B - Thimerosal

Oyewale Bello, RohitNavlani

[Because of its mercury content, the vaccine preservative, thimerosal, has been suggested as the agent linking vaccination with autism. This claim is now not taken seriously since extensive studies have failed to support such a relationship definitively. – Ed.]

Hypothesis

Thiomerosal, an organomercury compound found in certain vaccines, was once considered to have the potential to cause neurologic damage. Based on the known toxicity of mercury containing compounds, thimerosal has long been postulated as a precipitating factor in the development of autism.

Observations

Mercury (Hg) is a metallic compound and the principal potentially toxic element in thimerosal. The term, organomercuric compound, refers to mercury covalently bonded to carbon.

Thimerosal is 49.6% mercury by weight (1) and is rapidly degraded in the body (2). Several studies have been conducted that has shown that ethylmercury is a potential neurotoxin, especially in high doses.

The initial blood plasma half-life of ethylmercury in experimental monkey infants exposed to a similar dose of thimerosal contained in human vaccines was measured at 2.1 days, while the terminal half-life is 8.6 days, meaning that it initially takes 2 days for a newly vaccinated monkey infant to degrade half of the thimerosal administered to it (2,3). The increased terminal half-life shows that the metabolism is thimerosal gradually depreciates as the body metabolizes and excretes the chemical.

One of the dangers of ethylmercury is its ability to cross the blood-brain barrier. It is unknown at this point how much of it actually crosses the barrier (3). This barrier is a protective fortification composed of cells closely aligned in an adjacent fashion, designed to keep molecules of a certain size and polarity from accompanying the bloodstream that supplies the brain. Ethylmercury is oxidized to an inorganic cation in the red blood cells, lungs and liver in both humans and animals. The process of oxidation of mercury seems to have a protective effect against the passage of mercury into the brain. Because preterm infants may have a decreased ability to oxidize mercury due to their underdeveloped status, they may have a higher level of mercury in the brain if exposed than adults (4).

Ethylmercury also crosses through the placental barrier (3), a barricade similar to the blood-brain barrier but constituting different types of cells. Communication between the maternal circulation and the fetal bloodstream is tightly regulated. Substances that readily cross the barrier include immunoglobulin IgG, small drugs, ethanol, and some maternally acquired viruses such rubella and herpes simplex virus II. This is important to note because there is a chance that the fetus may be exposed to thimerosal during routine administration of the prophylactic flu vaccine to pregnant mothers. Fluzone is an example of such vaccines; it has a thimerosal content of 12.5 μg/dose (5), making it the highest thimerosal-containing vaccination administered in the United States today. It theoretically possesses the greatest risks of ethyl mercury poisoning. This vaccine is not administered to children less than 6 months of age.

The ability of ethylmercury to freely cross several body compartments throughout the body, especially to the brain, makes thimerosal a central subject in the ongoing debate associated with the etiology of autism. The first safety study on thimerosal (merthiolate) was conducted and published in 1930 by Powell and Jamieson, entitled "merthionate as a germicide." (6). It defined the chemical as safe. However, clinical research performed in the study was deeply flawed. A total of 22 patients dying of meningococcal meningitis were injected with 50 cm^3 (ml) of 1% solution of merthiolate, in order to evaluate human tissue response to the germicide and also to effect killing of the bacteria (6).The actual content of pure merthiolate from the solution was 0.5 ml (500,000 μg). According to the CDC, the maximum thimerosal content in vaccines after 2004, including the influenza vaccines, was about 40 μg for children over the age of 2 and 2.5 μg for neonates under the age of 6 months in which the influenza vaccine is not recommended (10).

These individuals were therefore exposed to 208,000 times more mercury than what is currently used in vaccines in children 6 months old and 12,500 times more than children 2 years old.

There were a number of details omitted in the publication of the study that cast enormous doubt as to the validity of this experiment, and also whether or not there was bias involved, especially since the conductors of the study were also the creators of the drug. The authors of this article failed initially to mention that the subjects were infected with meningitis. This is a fundamental flaw because proper evaluation of the safety of a drug should also be assessed on healthy individuals. The paper also failed to mention the fact that a large percentage of participants in this study died after administration of merthiolate, some only after a day 7, without indicating what share the meningitis had on the cause of death. The duration of time in which the subjects were exposed to merthiolate, the amount of time the researchers followed the participants, and the time that elapsed between the start of the study and subsequent deaths makes it impossible to truly evaluate any side effects of the medication. Geier et al., who reviewed the study, noted that $1/3^{rd}$ of the participants were only followed for one day, while the lengthiest follow-up period was 62 days. They note that the reason for the brief observation period was probably due to the rapid death of many of the participants in the study, making it difficult to actually evaluate mercury toxicity levels and also to allow for adequate time for mercury toxicity to manifest. This is significant because mercury toxicity typically takes months to develop (7).

Since the study was conducted only on persons already suffering from a life-threatening disease, it would have been difficult to ascertain whether or not the death was due to thimerosal or meningitis. This would have been the case even if the time parameters explained earlier were valid as healthy volunteers were not used in the study. These serious omissions would have rendered the study scientifically invalid, yet the chemical was declared safe to use. For a number of years, this was the only study conducted to evaluate the toxicity of thimerosal. This may be one of the main reasons that thimerosal was suspected as an etiological agent in the onset of increased autism incidence rates decades later. The nature of this poorly conducted experiment and the apparent attempt to conceal crucial information concerning its cogency certainly provided the public with a strong and valid skepticism as to the safety of the chemical.

In order to develop a proper understanding about the importance of using preservatives in vaccinations and why thimerosal was developed, it is important to consider the effects of administering non-preserved vaccines. Prior to the introduction of preservatives such as thimerosal in vaccines, the risk of microbial infections from vaccines was significant, especially from bacteria and fungi. In 1928, a diphtheria vaccine was developed and administered to 21 children. A preservative was not included in this injectable. Of the 21 children vaccinated, 12 children died. Further investigation of the cause of death revealed that all the children developed a staphylococcus infection that was determined to have developed from the vaccine itself (8). It became apparent that antimicrobial agents needed to be included in vaccines to prevent the growth of pathologic microbes causing infections. The efficacy and dimished toxicity of thimerosal in comparison to other preservatives such as phenol and cresol was the dominant reason thimerosal became widespread. It is estimated that thimerosal is 40-50 times more effective at preventing the replication of microorganisms in vaccines than phenol, while maintaining the efficacy of the vaccines itself (9).

The controversy surrounding thimerosal escalated, especially the 1970's and subsequent years to follow, during which the apparent incidence of diagnosed autism increased drastically. Thimerosal was used to prevent microbial contamination routinely until 1999, when the Center for Disease and Control (CDC) advised that the concentration of thimerosal should be reduced to trace amounts (<0.5 µg Hg per dose) or eliminated from vaccines (8). It is important to note that this was merely a recommendation and no official ban had been imposed. Table 7C-1 compares the relative exposure of children to mercury in 1999 and 2004 due to vaccinations. The table defines the exposure of mercury within the first 6 months and the first 2 years of life (10).

Table 1:

Estimated Exposure to Mercury from Vaccines in the United States in 1999 and 2004 (<6 months of age)		
Vaccines	1999 Maximum Mercury Dose (µg)	2004 Maximum Mercury Dose (µg)
3 doses of DTaP *	75.0	<0.9
3 doses of Hep B **	37.5	<1.5
3 doses of HIB	75	0
TOTAL	187.5	<2.4
Estimated Exposure to Mercury from Vaccines in 1999 and in 2004 (<2 years of age)		
Vaccines	1999 Maximum Mercury Dose (µg)	2004 Maximum Mercury Dose (µg)
4 doses of DTaP *	100	<1.2
3 doses of Hep B **	37.5	<1.5
4 doses of HIB	100	0
3 doses of Influenza	37.5	37.5
TOTAL	275	<40.2

*A trace amount of mercury is present in Tripedia (DTaP) thus, the maximum mercury dose following three doses of Tripedia following four doses of Tripedia is <1.2 µg

As evident from the table, the single greatest possible risk of complications based on concentration of thimerosal comes in the form of influenza vaccine. It should be noted that even though the influenza vaccine accounts for almost 90% of all mercury within vaccines, it is still below the level the United States Government considers to be safe. Currently, the EPA recommends that children who are in the 5th percentile of their body weight and under the age of 6 months should not be exposed to thimerosal in excess of 65µg (11).

In 2008, the CDC released a retrospective study on children who had received trivalent inactivated vaccines (TIV) to determine any adverse outcomes (12). The TIV vaccine contains virus that has been inactivated and no longer has the capability of being virulent. The study showed that delayed-type hypersensitivity at the site of injection was reported rarely. (A common side effect of thimerosal is its ability to act as an allergen (12)). A similar study was also conducted by the Food and Drug Administration, comparing similar side effects at the injection sites for both preservative-free and thimerosal-containing vaccines. They concluded that both medications produced similar side effects with insignificant differences in results (13). A delayed-type hypersensitivity reaction is a type IV hypersensitivity response mediated by T-lymphocytes cells, causing swelling, redness and some pain. A Type IV hypersensitivity reaction occurs when an antigen, in this case thimerosal, is processed by cells of the innate immune system such as macrophages and dendtitic cells, which then present specific proteins to the adaptive immune system T-lymphocytes. Through a series of communications between the cells, the T cells and macrophages facilitate the destruction of tissue around the affected area, creating inflammation and pain (14).

A common example of such a reaction is seen in patients reacting positively to a purified protein derivative (PPD) test, which involves injecting tuberculosis antigens under the skin to elucidate prior exposure to various strains of mycobacteria, specifically Mycobacterium tuberculosis or a positive tuberculosis vaccine history. Although this reaction can be painful and irritable, there is no evidence that suggest that the presence of this reaction at the site of injection correlates to the development of ASD. In addition, the American College of Obstetricians and Gynecologists and the American Academy of Family Physicians recommend that all women who are pregnant receive the TIV vaccination (15). This recommendation is based on the fact that neonates under the age of 6 months lack the humoral immune capacity to combat organisms such as influenza. Therefore, vaccinations of the mother can provide passive immunity to the fetus prior to parturition via the transfer of IgG antibodies across the placenta. Other than these reactions, no other side effects or links to ASD were reported. Even though the use of thimerosal has significantly declined recently in some developed countries, there are still high doses of thimerosal being used in vaccines in developing countries. It is still used today in double-dose influenza vaccines for children over 6 months and also in vaccines not routinely administered to young children, such as diphtheria and tetanus.

The general concern of the public to the safety of thimerosal is certainly not without merit. Thimerosal has chemical properties that may cause deleterious effects on the human body in high doses. As more vaccines were developed in the 1970's, an increasing number of young children were exposed to thimerosal. This contributed to the developing notion that thimerosal might be a contributor to the increase in the incidence rate of autism. Another reason for the public misconception was that the FDA decided promptly to advocate the removal of thimerosal from vaccine, even though there was no evidence directly or indirectly linking thimerosal to autism. This action simply advanced preconceived notions without any tangible proof. Nevertheless, these principles have caused numerous problems in terms of vaccination of children, especially when thimerosal was still in active use, as many parents chose not to vaccinate their children with thimerosal-containing vaccines.

To begin the rebuttal of this controversy, there are a couple of issues to address regarding the increase in incidence of autism in the 1970's and beyond. There are numerous factors that could have contributed to the rise. One of the major reasons autism incidence increased could be due to the methods and criteria to diagnose the disease became more inclusive. Environmental changes could have also played a role due to nationwide industrialization. Currently, the EPA sets the standard for the safe exposure to mercury at 0.1 µg/kg body weight/day (15). The environmental changes in mercury are reviewed in chapter 5D in particular.

Another important avenue to investigate is the incidence of autism after thimerosal was removed from most vaccines. Denmark discontinued thimerosal from vaccines in 1992, seven years prior to the United States, even though it had not experienced in increase in incidence of autism since 1971. Following this change, there was a study conducted on the incidence rate of autism from 1991 to 2000. Surprisingly, data did not support a decrease, but rather, an increase in autism diagnosis incidence in those years (16). These data are a weak negative correlation because ASD is potentially a disease of multifactorial origin and no single trend can included or exclude it an etiological agent, however; it may be an important clue supporting the exclusion of vaccination as a cause. A way to consider the possible effect of thimerosal on the onset of ASD would be to perform a case study on the incidence of autism in the developing countries which still administer vaccines containing higher levels of thimerosal currently, relative to the United States.

Results/Data

The toxicity of ethylmercury is not yet well understood; much of the data on risk assessment came from interpreting research done on methylmercury (17). Methylmercury is also an organometallic compound, which is structurally very similar to ethylmercury. Ethylmercury is the metabolic breakdown product of thimerosal, which is central to the vaccine controversy regarding autism spectrum disorders. Methylmercury is an extremely toxic in high enough concentrations. This is evident by the tragedy that occurred in Minamata Bay of Japan decades earlier (chapter 5D).

With such structure similarity, is it easy to see how one could conclude that the two organometallic compounds would illicit similar symptoms in patients. However, they do differ in one key component: bioaccumulation. Bioaccumulation refers to the simple accumulation of a substance, in this case methylmercury in the cells of an orgasm (19). Methylmercury is able to accumulate inside the shellfish at a pace that exceeds its elimination. As with the shellfish, humans who were exposed to the methylmercury have similar problems excreting the toxin.

Based on the neurotoxicology of methylmercury, ethylmercury is obviously a possible subject for research involving ASD. New studies have been conducted investigating the specific mechanisms of ethylmercury toxicity on nervous tissue. Much of this research provides a multifactorial explanation as to the etiology, some of which include genetics and environmental factors. These factors collectively produce a multifaceted presentation of symptoms seen in part in patient with autism disorders.

A new mechanism for the toxicity of ethylmercury has been proposed by Sharpe et al. indicating its possible role as a mitochondrial toxin (18). The study exposed astrocytes to varying levels of thimerosal in order to assess the neurological damage induced by the chemical and its byproducts, mainly ethylmercury. Thimerosal is very lipophilic and, hence, has the potential to cross the blood-brain barrier, as mentioned earlier. Once in the brain, it has the potential to easily impact growth and development in an infant, and in theory could cause damage resulting in symptoms similar to those seen in ASD. It should be noted, however, that no study has actually shown a direct relationship between thimerosal administration and subsequent development of autism. This particular study examined the compound's effects on astrocytes, the most abundant cell type present in the human brain.

Astrocytes normally become "activated" during infection and begin to produce glutathione peroxidase, a key enzyme involved in removing reactive oxygen species (ROS) (chapters 8B,8C). The presence of ethylmercury can increase ROS within the cell, as the exposed cells were found to generate four times as much ROS as the control sample. ROS are oxygen-derived molecules which are highly reactive. They can damage proteins which are part of the electron transport chain located inside the mitochondria, which are crucial for energy production in aerobic species. ROS have also been shown to damage DNA, RNA and cytoplasmic proteins (36). While they are a normal product of oxygen metabolism, increased levels of ROS leads to damage of intracellular structures. This process of oxidative stress can lead to death of the cell. The experimental increase in ROS induces a morphologic change in the cells including shrinkage and blebbing of the cell membrane. Evidence of DNA damage is also present within the cell, but the primary injury is in the cytosol (20).

The ethylmercury is preferentially taken up into the mitochondria by a factor of 1,000 fold, compared to the cytosolic concentration (20). This is due to the difference in electrical potentials across the cellular and mitochondrial membranes. The following describes the proposed mechanism elucidated during the studies conducted by Sharpe et al. (20): Initially, there is preferential absorption of ethylmercury into the astrocyte mitochondria due to the differences in resting membrane potential between the cytoplasmic cell membrane and the mitochondrial cell membrane (45 mV of the plasma membrane vs. 180 mV of the mitochondria membrane). Once inside the mitochondria the ethylmercury will react with iron-sulfur centers such as Rieske proteins involved in cytochrome complexes. This will cause inactivation of enzymes in the electron transport chain (ETC), which is the main source of energy transformation for the cell. In addition, the levels of free iron are increased inside the mitochondria, which ultimately leads to the formation of free radicals, specifically hydroxyl radical, •HO. High levels of hydroxyl radicals causes the release of cytochrome c from the mitochondria, which initiates the process of apoptosis. The death of the astrocytes strongly implicates ethylmercury as a mitochondrial toxin. Rapid death of astrocytes has the potential to cause damage during early development, leading to the type of neurologic defects seen in ASD. Increasing levels of free iron cause excess formation of ROS such as $O_2\bullet$ inside the mitochondria.

Due to the concerns emerging within the past decade regarding the safety of thimerosal, further studies were conducted on its effects on neuronal development. Olczak and coworkers demonstrated neuropathic changes after postnatal administration of thimerosal to young Wistar rats. "Dark neurons" were seen scattered throughout various regions of the brain, including the prefrontal cortex, temporal cortex, hippocampus and cerebellum. These areas correlate with others that would be expected to be damaged given the clinical presentation of ASD which include behavioral issues, deficits in communication, and social interactions, as well as motor dysfunctions (chapters 3B-3D). The "dark neurons" seen in those animals treated with thimerosal represent ischemic degeneration. Such changes occur when the cell is deprived of nutrients, mainly oxygen and glucose. The neurons appeared shrunken and hyperchromatic on microscopic examination due to the chronic exposure of neurons to the accumulating levels of ethylmercury resulting from the breakdown of injected thimerosal. The treated mice also showed changes in their reaction to pain stimulus, alluding to the possibility that thimerosal also has effects on the opioid system. In addition, the mice were noted to have enhanced anxiety and locomotor defects. The presence of the ischemic lesions is similar to the brain lesions seen in patients with Minamata disease, which is also due to mercury poisoning. (23) (chapter 5D).

The thimerosal-treated mice demonstrated a significant loss of the synaptophysin marker (23). The exact function of this molecule is not yet fully understood, but it is known to interact with synaptobrevin, an essential synaptic vessel protein needed to release the contents of the vessel into the neuromuscular junction. Recent research conducted by Schmitt et al. in which synaptophysin has been "knocked out" in experimental mice showed varied behavior changes and reduced spatial learning (24). The link between thimerosal and synaptophysin is an intriguing one and deserves further research to elucidate the interaction between the two.

Thimerosal-induced neuronal cell death appears to depend on many factors, including the concentration of mercury developmental stage of the animal, and the presence of neuroprotective molecules such as glutathione (and possibly dehydroepiandrosterone sulfate (DHEAS). Researchers believe neural cell death may also be due to mitochondrial injury and MtDNA damage, which leads to bioenergetic crisis and increased oxidative stress on the neural cells culminating in apoptosis and necrosis. MtDNA is the circular, double-stranded DNA found inside mitochondria, which encodes for many of the proteins involved in the ETC. Caspase-3-independent apoptosis has also been seen in methylmercury toxicity in cerebellar neurons and oxidative stress in cortical neurons. (23).

An interesting observation was made regarding the state of the astrocytes after thimerosal administration. Normally, when rats are exposed to methylmercury, the astrocytes change into their "reactive" form, where they express high levels of glutathione reductase (27). This enzyme is used to reduce the level of oxidative stress in times of infection or other pathologic processes (chapters 8B,8C). The rats exposed to ethylmercury (thimerosal) did not exhibit the normal reactive astrocytosis, but instead astrocytic atrophy, suggesting that they were better suited to defend against the toxicity of methylmercury. This atrophy noted due to the lack of glutathione reductase was the major factor leading to oxidative stress and, thereafter, apoptosis in an intrinsic, caspase-3-dependent mechanism (23).

Recent research conducted at the Institute of Psychiatry and Neurology in Poland indicated that thimerosal influences release of neuroactive amino acids in the prefrontal cortex. Experiments were conducted in rat models in which thimerosal was directed injected into the prefrontal cortex, the area of the brain responsible for planning complex cognitive behavior, personality expression, decision making, and moderating social behavior (27). The basic activity of this brain region is considered to be orchestration of thoughts and actions in accordance with internal goals. After administration of the compound containing thimerosal, there was a marked increase in glutamate and aspartate, accompanied by a decrease of glycine and alanine. Glutamate and aspartate are major excitatory transmitters in the brain, while glycine is a major inhibitory neurotransmitter; i.e., glutamate and aspartate turn things "ON" while glycine turns them "OFF." It is believed that this imbalance in these neuroactive amino acids leads to some of the behavioral symptoms seen in ASD and mercury-induced neurotoxicities. The balance is shifted in favor of neuronal stimulation, which will inevitably lead to excitotoxic neuronal injuries, are hypothesized to ultimately lead to the changes in behavior seen in neurodegenerative disorders such as ASD (28) (chapters 3E,3F). Excitotoxic injuries are defined as damage due to excessive stimulation by neurotransmitters, such as glutamate.

It should be noted that when mice were injected with low dose thimerosal (12.5ug/kg) no altered levels of glutamate or glycine were produced. These low levels correlate with those seen in normal full-term infants that receive vaccines containing thimerosal. When the mice were injected with higher doses of thimerosal (240 ug/kg), which is 20 times the levels normally employed with human infants, alterations in the levels of neuroactive amino acids released within the prefrontal cortex of the injected mice were seen. The mice were also administered injections of thimerosal 7, 9, 11, and 15 days post-natal during the experiment where a rise in the neurotransmitters was seen. In contrast, infants in the United States are exposed to thimerosal containing vaccines later in life (28). Mice may respond differently than human infants. Secondly, the exposure to thimerosal in these experiments occurs much earlier in the mice experiments than it typically does to human infants in the clinical setting.

This issue points out a large flaw in a majority of the studies conducted to date, which attempt to link vaccines with autism. The studies administer the thimerosal into the animal models just days after birth. As demonstrated by the chart below, infants are not exposed to any s vaccines containing thimerosal until they are at least 6 months. Even then, the dosage of thimerosal contained in the vaccines is just a fraction of the dose injected into the animal models used in these studies.

Table 2:

Age	1 month	2 months	4 months	6 months	9 months	12 months	24 months	36 months
Vaccines containing mercury								
DTaP						DTaP	DTaP	
Hep B				HepB	HepB	HepB	HepB	
Hib						Hib		
Influenza				Inlfuenza	Inlfuenza	Inlfuenza	Inlfuenza	Inlfuenza

The table above is a modified pediatric vaccination schedule for children up to 36 months old, showing only the vaccines that contain trace levels of mercury. (For exact mercury levels, see table 1 of this chapter) (36)). Note that the earliest possible exposure to any thimerosal from vaccines occurs at 6 months post-natal, not a few days old as in the studies conducted by Olczaket et al. (23,28).

An interesting discovery was made during the study conducted by Duszczyk-Budhathoki et al., indicating that a naturally produced neurosteroid may be a biologic defense mechanism against mercury-induced neurotoxicity (28). Dehydroepiandrosterone sulfate (DHEAS) is synthesized in the brain as well as other organs such as the adrenal glands, which has been shown to prevent the negative effects of thimerosal on the frontal cortex. Specifically, DHEAS prevents the excess release of glutamate and aspartate, avoiding excitotoxic neural injuries. It should be noted that this was the first study to identify a possible link between DHEAS and ASD. Further studies need to be conducted, but there may be a future role of DHEAS as a prenatal supplement to further improve the safety of thimerosal-containing vaccines, similar to the way folate is used to prevent neural tube defects such as spina bifida (28) (chapter 5A).

A related study was conducted by Sharpe et al. in children diagnosed with ASD and their siblings. B-lymphocytes, cells responsible for generating antibodies against foreign antigens, were taken from patients with ASD and their unaffected siblings. The B-lymphocytes from the affected children were then compared with normal controls. The cells were exposed to low dosage thimerosal (0.5-1 μM, the same as in some series vaccines) and the effects on cell proliferation and mitochondrial function were observed. Interestingly, a third of those sampled with ASD showed hypersensitivity to thimerosal as a mitochondrial toxin and a third of the siblings also exhibited the same hypersensitivity. This just serves to strengthen our hypothesis that ASD is a multifactorial disease involving genetics and a predisposition to mitochondrial hypersensitivity as well as environmental triggers.

These research data pose a few questions. What is the determinant factor causing only a third of patients with ASD to exhibit mitochondrial hypersensitivity to thimerosal, and if there is an actual link between low dose thimerosal and ASD, why do the siblings who also show the same hypersensitivity not develop the neurologic disease? This study demonstrates more correlation than causation, as it does not establish any connections or provide a specific etiology for ASD.

The controversy of vaccines and autism continues to polarize the American public (chapter 7A). While the Wakefield article brought the issue of vaccines and autism into the mainstream, thimerosal entered the conversation later. In 2003, an autism awareness group known as SafeMinds published a paper in the medical journal *Medical Hypotheses* (which was non-peer reviewed at that time) regarding the autism-mercury hypothesis. The paper tried to establish strong ties between autism and thimerosal based on similar symptoms with mercury exposure and autism. Although there were no scientific data to back the claim at that time, this story sparked the thimerosal controversy (33).

In 2008, there was the controversial case of Hannah Poling, a girl who developed symptoms similar to those seen in ASD after receiving a series of vaccines in a single day (34). She received the following vaccines: Diphtheria-Tetanus-Pertussis (DTaP), Haemophilus Influenza type B (Hib), Measles-Mumps-Rubella (MMR), varicella and inactivated polio vaccines. It should be noted that of those vaccines, only one may have contained low levels of thimerosal, the DTaP. Before receiving the vaccine, Hannah was able to communicate and play at the normal level of a 19 month old. Months later, she began to display deficits in her abilities to communicate as well as changes in her normal behavior. She was later diagnosed with a mitochondrial encephalopathy, for which her parents believed the vaccines were the trigger. Although Poling was awarded upwards of 1.5 million dollars for the perceived neurologic and cognitive damage done to the child, no connection between ASD and the vaccine was made and the Department of Health and Human Services (HHSS) simply conceded the case.

This details another event that provided a media frenzy, even though there were no scientific data to support the claim. The fact that the family was awarded damages also certainly implies a certain sense of guilt by the HHSS, which caused some members of the public to believe in a positive causative relation between vaccination and autism. The fact that Hannah Poling did have an underlying mitochondrial enzyme deficiency does relate to the hypothesis that ASD is a multifactorial disease in which mitochondrial genetics may play a role. However, there is no scientific evidence suggesting that her symptoms were brought about by the vaccinations (32). In fact, the research on mouse models that were administered thimerosal discussed earlier in this chapter suggests that the small dose of thimerosal (and the breakdown product, ethylmercury) that Hannah was exposed to would not be significant enough to evoke the neurologic and cognitive damages seen in her case, excluding it as the causative agent (23,28, 29).

Conclusions

As evident by the number of case studies presented in this chapter, thimerosal is extremely toxic to neuronal cells. Ethylmercury is now known to be a mitochondrial toxin, leading to increased oxidative stress and eventual apoptosis of neuronal cells. Ethylmercury toxicity demonstrates a very plausible mechanism which may lead to potential damages seen in ASD. As compelling as these findings might be, the important notion to understand is that as with any other medication, there is a therapeutic and a toxic level. The recognition of the two is the basis for pharmacology and treatment. Based on scientific experience and studies, the amount of thimerosal needed to elicit neurological changes that would predispose an infant to the development of autism-like characteristics 20 times greater than what is currently available in vaccines. To put this into perspective, the therapeutic range for acetaminophen in adults is about 5-20 mcg/ml and the potentially toxic range is 150 mcg/ml (14). This means that the amount of agent needed to produce a toxic effect is 7.5 times more than the maximum amount of drug that is considered therapeutic. By these measurements, acetominophen is nearly three times as toxic as thimerosal to the body. Prior to the discontinuation of thimerosal in most vaccines, the amount of exposure was not at a level that put its recipients at risk.

Currently there are no data detailing the bioavailability of ethylmercury across the blood-brain barrier. Such knowledge could provide a better assessment and estimation of the risk that ethylmercury could pose in inducing neurological damage. The implication of this gap in knowledge is inconsequential, as numerous studies have been successfully conducted to evaluate the efficacy and safety without this information. A majority of these studies found no positive correlations. The media has presented this issue to the public in a manner that has created uninformed skeptics, which has proved to be detrimental on several occasions in the protection of our young children from deadly diseases. It is important to be well informed and to engage in proper research and physician consultation in order to make the decision whether or not to vaccinate.

GENETICS; REDOX

Chapter 8A: Genetic Errors

Corina Din-Lovinescu, Christopher Shackles, Sina Zomorrodian

[While several genetic mutations and alterations have been identified in autistic individuals, none has been found uniformly and consistently. While these errors may represent several potential preconditioned factors setting the stage for a neurologic anomaly under the right environmental trigger, no recurrent theme is found in all such cases. – Ed.]

Hypothesis

Autism was first identified and described by the psychiatrist Leo Kanner in 1943 after he observed eleven children who exhibited social withdrawal from the age of one (1). One theory that arose at the time to describe the cause of this condition was aloof parenting (chapter 2D). Since then, clinicians and researchers have come a long way in understanding autism and its apparent etiology. It is now thought that autism is the result of the interaction of a combination of abnormal genes awith multiple non-genetic environmental risk factors.

Observations

The first study that suggested a genetic component of autism was published in the 1970s and examined the prevalence of autism among monozygotic twins (MZ) and dizygotic (DZ) twins (2). The study found a significantly higher rate of duplicate autism in MZ than in DZ twins. In the field of genetics, twin studies generally provide the first line of evidence suggesting a genetic contribution to a disease (chapter 1C). Subsequently, epidemiological research revealed that the relative risk of developing autism in the sibling of an affected individual is up to 20 times greater than in the general population (3).

These and other similar studies lead researchers to believe that autism is a heritable trait. Initial investigations estimated the heritability of autism to be up to 90% (i.e. 90% of the difference between autistic and non-autistic individuals can be attributed to a genetic component) (4). However, more recent studies have challenged this degree of heritability, estimating that it is only around 55%, leaving another 45% to be determined by non-genetic risk factors (5,6). These studies have generated considerable discussion about the genetic component of autism. Nonetheless, autism is still considered to be one of the most heritable neuropsychiatric disorders. Researchers continue to seek answers lying in the genetic code (7).

Despite the suggestive evidence that genetic factors contribute to autism, the exact genes and mechanisms contributing to its pathophysiology are still being elucidated. Unlike Mendelian (monogenic) human diseases, such as Huntington's disease and sickle cell anemia, which tend to have one causal gene variant, autism seems to be a genetically heterogeneous condition; similar autistic phenotypes arise from variants on multiple genes. In the case of autism, hundreds of genetic dissimilarities have been found on numerous genes. This means that one individual with autism may have a completely different genomic profile than another affected individual, making it more difficult to pinpoint predisposing genetic risk factors. For this reason, many genetic variants are referred to as "risk factors" for autism, rather than "causes" of autism, indicating that no single genetic variant is necessary or sufficient to predict a disease outcome (8).

With the advancement of genetic assaying techniques in the past few decades, several approaches and methodologies have been developed to explore the genetic architecture of autism. In addition to developing new physical tools, researchers have also developed new approaches to study autism. For example, one problem not limited to the field of autism research but encountered by autism investigators is selecting cases for studies. Autism patients have diverse clinical manifestations, ranging from absent speech to fluent language, and from profound intellectual disability to normal intellectual functioning. One technique used to reduce the effect of clinical or phenotypic heterogeneity is to define autism using specific parameters, such as head circumference, in order to narrow down the degree of genetic variation and pinpoint relevant genes.

The following sections will describe several theories proposed to explain the genetic component of autism, and the respective studies that were performed by hundreds of researchers around the world in order to elucidate the underlying genetic mechanisms of autism.

Rare vs. common mutations

When looking for genetic variation in disease states, a spectrum of genetic mutation frequency exists on which researchers can investigate. On one end of the spectrum are rare variations, which are found in roughly 1% of the affected population. These are genetic mutations that are potentially harmful to a carrier's fitness; if one carries a deleterious gene mutation that decreases a carrier's ability to survive, mate, and pass his/her genes on to the next generation, the mutation would likely not proliferate amongst the population. One explanation for the persistence of a rare mutation is that it appeared recently in a population so that natural selection did not have time to weed it out. In genetic studies, it is only feasible to look for rare gene mutations with strong effects, as rare gene mutations with lesser effects are exceedingly difficult to identify (due to their rare frequency in the population) and require a high degree of statistical power.

By direct contrast, common genetic variations are found in more than 5% of the population. Searching for unexceptional deviations requires a large study sample size in order to increase the statistical power. For example, by increasing the number of autistic individuals studied from hundreds to thousands, it is possible to find common genetic variations possibly contributing to the disease. Such modifications can contribute to disease through several mechanisms. One hypothesis is that common genetic variants enhance fitness by coding for an adaptive trait. For example, it was first observed in the 1940s that sickle cell anemia occurred at a greater rate among people from Africa and in other malaria-stricken areas (9). Individuals who are heterozygous for the sickle cell allele have a protective advantage against malaria, which explains its relatively high frequency among the African population and those with African ancestry. However, those who are homozygous for the allele develop sickle cell disease. This explains how relatively common genes can proliferate in a population while still causing a predisposition for disease states. Other reasons for the phenomena of common genetic variants leading to disease are that they have a neutral effect on overall fitness of the carrier, their tendency to lead to disease has a late onset in the carrier's life (after reproductive age), or the allele is located near another gene that has been positively selected (10). By virtue of the gene's location, replication over time leads to an increase in the allele's frequency in the population.

When searching for genetic mutations that might predispose individuals to ASDs, researchers are faced with the decision of either looking for rare or common genetic variations. This dilemma ultimately raises the issue of a paradigm of autism:

1) Is autism a disorder made up of a few rare genetic variations of sizable effect?
2) Is it caused by many common genetic variations each imparting a small effect, until a certain threshold for disease is reached? or
3) Is it a combination of the two?

The following sections will describe the approaches that researchers have used to attempt to answer these questions.

Cytogenetic and microarray studies

Cytogenetic studies and chromosomal microarrays (CMAs) have been used since the 1990s to identify chromosomal defects in many diseases and provide researchers with some of the first clues about autism-associated genes. These studies employ various stains and probes to analyze chromosomes for breakpoints, translocations, deletions, and duplications. The technology for CMAs has improved so much in the past decade that the American College of Medical Genetics now recommends that CMA be used as first-tier test for diagnosis of individuals with developmental disabilities or congenital anomalies (11).

Using these technologies, researchers have found abnormalities on almost every chromosome consistently associated with autism (11). By examining the disrupted genes on these chromosomes more closely, we have learned that many of the genes associated with autism to date are implicated in biological pathways of neuronal synapses. Of the genes discovered to be associated with autism, some of the most interesting are the neuroligin genes, *NLGN3* and *NLGN4*, encoded on the X chromosome, which code for proteins involved in the neuronal synapse and have been previously associated with autism in several studies (12,13).

Another gene implicated in synaptic pathways was discovered in 22q13.3 deletion syndrome, which has been associated with the development of autistic features such as delayed speech. Of the genes located at 22q13.3, *Shank3* was identified as the candidate gene most likely relevant to autism spectrum disorders (ASDs) due to its role in encoding scaffolding proteins at the post-synaptic membrane (14). Bozdagi et al. expanded upon this research by studying mice heterozygous for *Shank3* disruptions (chapter 3F) (15). These mice were compared with wild-type and homozygous *Shank3*-deleted mice for synaptic function, plasticity and social behavior. Heterozygosity was purposefully studied because it is the heterozygotic genotypes that are implicated in disease states, not the knock-outs. Bozdagi et al. found a decrease in excitatory postsynaptic potential and long-term potentiation in heterozygotes compared to controls. Moreover, given the previously established connection between α-amino-3-hydroxyl-5-methyl-4-isoxazole-propionic acid (AMPA) receptor subunit trafficking and synaptic strength (16), antibodies to glutamate receptors were used to quantify puncta for GluR1-immunoreactivity (since GluR1 is a subunit of the AMPA receptor). Heterozygotes for *Shank3* exhibited fewer puncta with GluR1-immunoreactivity. Lastly, social behavior was characterized in the mice as a model for autistic behavior. This was accomplished by measuring social interactions between wild-type or heterozygous *Shank3* mice and estrus B6 female mice (15). *Shank3* heterozygotes spent less time engaged in social sniffing of the female mice when compared to wild-types, and they emitted less ultrasonic vocalizations (as measured by an ultrasonic microphone) in comparison to wild-types. Ultimately, the significance of *Shank3* in autism was deduced by showing decreased synaptic transmission and plasticity in glutamatergic neurons, a reduction in GluR1 concentration in spinal puncta, and less social interaction of heterozygotes with females compared to wild-type mice. The findings point to *Shank3* haploinsufficiency as a cause for neurodevelopmental disorder due to retardation of synaptic development and maturation.

These and other functional studies are not only important in identifying diagnostic biomarkers for autism, but also help point to possible therapeutic interventions. Functional and animal-model studies have shown that changing the levels of proteins, such as those encoded by the neuroligin genes or *Shank3* alters the function and plasticity of synapses. Many of the associated phenotypes can be reversed once the level of decreased protein has been restored (17). Possible therapeutic interventions could target these specific neuronal synapses and increase neuronal transmission signals.

Related disorders

As many as 300 different genetic syndromes have been associated with the onset of ASD. The utility of investigating ASD-related disorders lies in identifying genes that predispose individuals to varying degrees of autism. As autism is represented along a spectrum of conditions, it has been associated with several autism-like disorders. One such disorder is Asperger syndrome, which shares many traits with autism, however is not characterized by language impairment. Autism shares similar traits with Rett Syndrome (RS) as well, in which patients typically exhibit motor and language skills regression during early childhood (18) (chapter 1D). RS is found almost exclusively in females, affecting one out of every ten thousand newborns. The symptoms of the disorder are marked by repetitive behavioral patterns in addition to sudden loss of social and cognitive skills. Children suffering from RS typically develop normally for the first six months to one year of age and then start to show dramatic decreases in cognitive and motor functioning.

RS is an X-linked chromosomal disorder that has been correlated with the paternal X chromosome. RS is apparently caused by a mutation in the methyl CpG binding protein 2 (MECP2) gene, resulting in a decrease in overall protein production (19). MeCP2 serves to activate and deactivate the production of other proteins in the cell by the methylation of their concordant genes. A decrease in MeCP2 protein production leaves cells with an excess of some proteins and a deficit of others, creating a significant change in "normal" biochemistry. Although MeCP2 is present in all cells and contributes on multiple levels of cellular activation and deactivation, neurons are most affected by a change in the MeCP2 gene. A study used immunofluorescence to compare overall MeCP2 protein concentration in the frontal cortex of children with autism compared to that of unaffected aged-matched controls (18). These findings showed a significant decrease in overall MeCP2 protein concentrations in addition to the presence of aberrant promoter methylation of the MeCP2 gene. Mutations in this gene can result in a range of neurobehavioral abnormalities, resembling autism. MECP2 mutations have been reported in about 1% of children with autism making it a possible comorbidity.

Table 1: Key Differences between Rett Syndrome and Autism (47)

	Rett Syndrome	*Autism*
Cranial abnormalities	Microcephaly	Macrocephaly
Primarily effects	Cholinergic neurons	Serotonergic neurons
Cerebral abnormalities	Frontal cortex pathology	Cerebellum/Hippocampus
Age of onset	Postnatal	Early prenatal
Mutation site	MECP2	Variable/Undetermined
Gender association	Almost all female	Predominantly male

As previously established, most cases of autism are not associated with single genetic mutations. In fact, about 10% of autism cases co-occur with another known genetic condition. Examples of these diseases are tuberous sclerosis and Fragile X Syndrome (FXS), which are monogenic and can be concurrent with autism (19) (chapter 1D). Up to 50% of children affected with tuberous sclerosis show autistic symptoms, most with intellectual disability. FXS is an X-linked genetic disorder characterized by cognitive impairment, macro-orchidism, and facial abnormalities. Up to 30% of individuals with FXS also have an ASD. Other ASD-associated diseases that are either monogenic or due to rare microdeletions include Cowden, Timothy, Smith-Lemli-Opitz, Williams-Beuren, Moebius and Sotos syndromes. It should be noted, however, that more than 90% of autistic individuals do not have one of these infrequent monogenetic diseases. Still due to their similarity, understanding the nature of these conditions and what causes them may provide insight on autism.

Genome-wide association studies

A different approach for studying genotype-phenotype correlations is the Genome Wide Association Study (GWAS). GWASs are powerful research tools for testing associations between millions of genetic variants and disease phenotypes without having a prior hypothesis about the genes implicated in the condition. Automated genome sequence analysis has made possible rapid determination by microassay of many candidate genes in a short period of time. The theory behind GWASs is that common genetic variants (found in more than 5% of the population) contribute significantly to the risk of complex diseases. Single Nucleotide Polymorphisms (SNPs) are the most simple and common type of polymorphism between individuals. SNPs refer to variation in only one base pair of the same gene when comparing the DNA sequences of two people. These are often used in forensic studies, such as paternity cases, to distinguish genetic similarities and differences between individuals. By comparing millions of SNPs between a control population and a disease population, GWASs allow researchers to look for variants that are found more frequently in one group over another. If the presence of a particular allele is increased or decreased in affected individuals, one can say that the allele is statistically associated with the disease. Each case-control based GWAS reports an odds ratio (OR) to assess the strength of the association. An OR above 1 indicates a positive association, while an OR below 1 indicates a negative association.

In the past decade, advancements in genetic assaying technologies have made GWASs a feasible choice for investigating the underlying causes of complex diseases. Since early GWASs showed promising results in finding common genetic variants associated with conditions such as type 1 diabetes and age-related macular degeneration, hundreds of genetic variants have been linked with a wide variety of diseases (20).

As of January, 2014, just under ten SNPs have shown a statistically significant correlation with autism, and seventy-five more have been associated with a cohort of ASD, bipolar disorder, schizophrenia, and ADHD subjects combined (20). Several of these SNPs were found in intergenic regions, while others were found in genes implicated in neuronal signaling pathways (including *CDH9*, *CDH10*, and *SEMA5A*), as well as in non-autism-related pathways (e.g. *TAS2R1* is a taste receptor gene) (chapter 3E). One autism study used a GWAS to identify multiple SNPs in the 5p14.1 region (21). The 5p14.1 region is located near the *CDH9* and *CDH10* genes, which code for the cadherin proteins involved in neuronal attachment and neural tube closure in the early fetus, similar to the previously mentioned SHANK scaffolding proteins. The study further points to a possible defect in the connection of neuronal synapses in autistic brains (chapter 3F). Despite the known functional relevance of some SNPs, many of them only show a modest contribution to the risk for developing autism, with reported ORs below 2.

A subsequent review study suggested that finding any genetic variants with an OR greater than 1.5 for autism is extraordinarily unlikely (22). The conclusion drawn from these studies, along with GWASs in other neuropsychiatric disorders, is that common variants contribute to only a small portion of the estimated heritability of autism, and that much of the genetic contribution of autism is still unknown.

Because GWASs are grounded in the general hypothesis that common genetic variants are responsible for complex diseases, one fallacy of these studies is that they do not have the power to detect rare SNPs (found in less than 1% of the population) that could contribute to the deleterious changes in certain diseases. Proposed methods for studying rare mutations include increasing the size of study samples and using deeper sequencing techniques, such as whole-genome sequencing in order to capture the rare variants. In the past several years, several groups such as the Psychiatric GWAS Consortium (PGC) and the Autism Genome Project have started to tackle these problems (23,24). The goal of these groups is to pool together autism research cohorts and analysis tools from researchers around the world in order to increase the sample size and power of each study, and to begin sequencing deeper into the genome in order to find rare mutations contributing to autism risk.

Next generation sequencing

Next generation sequencing is the newest and most promising type of genetic assaying tool thusfar. Several methods exist for genome sequencing, two of the most popular being whole-genome and whole-exome sequencing. The first whole-genome sequencing study was the Human Genome Project (HGP) completed in 2003 (25). In the HGP, researchers determined the exact sequence of every DNA base within the human body, which can now be used as a reference, or "normal" sequence to which one can compare diseased or "abnormal" sequences. In contrast, whole-exome sequencing studies only sequence the 1% of the genome that codes for proteins, leaving out the areas of the genome that do not have a known functional significance, as of yet. Next generation sequencing can also be used to sequence selected parts of the genome, such as specific candidate genes, or intergenic regions, depending on the interest of the investigators.

Since the completion of the HGP, the cost of sequencing an entire genome has dropped considerably from millions of dollars spent on the first HGP, to the $5000 genome available today (26). The decrease in cost has made it feasible for several groups of researchers to complete whole-exome and whole-genome sequencing studies in autism (27-34). These investigations have identified that the majority of the genetic mutations in autism individuals are *de novo*, meaning that they are spontaneous mutations not seen in other family members. These novel mutations are found in a two-fold to four-fold increase among affected subjects over that expected by chance (although it should be noted that researchers are still debating the average mutation rate in normal genomes).

De novo mutations associated with autism have been found in hundreds of different genes across the genome. Through each new discovery, we gain more insight into the biology of this complex disease and learn the extent of its extreme genetic diversity. Interestingly, many of the newly discovered mutations were found in genes known to be involved in synaptic plasticity pathways and chromatin remodeling during brain development (chapter 3F). Furthermore, several of the *de novo* mutations were found in genes previously implicated in other neurodevelopmental disorders and in intellectual disability. For example, *de novo* mutations were discovered in the gene, *NTNG1,* which plays a role in the organization of nerve cells. Similarly, mutations were identified in the *FOXP1* gene, which has been associated with intellectual disability, autism, and language development (35).

In addition to finding mutations in genes implicated in brain development pathways, other novel candidate genes were also discovered. Going forward, many studies still need to be performed in order to understand how the mutations in these genes affect brain development in autistic individuals. As the technology for genetic sequencing and functional analysis continues to develop over the next few years, we will likely see more whole-genome sequencing studies identifying new and exciting genetic contributions to autism.

Copy number variations (CNVs)

Rapid advancements in DNA microarray and sequencing techniques in the past two decades have also opened the door to the analysis of Copy Number Variations (CNVs) in autism. CNVs refer to duplications or deletions in the genome of at least 1000 base pairs that result in either a greater or decreased amount of DNA. Perhaps one of the most interesting discoveries in the field of genetics over the past several years has been that many neuropsychiatric disorders such as autism, schizophrenia, and bipolar disorder have an excess of *de novo* CNVs in comparison to controls (36). Some researchers have reported that up to twenty percent of ASD cases could be due to CNVs, although this number is most likely more modest than reported here (37). Just about ten CNVs have been strongly associated with autism, but each individual CNV is rare and accounts for less than one percent of all cases of autism. When multiple rare CNVs are combined, however, together they can significantly increase the risk of developing autism, suggesting that hundreds of different genes across the genome are implicated in the onset of this condition. CNVs have been associated with a variety of clinical features in autism, ranging from mild to full-blown autism. Thus, the phenotypic heterogeneity seen associated with CNVs makes it difficult to determine whether a CNV is the sole cause of autism or if a combination of factors contribute to the disease.

Epigenetic studies

MZ and DZ twin studies have been used as an important means of identifying causes that play a role in disease processes (chapter 1C). Disease discordant MZ twins represent an ideal model for investigation of factors other than genetics that contribute to neurocognitive development as they inherently control for a plethora of possible confounding variables including genotype, age, sex, maternal environment, and many influential environmental exposures. Recent work has demonstrated discordance within MZ twin pairs for diagnosed autism, as well as a variable symptomatology and severity in concordant twins (38,39).

This evidence strongly supports the role for factors other than genetic sequence contributing to the onset of autism. One proposed alternative mechanism is through epigenetic modifications of DNA. Epigenetic modifications are alterations in DNA methylation and chromatin structure, which results in a variation in DNA expression (on/off), thus changing the way a cell functions. In 2010, Nguyen et al. conducted an investigation through global methylation profiling of lympho-blastoid cell lines from phenotypically discordant MZ twins and non-autistic siblings (40). The data collected suggested that increased methylation resulted in gene silencing and decreased protein expression in the brains of autistic patients.

More recently, Wong et al. conducted the first systematic epigenomic analyses of MZ twins discordant for ASD and found a role for altered DNA methylation in autism (41). The study investigated 50 MZ twin pairs through a genome-wide analysis of DNA methylation among disease discordant and concordant twin pairs. The results identified numerous DNA methylation differences between MZ twins discordant for ASD and ASD-related traits, as well as between autistic individuals and control samples. In addition, many of these differences were seen in locations that have been previously implicated in autism. As epigenetic studies continue to grow in number, we will likely see more correlations between autism and changes in DNA expression.

Gene-environment interactions

Yet another approach to studying the genome and its relation to disease is to look for the interaction between genes and environmental triggers (Conclusions and Prospectus). These investigations, called gene by environment interaction studies, come in two forms:

1) One approach is to investigate how different genetic profiles affect an individual's reaction to environmental exposures.
2) The other is to investigate how an environmental trigger alters the expression of an individual's genetic profile.

Recently, several autism research groups have focused on how infections and immune activators alter the expression of genes involved in immunity, and how those genes are implicated in the pathophysiology of autism (chapters 6B,6C). For example, a study in 2010 showed that bacterial and viral infection-related hospitalization during early pregnancy increased the risk of developing autism (42). Interestingly, the risk of developing ASD was not associated with any particular kind of infection, suggesting that the change in general immune mechanisms was responsible. Although it is still unclear how maternal immune activation increases the risk for developing ASD in offspring, one hypothesis is that the hyperactive maternal immune system increases cytokines (e.g., IL6) that cross the placenta and alter gene expression (such as IGF production) in the developing fetus, especially in its brain. Furthermore, a growing number of studies have observed mutations in the Major Histocompatibility Complex (MHC)—a cluster of genes coding for proteins involved in the activation of immune cells— in patients with ASD, suggesting a potential link between immune signaling and autism (43). Because the MHC region is highly polymorphic and translation of these genes into proteins depends of a variety of environmental triggers, including different infections, it will be interesting to continue investigating the role of immune complexes and environmental exposures in the onset of autism.

Another example of a gene by environment interaction hypothesis for autism is the interaction of air pollution with the MET receptor tyrosine kinase gene (chapters 3F,4E). One study found that subjects with a risk allele in the MET gene and high exposure to air pollution were more at risk for developing autism compared to subjects with a protective allele in the same gene and the same amount of air pollution exposure (44). The authors hypothesize that having either the risk allele or the protective allele changes the subject's reaction to air pollution exposure, which in turn changes his/her risk for developing autism. This study has yet to be replicated, and much still needs to be learned about the underlying biology of this hypothesis. Still, the study demonstrates a novel approach to uncovering new risks for developing autism. Future researchers will need to leverage similar creative abilities in order to come up with new and testable hypotheses for studying autism.

Insulin-like growth factor-1

Extensive studies provide a basis for the potential link between insulin-like growth factor-1 (IGF-1) and autism (45). IGF-1 is an anabolic polypeptide produced by the antepartum placenta and the neonatal liver that mediates growth. The involvement of IGF-1 in ASD is plausible as an etiologic agent due its role in axon myelination through switching on oligodendrocyte gene expression in fetuses and neonates (see chapters 6A,6D) (46). IGF-1 is also known to promote astrocyte proliferation, the regeneration of axons, and the germination of neurites in motor neurons (45). It follows that a deficiency in the growth factor might lead to abnormal neurogenesis or defective neural communication in the brain. In fact, one study found cerebrospinal fluid (CSF) samples of autistic children to contain lower levels of IGF in comparison to controls (47). Furthermore, Zikopoulos and Barbas found on biopsy that various regions of the autistic brain revealed hypomyelination (48).

An etiologic explanation for these abovementioned occurrences is the existence of a polymorphism that downregulates the production of IGF-1 (chapter 6D). By decreasing IGF synthesis, such polymorphisms could increase the risk of autism (49). For example, this may enhance CNS (central nervous system) myelination defects characteristic of this disease. Although no specific genetic mutation has yet been reported in the IGF-1 gene of ASD patients, previous studies have demonstrated a relationship between an IGF-1 gene polymorphism and lower levels of serum IGF-1 in children born small-for-gestational-age (SGA) (50). This is relevant to ASD because of the fact that the incidence of autism rises in very small for gestational age (VSGA) newborns in comparison to normal-weight ones (51).

Along with short stature, increased head circumference is observed in 15-35% of autistic children, which might be explained by low CSF levels in young autistic children causing a subsequent "compensatory overgrowth of the brain" (52). Although it is quite possible that lower levels of IGF-1 instigate the manifestations of autism, the reason for altered levels of this growth factor could be anything from genetic polymorphisms to antepartum chorioamnionitis.

Notwithstanding, it is reasonable to ask that if decreased IGF-1 levels are involved in the pathophysiology of ASD, would restoration of IGF-1 levels be therapeutic? This hypothesis was tested in murine models and it was found that administration of IGF-1 to mice with *Shank3*-haploinsufficiency exhibited improvement in previously deficient motor skills, AMPA signaling (an agonist which mimics the effects of glutamate in neurotransmission), and long-term potentiation (52). Since IGF-1 is already available to treat children with short stature, it is not unreasonable to think that clinical trials using IGF-1 to treat autistic children are on the horizon. Also, as noted in chapter 9A, prolonged feeding of neonates with breast milk, a known abundant source of IGF, is correlated with reduced incidence of autism.

Maternal/paternal age

Several epidemiological studies have been performed to explore the link between paternal age and the neurodevelopment of children after a theory was proposed associating increasing parental age with the risk of developing ASD in offspring. For years, increasing maternal age was considered one of the most significant predisposing variables linked to dysfunctional neurodevelopment in children. However, recent analysis has shown that increased paternal age may be even more highly associated with developmental delays. Proposed mechanisms for this disposition are based on the production of the male and female sex cells. Although most human cells undergo mitosis to replace injured cells, only specialized sex cells (sperm and eggs) undertake meiosis to create reproductive cells. In both meiosis and mitosis, cells experience a series of cell divisions to replicate and divide their genetic material among the new duplicated cells. During meiosis, however, gametes in the male and female reproductive organs decrease the total number of chromosomes per cell in half. This allows for one "complete cell" of 46 chromosomes to be formed during fertilization.

As age increases, so does the susceptibility to genetic irregularity and occurrence of genetic mutations (53). Many of these genetic mutations arise while the cell is replicating its DNA during mitosis and meiosis. If small changes go unnoticed by the cell and escape organism-induced apoptosis during meiosis, a child can be conceived with chromosomal aberrations that can manifest into debilitating disorders later in life. As the number of cell divisions increase, so do the chances of developing new mutations. There are inherent differences in cell division between oogenesis and spermatogenesis. Throughout oogenesis, there is a much smaller number of germ cell divisions compared to spermatogenesis, creating a greater opportunity for mutation and variability stemming from male gamete formation (53). Furthermore, oogenesis is completed early in life in the female, with division arrested for many years, while males continue spermatogenesis throughout their lives. With the possibility of genetic deterioration or damage as we age, this can lead to increased chance for genetic mutation from paternal division.

Recent research has correlated an increase in paternal age with below average scores on neurocognitive and developmental measures in children, while demonstrating maternal age to be associated with higher scores in these same areas (54). These studies also show that advanced paternal age increases the risk of neurodevelopmental disorders, especially autism. A study reported by Durkin et al. illustrated a significant increase in the risk of the development of ASD with parental age of 40 or above (chapter 2A) (55). Reichenberg et al. investigated the relationship between advancing paternal age at birth of offspring and their risk of ASD (56). The data were collected from the Israeli Draft Board Medical Registry and consisted of over one hundred and thirty thousand participants. This information illustrated that children born from fathers of age forty or older were 5.75 times more likely to develop autism compared to the group of children with fathers lower than 30, while controlling for possible confounders such as socioeconomic status, maternal age and year of birth. In the end, investigators concluded that paternal age was correlated with an increase in the risk of ASD development possibly due to genetic mutation. However, considering the small number of cases of autism in the study, especially in that of the older fathers, the analyses did not have enough power to reach definitive conclusions in some of the strata. In general, fathers over 40 sire about 4% of neonates presently. These studies suggest that there is an association between the increasing risk of autism and an increase in paternal age. The bigger question remains if the possibility of ASD development increases in an accelerating manner, as some of these studies suggest, especially since the average age of new parents is currently increasing in Western countries.

Conclusions
Implications for individuals and families

Despite the hundreds of research studies that have been described in the previous sections, many of the findings have yet to be useful clinically. The process of taking a research finding, such as a genetic test, and turning it into a clinically validated and useful tool can take many years. Not only does the research need to be replicated in numerous studies, but laboratories need to demonstrate the usefulness and cost-effectiveness of a test before it can be used for clinical purposes. For example, many CNVs may be associated with a variety of autistic features in research studies, but genetic testing for CNVs has not yet been established as the nationwide standard of care for ASDs (36). Even so, genetic testing does have a value in establishing a diagnosis in many diseases, including autism. It is likely that the aforementioned genetic discoveries will play a role in clinical diagnosis and management of autism in the near future.

Besides genetic testing, another product of the genetic boom since the HGP has been the rise in availability of clinical geneticists and genetic counselors, who have been increasingly sought out by families with autism. This may be due to the fact that the prevalence of autism has increased greatly over the past decade (from 1-in-150 in 2000 to 1-in-88 in 2008, according to the Centers for Disease Control) (57), or because there has been an increase in new diagnostic options available to identify autism patients. This would amount to about 730,000 new cases in the United States each year (chapter 1C).

In general, the role of the clinical geneticist is to determine if there is a genetic component to a patient's autistic condition, and to help provide counseling for the family. Although a psychiatrist can diagnose autism clinically, a geneticist can uncover any plausible underlying genetic causes of the disease, if they exist. As previously mentioned, about 10% of ASD cases tend to occur in children who have other chromosomal anomalies such as Down syndrome, Fragile X, or tuberous sclerosis, among others. The remainder of autism cases may also have genetic factors that predispose them to the condition. Genetic counselors can provide this information to families, which can help them in several different ways.

For the most part, knowing a patient's genetic profile nowadays does not mean that anything specific can be done therapeutically. We do not know enough about the therapeutic targets of autism or the methods to implement such treatments. However, many families have found it helpful and empowering to know if there is an underlying genetic component, as this information can be looked at as a sort of diagnosis or explanation for the condition. In addition, specific recurrence risk counseling can be provided and family members can be tested for similar genetic components. However, obtaining a prenatal genetic test for autism generally raises unrealistic expectations in parents of autistic children (chapter 2A) because most of the genetic abnormalities associated with ASDs, with the exception of large chromosomal rearrangements, cannot be detected with current prenatal screening.

The explosion in genetic research over the past two decades has made it possible to come closer to understanding the genetic underpinnings of autism. Although the etiology of autism is still not completely understood, the majority of researchers believe that autism is a largely a complex genetic disease characterized by much heterogeneity. Data from GWASs, next-generation sequencing, and CNV studies point to the ever-increasing importance of rare *de novo* mutations in the etiology of autism and less to a role for common genetic variants. For example, a study in 2011 identified 103 ASD-related genetic abnormalities (58). Moreover, candidate gene and functional studies report that many genetic mutations seen in autism cases affect synaptic connections and signaling pathways, which might play a role in the cognitive deficits and phenotypic behaviors displayed by ASD children (chapters 3E,3F). However, the unusual mutations found so far in some cases of autism have not been documented by GWAS as common variations in this disorder (58). This is in contrast to cystic fibrosis, for example, where the ΔF508 mutation, involving a three nucleotide deletion, is found in 90% of cases in the United States (59).

Others are investigating different functional pathways, such as those mentioned in the section about IGF-1. If future research corroborates the hypothesis that genetic polymorphisms decrease the production of IGF, causing hampered neonatal myelination, an improved approach to autism therapy and prevention could result. Additional approaches to investigate autism through gene-environment interactions, epigenetics, and maternal/paternal age provide new and exciting plausible directions to be tested in the future of autism research. With the identification of new susceptibility genes and biomarkers will come the ability to develop a deeper understanding of the etiology and pathophysiology of ASDs. This will, in turn, help patients and families make more informed healthcare and lifestyle choices (chapters 2A,2B). As susceptibility genes and molecular pathways are increasingly identified, it is reasonable to anticipate that therapies targeting these genes and pathways will follow.

Chapter 8B – Oxidative Stress
Marissa Botwinick, Marissa Opilas

[The failure of the body's defense mechanisms to deal with oxidative insults
may hold the key to explaining some pathologic aspects of autism and
autism-like disorders. – Ed.]

Hypothesis

Reactive oxygen species are normal products of cellular metabolism that can pose a threat to proper cell function and integrity. Free radicals, such as superoxide and hydroxyl radicals, are known to damage fatty acids in the cell membrane, DNA, and amino acids in proteins (1). Fortunately, the body has built-in mechanisms to combat oxidative stress. For example, glutathione contains thiol groups that serve as reducing agents to neutralize free radicals. In addition, superoxide dismutase catalyzes superoxide's transformation into oxygen and hydrogen peroxide.

Recent studies have noted that these essential metabolic mechanisms in the cell are decreased in autistic patients. These mechanisms also seem to be dysfunctional in other genetic conditions that resemble autism clinically. As a result, therapies that increase glutathione and superoxide dismutase are topics of current research in the quest to treat autism. In addition, disorders due to mitochondrial dysfunction and their possible link to autism are under investigation, since many of the metabolic reactive oxygen products come from mitochondria (chapter 8C).

Finally, many antioxidants in our bodies, such as ascorbic acid, α-tocopherol and β-carotene are already commonly consumed in our diet (1), so a lifestyle change as simple as diet alteration may be beneficial for autism patients. Though oxidative stress appears to be a co-morbidity of autism, the reduced ability to rid the body of reactive oxygen species seems to be associated with autistic patients (chapter 8C). By preventing exposure to certain exogenous agents, such as toxic chemicals, pollutants, and microorganisms, one can decrease the potential amount of oxidative destruction within the body (chapter 4E).

Observations

Current research indicates that autism seems to be a multi-factorial disease (2). There is not a single gene mutation or malformed protein that leads to the disorder by itself. A combination of genetics, environment, and defects in cellular metabolism may contribute. It is necessary to examine each piece of the puzzle to better understand what is occurring within an autistic psychological and physiological makeup. Here we will take a look at the cellular level and what is possibly malfunctioning microscopically to result in autism.

Cellular metabolism is the process by which chemical bond energy is made. Along with the conversion of energy comes the creation of certain metabolic byproducts that must be discarded. For example, ammonia is normally excreted in the urine because it is a neurotoxin if it remains in the body. Similarly, hormones must be activated or disposed of if they are not needed. Finally, for example, acetaldehyde from alcohol metabolism could damage DNA if not eliminated properly (3). Without the removal of such toxic byproducts, these wastes would remain in the body, often causing biological dysfunction.

Glutathione (GSH) is the primary metabolic factor in the body that functions to remove oxidative stress (chapter 8C). The amino acid, cysteine, in glutathione has a sulfhydryl (SH) group, which serves as a reducing agent (2). The molecule exists in proportion to an oxidized disulfide (GSSG), together maintaining homeostasis between oxidizing and reducing compounds in the body. The GSH/GSSG mechanism removes free radicals produced inside the cell. In more than half of autistic patients, there is a decreased level of glutathione and increased oxidized disulfide, leading to increased oxidative stress due to free radicals. Glutathione-related oxidative stress is also apparently linked to gastrointestinal pathology experienced in autistic patients.

A redox precursor to the cysteine residue in GSH is S-adenosylmethionine (SAM). SAM is a molecule in a mechanism of epigenetic methylation (2) (chapter 8A). When DNA is methylated, gene expression is repressed or activated, depending on the molecule. Epigenetics provides important regulatory mechanisms used by the cells to make sure proper amounts of active DNA is present at the appropriate time.

The mechanism for SAM metabolism is interconnected with both glutathione and folate (vitamin B9) metabolism (chapter 5A). Similar to an integrated chain reaction, the quantity of each reactant impacts the amounts of the others; therefore, the abnormal glutathione synthesis in autistic patients discussed above causes decreased SAM, methionine, and the biologically active form of folate, tetrahydrofolate (THF). As a result, the processes that depend on these products do not function properly (2). SAM, for example, is the major methyl group donor in 1-carbon metabolism, used in the synthesis of phosphatidylcholine from phosphatidlyserine, the conversion of norepinephrine to epinephrine, creatine synthesis, adding the 5' cap during the transcription of eukaryotic mRNA, and the methylation of cytosine bases of DNA that distinguishes active from inactive DNA strands (1). THF is also a carrier of 1-carbon units. It is essential for the degradation and synthesis of the amino acid, methionine, and serves as an atom donor to the heterocylic ring during the synthesis of purine nucleotides. All of these molecules are essential for proper cell function, and an imbalance in their mechanisms could result in impaired protein translation, decreased synthesis of phospholipids for cell membranes, and poor regulation of amino acids.

While oxidative stress contributes to a variety of the pathologic manifestations of ASD, certain aspects of it have been attributed to specific symptoms. For example, the regression of language in autistic children is often one of the more devastating symptoms for parents. Transferrin and ceruloplasmin are two anti-oxidant proteins found in the blood that bind iron and copper, respectively. Ceruloplasmin protects membrane lipids and red blood cell membranes from free radicals (4). Similarly, transferrin reduces the amount of iron in the ferrous form (Fe^{+2}), which produces free radicals. Decreased levels of these essential proteins resulting in increased oxidative demand on the cell have been found in ASD. In fact, a 2006 study shows 84% of autistic patients have lower levels of transferrin and 68% have lower levels of ceruloplasmin compared to their unaffected siblings. Furthermore, autistic children who had not lost previously acquired language skills had similar antioxidant protein levels to their unaffected siblings. Though further investigation must be done, these statistics suggest a link between decreased transferrin and ceruloplasmin, and loss of language in autistic children.

Hyperactivity is another common symptom in people with autism. A correlation between hyperactivity and abnormal red blood cell (RBC) membrane fluidity has been observed. RBC membrane fatty acid composition is an indicator of lipid composition of other tissues, such as the brain; it is likely that hyperactivity may be due to the same abnormal concentrations that cause the reduced fluidity of the RBC membranes. A study comparing autistic and non-autistic children found the higher the fluidity of the RBC membrane and the lower the polyunsaturated fatty acid (PUFA) concentration, the greater the hyperactivity level (5).

An increase in mono-unsaturated fatty acids and a decrease in omega-3 fatty acids, such as eicosapentaenoic acid (EPA) and docosahexaenoic acid (DHA), have also been found in autistic patients. This increase in monounsaturated fatty acids leads to up-regulation of fatty acid oxidation, thus raising the level of oxidative species in the body. This further decreases membrane integrity (5). In addition to the maintenance of cell membranes, fatty acids are important in signal transduction (chapter 5D), regulation of inflammation (chapter 6C), and neuron repair and survival. Abnormal amounts could lead to neurological consequences such as hyperactivity. Many metabolic processes take place inside the mitochondria of the cell, including those that produce reactive oxygen and nitrogen species. One of these is oxidative phosphorylation (6). A defect in this process is believed to predispose patients to risks from other exposures that may cause oxidative stress, such as drugs, environmental toxins, and LDL-cholesterol.

Mitochondrial dysfunction itself is known to cause oxidative stress and thus may contribute to the pathology of autism. Specifically, the level of lactic acid is elevated in some autistic patients. This often indicates abnormal mitochondrial function and it has been linked, in particular, to the neurodegenerative effects of the disease (7). There is growing evidence that autism and mitochondrial disorders, which produce free radicals, are related. Studying patients with both disorders may help us understand the underlying biochemical mechanisms of ASD.

Certain single-gene disorders which seem unrelated to ASD overall, share some of the features of the autistic phenotype. Most notable are tuberous sclerosis (TS), Rett syndrome, Down syndrome, and Fragile X syndrome (chapters 1D,8A). The commonality suggests a correlation between oxidative stress, altered methylation capacity, and autism because each of these disorders shows evidence of similar neurologic and metabolic dysfunctions (2). It does not, however, necessarily define the cause of autism.

Tuberous sclerosis (TS) is an infrequent genetic disorder that results in benign tumors growing on the skin, brain, kidneys, and heart (8). Seizures and behavioral problems are common in TS patients as well. Autism-like characteristics are not uncommon in cases of TS.

In a study with young twins, only one of whom had diagnosed autism, the affected twin also experienced the seizures. As a result, the twin with full-blown autism would apparently be subjected to greater oxidative stress than the healthy twin because concurrent chronic seizures are know to enhance reduced glutathione levels in the body. The depletion of glutathione from repeated seizures increases oxidative stress. The degree of oxidative stress is proportional to the severity of neurological dysfunction that appears clinically (10). This supports the proposal of a positive correlation between oxidative stress and the development of autistic symptoms in some patients (2).

Rett syndrome is a neurological disorder found almost exclusively in females. It is most commonly related to a spontaneous mutation on the X chromosome, leading to a defect in methyl-binding protein (MeCP2), thereby preventing it from binding to the DNA methyl groups (2) (chapter 8A). When MeCP2 fails to unite with DNA promoter regions, there is an up-regulation of genes that are normally silenced. Though the exact genes MeCP2 silences are not fully known, they apparently play a role in maintaining signaling at neuron synapses (9) (chapter 3F). MeCP2 protein is found in high concentration in the central nervous system and defects lead to severe problems with learning, coordination, breathing abnormalities and seizures. Many of these symptoms emulate autism, and the two conditions are often confused. This conclusion suggests a correlation between increased reactive oxygen species and the behaviors exhibited by autism patients in many cases.

Fragile X syndrome is similar to Rett syndrome, in that a methylation defect from an abnormal nucleotide expansion leads to gene silencing and, ultimately, disease. It is the most common comorbidity of Down syndrome with a single gene mutation (2). Normally, the Fragile X mental retardation-1 (FMR1) gene on the X chromosome has 5-44 CGG expansions. An FMR1 gene with a CGG trinucleotide expansion greater than 200 is considered to be fully mutated, and results in the silencing of this portion of the gene. If the FMR1 gene is stilled, the fragile X mental retardation protein (FMRP) cannot be produced. The FMRP protein is found in large quantities in brain cells, functioning as a regulator of the neurotransmitter glutamate and an RNA-binding protein. A deficiency in FMRP has been found in certain psychiatric disorders without a mutation in the FMR1 gene (11). Loss of FMRP results in an increased production of reactive oxygen species in the mitochondria. The glutathione detoxification system is deficient in Fragile X patients as well. Oxidative stress in these patients may result in altered neural pathways leading to mental retardation, abnormal facial features, seizures, and irregular hand movements.

Down syndrome (DS), on the other hand, has a slightly different mechanism. An extra copy of chromosome 21 leads to an increase in hydrogen peroxide, which is beyond the capacity that can be readily removed by the body. This exhausts the glutathione supply, resulting in oxidative stress-induced cell damage (2). Furthermore, in conjunction with the discussion above regarding mitochondrial dysfunction leading to oxidative stress and autistic behaviors, DS patients have also been shown to have mitochondrial dysfunction and defects in DNA methylation (12). Down syndrome results in distinct physical features such as flattened nose, small ears, upward slanting eyes, short hands and fingers, as well as a range in severity of mental retardation. About 10% of patients with DS display autistic behaviors (2), which may suggest a correlation in the mechanisms leading to both conditions. This is further supported by the overlap in increased oxidative stress in DS and autism resulting from dysfunctions in epigenetics and mitochondria.

In addition to the endogenous mechanisms that produce excess free radials and fail to get rid of excess oxidative stress, there are exogenous factors that increase oxidative products in the body. Exposure to toxins in our environment can exacerbate oxidative stress in patients with autism (chapter 4E). The increase in free radicals can lead to cell damage and worsen the effects of autism, such as problems with the gastrointestinal system and possible inflammation of the brain (13). By preventing exposure to certain exogenous agents, such as toxic chemicals and microorganisms, one can decrease the potential amount of oxidative destruction within the body (7).

Exposure to teratogenic drugs prenatally, specifically valproate and thalidomide (chapter 4D), can affect the neonate and pose possible risk factors for autism (13). Valproic acid, which is found in many mood-stabilizing drugs for treating epilepsy, depression and bipolar disorders, induces decreasing fetal glutathionine and methionine levels when given during the gestation period. It also increases DNA hypo-methylation, thereby decreasing the body's natural way of detoxifying itself through epigenetic mechanisms (chapter 8A). Furthermore, valproic acid is a histone deacetylase inhibitor. Histones are proteins that package and organize DNA into functional units. If histones fail to deacetylate, DNA can become more vulnerable to oxidative damage and can induce abnormally expressed proteins.

Maternal exposure to thalidomide and ethylmercury can be related to increased environmental risk for autism. Thalidomide toxicity, especially if encountered before fetal limb development, generates free radicals and depletes glutathione stores. This combination promotes high oxidative stress during a critical developmental time frame in fetal growth (chapter 4F). Ethylmercury in elevated amounts in gravidas has demonstrated some putative risk factors in the development of autism (2) (chapter 5D). The neurotoxin, mercury, may induce glutathione depletion and produce oxygen free radicals, which causes apoptosis in human brain cells. These environmental exposures may be associated with autism-like characteristics as well.

Although not well established, other exogenous causes, such as pro-oxidant metals, food additives, and microorganisms, are thought by some to possibly enhance development of neuropathology when associated with postnatal exposure (2). For example, pro-oxidant metals such as cadmium, arsenic, lead and nickel, as well as solvents such as benzenes, alcohol and chlorinated organo-compounds, generate oxidative stress (chapters 4A,4B). These compounds induce the creation of reactive oxidative species and promote the depletion of glutathione. Since many children with autism already have low levels of glutathione, exposure to these particular chemicals will lead to an accumulation of damaging molecules, potentially causing more injury to the child's nervous system in many cases.

Studies have also shown that certain food additives and microorganisms are toxic to the metabolic homeostasis of ASD patients. Food colorings, preservatives, monosodium glutamate (MSG), and aspartame are common ingredients in processed foods known to impact cell function negatively. Similarly, microorganisms that invade the body such as bacteria, viruses, and fungi proliferate internally to detrimental levels, causing the depletion of glutathione (2). Often the presence of these additives and microorganisms are more harmful to autistic patients than healthy individuals because of their impaired detoxification processes. It may be prudent to keep these particular chemicals to a minimum to avoid possible harmful effects.

Finally, aside from particular exogenous factors associated with the development of autism, there has been a noticeable gender disparity implicated in the disorder. The causation for the preponderance of autism in male over female patients is unknown; however, there are some possible explanations. Estrogen is a known anti-oxidant and the higher concentration of this hormone in females allows for an increase in reduced glutathione in their plasma and mitochondria. Additionally, the lower levels of glutathione in male infants leave their cells more prone to oxidative damage than their female counterparts. Furthermore, until females reach menopause, they have a faster turnover of the methionine cycle, leading to lower homocysteine levels. Therefore, there is increased cellular methylation in females allowing for better detoxification to occur. Males with lower estrogen levels have lower glutathione levels, causing a more vulnerable state in response to oxidative stress (2).

Now that the mechanisms leading to oxidative stress have been summarized here, it is important to specify which biological effects in autism may be due to proliferation of free radicals. They can be divided into prenatal damage to the growing fetus and postnatal changes in the affected child and adult.

One of the most significant aspects of fetal development is the maturation of the nervous system. Reactive oxygen and nitrogen species are known to impede this critical process. The blood-brain-barrier (BBB) is a specialized endothelial structure in the blood vessels permeating the brain that allows only small, hydrophobic molecules to diffuse through it. In a healthy adult, the BBB would restrict passage of free radicals. However, the barrier is not fully formed until about six months of age postpartum. As a result, infants have less protection, and the increase in number of oxidative species in neurologically affected patients leaves their central nervous system more vulnerable to additional oxidative damage.

Furthermore, the detoxification enzyme, glutathione-S-transferase (GST), functions at the BBB (chapter 8C). This enzyme requires glutathione to function properly for full effect. As discussed previously, in autistic children there is often a decrease in glutathione production. Therefore, in autism the developing brain of the fetus is not maximally protected by the BBB (2). In addition, the reduced glutathione reduces the transmission of signals from one brain area to the next. The conduction difficulty can contribute to the pathology of autism (3).

Microglia are unique cells in the brain and spinal cord that remove matter such as damaged cell fragments and infectious agents. Similar to the BBB, microglia are not finished maturing until late childhood. In addition, they are very sensitive to oxidation because they require high levels of iron to do their job. Redox stress on these cells impedes neurological development. The combination of non-optimal BBB function, decrease in GST, and underdeveloped microglia appears to contribute to the autistic characteristics (2).

Another common problem among autistic individuals is gastrointestinal (GI) pathology. A 2011 study titled, "The Prevalence of Gastrointestinal Problems in Children across the United States with Autism Spectrum Disorders from Families with Multiple Affected Members", demonstrated significantly more gastrointestinal problems in children with ASD than their unaffected sibling. The most common symptoms were chronic diarrhea and constipation (13). Inflammation of the intestinal mucosa that leads to such conditions may be attributed to oxidative injury. Additionally, decreased glutathione levels promote chronic inflammation, causing mucosal degeneration as well (2).

Finally, there is a putative link between autism and impaired immune status. A functionally important group of molecules in the immune system is the cytokines (chapter 6C). Cytokines come in a variety of types to regulate the body's response to endogenous and exogenous stressors. One such stressor is the type of dysregulated inflammatory response recognized in ASD. Studies have shown that T_H1-type T-cells, which secrete cytokines involved in inflammation, such as interferon gamma (IFN-γ), function abnormally in autistic patients (6). These cytokines act in both the digestive and the nervous systems, and could play a role in the pathology experienced in these biological systems. Specifically, in the GI tract cytokines operate in pathogen protection of the gut-associated lymphoid tissue (GALT) (2). Malfunctioning cytokines could contribute to the inflammatory disease autistic patients often experience.

Low glutathione promotes an abnormal T_H2-type T cell response to antigens. The T_H2 response is important in the allergic reaction to pathogens by stimulating IgE production, and the activation of mast cells and eosinophils. In some cases, autistic patients experience an autoimmune attack on the GI tract when they encounter certain food and environmental allergens suggesting their T_H2 response is not working optimally (3).

In the nervous system, cytokines activate microglia in the brain. Additionally, a positive correlation has been shown between increased levels of the free radical nitric oxide (NO) and increased IFN-γ in autism. NO is a free radical gas that affects the release of neurotransmitters, neuron growth, and learning (6). Consequently, high levels of NO could contribute to reperfusion injury leading to brain trauma and may play a role in the pathology of autism. Overall, the immunological homeostasis in the GI and nervous systems impacts the entire body, so an imbalance could prove detrimental to the patient (2) and cause psychological dysfunction.

Conclusions

When outlining the mechanism of a multifactorial disease such as autism, it is important to weigh the significance of each component. While oxidative stress appears to be a co-morbidity of autism and not what causes it, an increase in free radicals plays a compelling role in the metabolic dysfunction of autistic patients that contributes to many of the associated symptoms. The reduction of important biochemicals such as glutathione, SAM/SAH, methionine, and folate, in conjunction with mitochondria dysfunction and alteration in serum proteins, all decrease the detoxification capacity in ASD (chapter 4A). Furthermore, an individual who already has an excess of oxidative products in his/her system is more prone to injury from exogenous stresses that a normal individual would be able to eliminate. Consequently, exposure of autistic patients to certain environmental chemicals, metals, antigens, and food additives may possibly increase the oxidative demand on their bodies. When the load becomes overwhelming, damage occurs to specific body systems.

The pattern of pathology is relatively uniform across the autistic patient population. Most commonly, gastrointestinal, neurological, and immunological problems present clinically. This is consistent with the fact that these systems live in homeostasis with one another. Therefore, targeting the reduction of oxidative stress and the increase in detoxification enzymes should decrease a variety of autistic symptoms.

Additional research into the correlation between oxidative stress and ASD could have a meaningful influence on the future of autism control. Primarily, the more we know about what causes or promotes the disease, the earlier we can identify individuals who are at high risk for autism. Perhaps this classification can be accomplished even before birth. Furthermore, discovering a tendency to autism soon after birth and treating it prophylacticly could reduce the symptoms patients experience in their lifetime and eventually prevent the initial prodomal diagnosis from progressing into autism all together (chapter 9A). (The means for doing this remain to be discovered.) The more we know about how the symptoms correlate with metabolic processes, the more accurate diagnostic tests and treatments will be. There is exciting potential in this area of research (2).

GLOSSARY

BBB – blood brain barrier

DHA - docosahexaenoic acid

EPA - eicosapentaenoic acid

FMR1 – Fragile X mental retardation 1

GALT – gut-associated lymphoid tissue

GSH – glutathione (reduced)

Chapter 8C - Detoxification

Lidianny Polanco, Paola Reveco, Karen Justiniano

[The capacity of the body to deal with toxic insults, such as oxidative stress and inflammation, are described. As an introduction to factors in the environment which may negatively affect normal neural function, the methods the body uses to deal with these situations are reviewed. – Ed.]

Introduction

Under the umbrella of developmental disorders, autism still has no defined etiology. Current theories suggest that autism is a disease of early development, as younger children are more vulnerable to oxidative stress due to environmental exposures (chapter 3G). Furthermore, there have been studies that endeavor to explain a link in the pathophysiology of autism with increased oxidative stress and abnormal DNA methylation (chapters 8A,8B).

The body's detoxification system is responsible for quickly disposing of metabolites when produced in low quantities. Reactive oxygen species are normally formed during the energy production of mitochondria and in the breakdown of organic molecules (1). Through their reduction, these metabolites are converted into water. A deficit in the detoxification system can promote an increased level of reactive oxygen species causing the body's capacity to eliminate metabolites to become overwhelmed. Through this, cellular damage can develop, as well as altered gene expression.

This strives to make a connection between deficiencies in the detoxifying mechanisms and impairment in neurological development that ultimately increases the likelihood of autism in children. A detailed literature examination on recent studies about these detoxifying enzymes will be explored.

Observations

Mitochondria generate most of the cell supply of adenosine triphosphate (ATP), which is used as a primary source of chemical energy (1). Every time energy is produced in the mitochondria, a small amount of mitochondrial superoxide is produced. The mitochondria rely on glutathione to maintain the oxidation-reduction balance and limit the superoxide, therefore preventing mitochondrial damage. Glutathione is an antioxidant that is produced from the amino acids cysteine, glycine and glutamine. The free thiol group in glutathione is responsible for the majority of its protective action such as storing cysteine and assisting in cellular proliferation. Glutathione recovers antioxidants, protecting the cell from reactive oxygen species and detoxifying it from foreign compounds to which our bodies are exposed.

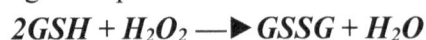

$$2GSH + H_2O_2 \longrightarrow GSSG + H_2O$$

The conversion of peroxide to water is achieved by the production of oxidized glutathione (GSSG) from reduced gluatathione (GSH) by the enzyme, glutathione peroxidase. Overproduction of superoxides can impair the function of glutathione, leading to mitochondrial damage.

In healthy cells, the mitochondria normally contain low levels of glutathione. Increased synthesis of glutathione occurs in the cellular cytoplasm, regulated by two enzymes, glycine cysteine ligase, the rate-limiting enzyme, and glutathione synthase. Depletion of these enzymes and, thus, glutathione during the developmental period of an infant can produce developmental abnormalities through oxidative stress and mitochondrial damage.

Decreased levels of glutathione and increased levels of its reduced form, glutathione disulfide, have been suspected to be a contributing factor of the neurodevelopmental manifestations in autism. James and colleagues theorized that these decreased levels of glutathione can cause mitochondrial damage and such individuals will present with dysfunctional energy metabolism. In their study, lymphoblastoid cells from autistic and normal individuals were assessed for oxidative stress, the generation of free radicals, mitochondrial damage, and ATP (2). The levels of glutathione (GSH), glutathione disulfide (GSSG), and the glutathione redox ratio were measured in whole cell extracts and in the isolated mitochondria of the lymphoblastoid cells of both autistic and control groups. The intracellular levels of GSH were decreased and the levels of GSSG were increased in autistic individuals, when compared to the control (non-autistic) group. In the autistic individuals GSH/GSSG redox ratio was decreased by approximately 60% of that in the control group. The levels of GSH in the mitochondria of autistic individuals were also decreased and the GSSH was increased when compared to the control group, resulting in the decreased redox ratio.

Unlike the cytosol, which can remove GSSG, the mitochondria rely on NADPH and glutathione reductase enzyme to reduce GSSG back to GSH. The mitochondria normally produces reactive oxygen species in the production of ATP. Because autistic individuals lack the reducing capacity due to the decreased levels of GSH, they are predisposed to mitochondrial damage by the reactive oxygen species.

In order to access the actions of GSH under increased oxidation, thimerosal reagent was administered to both autistic subjects and control group. Thimerosal reagent is a sulfyhydryl reagent that is normally found in some vaccines as an antimicrobial preservative, such as in the influenza vaccine (chapter 7B). The administration of thimerosal causes levels of GSH to decrease to even lower levels than baseline in both the autistic subjects and control groups. Even though some normal groups displayed decreasing levels of GSH, autistic subjects reached a lower level much faster, making affected subjects more susceptible to reactive oxygen species caused by exogenous exposure of chemicals (2). These findings lead to the hypothesis that autistic individuals, having decreased levels of GSH, are most affected by environmental exposures to chemicals that cause oxidative stress, than healthy persons who have higher levels of GSH.

Another study assessed the difference in the levels of GSH, GSSG and GSH/GSSH redox ratio among autistic children when compared to control unaffected groups. The decrease in the enzymatic activities of glutathione peroxidase (GPX), superoxide dimutase (SOD) and the detoxification imbalance, and susceptibility of cellular damage (3) reduced levels of total

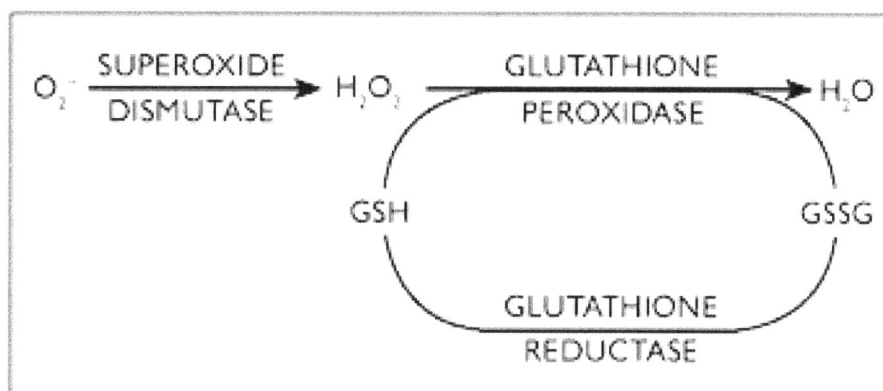

glutathione (GSH) in the plasma of autistic children is an indication of cellular oxidative status. Because GSH/GSSG ratio is important in maintaining the intracellular environment, reduced levels of this ratio can predispose autistic individuals to cellular damage through the production of free oxygen radicals and impairment of the detoxification system. All of the autistic children were found to have decreased level of GSH when compared to that of the control group, a decrease of approximately 46%. Unlike the GSH levels, the GSSG was increased among autistic children, contributing to a decrease in the GSH/GSSG redox ratio when compared to those of the control, with a percentage decrease of GSH/GSSG ratio of approximately 70% (3).

It was further theorized that the increased level of oxidized glutathione, GSSG, is an indication of oxidative stress in the cells of autistic children. This decline of the total GSH is further supported by the other studies that have found decreased levels of total glutathione in autistic children. The increased levels of both mitochondrial and intracellular GSSG are indications of apparent oxidative cellular damage. Furthermore, this study also observed decreased levels of glutathione–S-transferase (GSTP), an important enzyme which assists in the conjugation of GSH to a nontoxic form for cellular detoxification. The decreased levels of glutathione-S-transferase in the plasma of autistic children can correspond to the decreased levels of GSH in the plasma. This research has demonstrated decreased levels of glutathione as one of the contributing factors of the development of autism due to the accumulation and damage of cells, but the findings do not ascertain that it is the causative factor.

An investigation was conducted to evaluate pregnant mothers with glutathione-S-transferase P1 gene (GSTP1) haplotype and their risk of having an autistic child (8). GSTP acts in preventing oxidative stress by conjugating GSH into a nontoxic product for excretion. It is also important in regulating Jun N-terminal kinase (JNK), a protein kinase that phosphorylates genes involved in cellular functions such as mitosis and apoptosis, which in turn affects brain development and differentiation. Deficits in these cellular pathways may make a person susceptible to autism.

Transmission dysequilibrium testing, a way to assess for linkage between alleles and phenotypes, was performed on 137 autistic members from 49 families. It was seen that the GSTP1 haplotype was significantly transmitted to mothers of individuals with autism, suggesting that it may be acting in mothers during pregnancy to contribute to the phenotype of autism in the fetus (8). This mutation is not found in all autism cases; therefore, it does not define universal cause. Despite this, it is one of the first studies addressing this subject matter. Consequently, more experiments need to be conducted to validate its significance.

Chapter 8A offers a further review of genetic errors and their potential association with autism. An experiment was conducted by New York State Institute for Basic Research in Developmental Disabilities using tissue from the postmortem cerebellum of autistic children, in which they assessed if a defect in the synthesis or consumption of glutathione plays a role in the generation of autism. In this experiment, the activity and concentration of gluthathione peroxidase (GPx), gluthathione reductase (GR), glutathione-S-transferase (GST), and glycine cysteine ligase (GCL) in the brains of autistic children was comparable to the brains of control

1)GLUTAMATE + GLYCINE + CYSTEINE ————▶ GLUTATHIONE (GHS)
                                            GLUT.SYNTHASE

2)GLUTATHIONE ————▶ GLUTATHIONE CONJUGATE————▶ EXCRETION
        GLUT.-S-TRANSFERASE

3)GLUTATHIONE ————————▶ GSSH————————▶ GLUTATHIONE
        GLUT.PEROXIDASE   GLUT.REDUCTASE

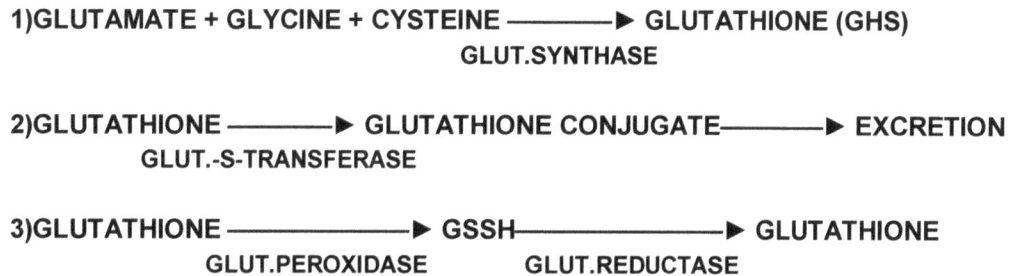

group. The levels of the proteins glutamate-cystein ligase modifier protein (GCLM) and glutamate-cystein ligase catalytic subunit (GCLC), two enzymes responsible in the regulation of glutamate-cystein ligase, were also measured. Compared to the control group in this study, it was found that the levels of GPx, an important enzyme in the prevention of oxidative stress (chapter 8B), were lower by 14.1% in the autistic subjects, with 70% of them with activities below the 95% confidence interval of the control group. GST is an important enzyme that is involved in the conjugation of GSH into a nontoxic product for excretion; in autistic subjects it was found to be lower than the 95% confidence interval in 50% of the autistic subjects when compared to the control group. The activities of GR had no significant difference between the autistic subjects and the control group with 20% of the autistic group with unusually elevated levels and 40% with decreased levels. In the autistic subject, the activities of GCL was reduced by 38.7% when compared to the control group, 80% of them presenting with values lower than the 95% confidence interval of the control group. The activity of GCLC was also found to be reduced further confirming the reduced levels of GCL activities (9).

As noted, GSH is very important in the detoxification of the cell. Consequently, the decrease of this molecule and the enzymes involved in its synthesis might be a contributing factor for the development of autism. The decrease in GSH can lead to the accumulation of reactive oxygen species and hydrogen peroxide, causing protein abnormalities, cellular damage, and cellular apoptosis. Because the mitochondria is not capable of producing its own GSH, reduced levels of GSH can make it more susceptible to damage by reactive oxygen species. The administration of GSH has been implemented in the therapy of other diseases, but this resulted in an ineffective treatment because GSH proved to have poor stabililty, solubility, and absorption. The conclusion of this study demonstrated the decreased levels of GSH found in autistic infants, but failed to find a certain pathway for the cause and development of autism.

Glutathione and reactive oxygen species were also the focus of a study conducted by Rose (4). This study focused primarily on the cerebellum and Brodmann area 22 in the brains of autistic infants. It was hypothesized that glutathione redox imbalance and oxidative stress play roles in the neurological deficits of autism. To assess protein oxidative damage, the tyrosine residue 3-nitrotyrosine (3-NT) was monitored. 3-NT is a product of peroxynitrate, an oxidant and nitrating agent produced from nitric oxide (NO) and superoxide. To determine the levels of inflammation, the tyrosine derivative, 3-chlorotyrosine (3-CT) was measured. 3-CT is a product of myeloperoxidase synthesized as a product of persistent activation of inflammation due to innate immune cells. 8-oxo-deoxyguanosine, a strong marker of oxidative damage of DNA during inflammation, was also measured. This study found altered levels of GSH, GSSG, 3-NT, 3-CT and 8-oxo-deoxyguanosine in both the cerebellum and Brodmann area 22 of autistic children compared to that of the control groups. GSH was decreased by 43% in the cerebellum and 32% in Brodmann 22 of autistic children compared to that of the control group (chapters 3B-3D). Along with this decrease, there was also an increase of GSSH in the cerebellum by 18% and in Brodmann area 22 by 19% in autistic subjects compared to the control. This decrease in reduced glutathione (GSH) and increase of the oxidized form of glutathione (GSSG) do support the hypothesis of decreased levels of GSH/GSSG redox ratio of autistic children compared to control group and, thus, increased risk of oxidative stress. The GSH/GSSG redox ration proved to be reduced by 52% in the cerebellum and 43% in Brodmann 22 area of autistic subjects. The concentrations of 3-CT and 3-NT were also elevated in autistic children compared to the control group. This further supported the hypothesis of increase in oxidative stress, protein damage, DNA damage, and increased inflammation, along with mitochondrial superoxide development in the autistic children (4).

At the same time the levels of 3-NT were increased by 42% in the cerebellum and 72% in Brodmann 22, indicating persistent inflammation. The levels of 3-CT were increased by even higher proportions than 3-NT, 95% in the cerebellum and 38% in Brodmann 22. Rose related the high levels of 3-NT as an indication of increased levels of nitric oxide (NO) production. NO promotes the generation of peroxynitrate which may result in inactivation of complexes 1, 3, and 5 in the mitochondrial membrane. These complexes are important for the transfer of electrons creating an electrochemical gradient driving the synthesis of ATP, the inactivation of these complexes leads to reduced ability to maintain normal neuronal function due to the decreases in ATP. 8-oxo-deoxyguanosine is used in order to assess DNA oxidative damage in the autistic compared to the control. 8-oxo-deoxyguanosine is made when a lesion is produced in the DNA by an attack by hydroxyl radicals. In this study a negative correlation between 8-oxy-deoxyguanosine and GSH/GSSH was found in the cerebellum. There were higher levels of 8-oxy-deoxyguanosine and lower levels of GSH/GSSH. This relationship is a sign of the importance of decreased levels GSH/GSSG in the autistic and the production of mitochondrial superoxide (4).

Aconitase was used in order to measure mitochondrial reactive oxygen species and oxidative damage. This enzyme is important in the tricarboxylic acid cycle, converting citrate to isocitrate. Aconitase also acts as iron regulatory protein-1 in the cytosol which increases the absorption of transferrin and iron out of the blood in the event that there are decreased levels of iron in the cells. A decrease of 45% in aconitase activity was demonstrated in the brains of autistic children compared to the control group (4). Because most aconitase is typically in the mitochondria and is very sensitive to superoxide radicals. Decreased levels of this enzyme serve as an indication of mitochondrial dysfunction and the production of excess mitochondrial superoxide resulting in mitochondrial damage. Aconitase inactivated by superoxides can be restored under the presence of sufficient reducing agents such as GSH or NADPH.

Damage specifically to the superior temporal lobe on the left side where Wernicke's area is located could be the contributing factor to the impaired verbal communication in autistic children. However, there has been no evidence that the decrease of antioxidants and the accumulation reactive oxygen species are the cause of the verbal impairment in autistic individuals. Rose demonstrated that the formation of mitochondrial superoxide might be elevated in certain regions of the brain. This, coupled with inflammation of these regions due to oxidative stress, can cause damage to cells and ultimately exhibit the characteristic neurodegenerative pattern seen in autistic children (chapter 8B).

Another investigation measured the levels of the antioxidant enzymes, superoxide dismutase (SOD) and glutathione peroxidase (GSH-Px), as well as levels of malondialdehyde (MDA) in autistic children. The study analyzed 20 children with autism and compared them to 25 age-matched control children. Superoxide dismutase (SOD), an important enzyme in protecting the body against oxidative stress, was found to be decreased in individuals with autism compared to the control group. The levels of glutathione peroxidase (GPX), a powerful antioxidant which converts hydrogen peroxide to water and oxygen (see equation above), was also found to be lower in autistic individuals. This decrease was only noted in autistic children younger than 6 years old. Younger children tend to have a lower level of glutathione when compared to older children. Therefore, it was theorized that the difference in age groups is due to the vulnerability of younger children to oxidative stress. Malondialdehyde (MDA), an indicator of lipid peroxidation and oxidative stress, was also found to be significantly high amongst autistic children when compared to control group. Lipid peroxidation occurs when the lipid membranes of cells are attacked by free radicals causing cellular damage (1).

The conclusion of this study was that the decreased levels of the antioxidant enzymes, superoxide dismutase and glutathione peroxidase, can produce increased susceptibility to cellular damage. Therefore, it might play a role in the development of autism in children. The decreased SOD is apparently involved in the reduction of neuronal growth and migration due to DNA damage through the production of high levels of superoxides. Because of these results, the supplementation of antioxidant along with polyunsaturated fatty acids is recommended for autistic children. Even though there is a significant difference in the levels of SOD and GPX, to

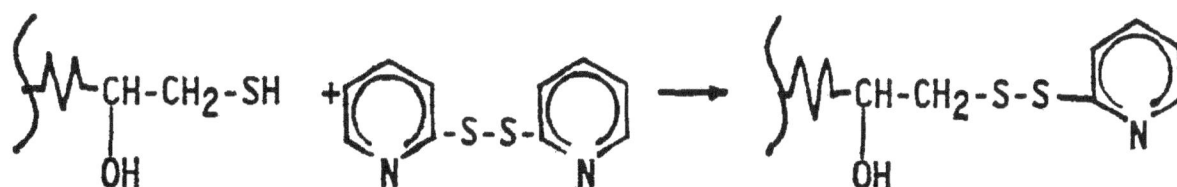

date there has not been found a direct link supporting changes in the levels of these enzymes as being due to enzymatic impairment caused by increased levels of reactive oxygen species or of the elevated levels of these radicals. However, this study did support the hypothesis that the increased susceptibility to oxidative damage and, thus, cellular damage can increase the chance of the development of autism (1).

Thioredoxin is an antioxidant important in the removal of oxygen radicals, balancing inflammation, and anti-apoptosis preventing cellular damage. Thioredoxin contains a thiol group in which it is oxidized by compounds such as hydrogen peroxide to form disulfide bonds. Thioredoxin (Trx) is kept in the reduced state by the enzyme thioredoxin reductase (TrxR). In one study, half of the autistic children presented with increased levels of thiorexin reductase activity in plasma when compared to a control group. The mean level of thioredoxin-1 was increased by 67% in autistic children when compared to a control group; this apparently supports the hypothesis of increased oxidative stress in the development of autism.

The levels of both peroxiredoxin-1 and peroxiredoxin-3 were overexpressed in autistic patients. Peroxiredoxin was markedly elevated in autistic children when compared to controls, with an increase of 101%. Peroxiredoxins are proteins in the cell that have an antioxidant role in the reduction of hydrogen peroxide into water and have also resulted in playing a role in cellular differentiation and proliferation. In high amounts, hydrogen peroxide can cause cellular damage and can cause cellular apoptosis (3). Since not all autistic subjects demonstrated this presentation, it may be that it is a co-morbid factor rather than a causative agent.

Oxidative stress alone may not be the only potential cause of autism. The idea that it may part of an autism presentation has been supported by several small studies. The combination of DNA methylation and oxidative stress has been suspected in the pathophysiology of autism. Methionine, a sulfur-containing essential amino acid, is important in many body functions. Methionine, activated by methionine adenosyltransferase, forms S-adenosylmethionine (SAM). SAM is a co-substrate involved in methyl group transfers. SAM is the primary donor for DNA methylation. A methyl group from SAM is transferred to many enzyme specific methyl acceptors, which results in the formation of S-adenosylhomocysteine (SAH). The ratio of SAM to SAH is a reflection of trans-methylation efficiency and cellular methylation potential. A decrease in the synthesis of SAM would be involved in a decrease in methylation activity.

In a study with 68 children with autism, 40 unaffected siblings, and 54 age-matched control children, the combined metabolic pathway of DNA methylation and cellular antioxidants was investigated (6). When compared to their unaffected siblings, both methionine and SAM were decreased significantly in children with autism, thereby indicating a possible correlation with increased oxidative stress. When the unaffected siblings were compared to the age-matched control group, there was no difference in methionine or SAM. Methylation inhibitor, SAH, was significantly increased in the children with autism compared to their unaffected siblings. The sibling SAH levels were intermediate between their affected siblings and the control group. The ratio of SAM to SAH was decreased in children with autism compared to their siblings and the age-matched control group. The unaffected siblings and the age-matched control SAM/SAH ratios were no different.

In a comparable investigation on 20 children with autism and 33 control children, concentrations of methionine, SAM, and homocysteine were significantly lower in autistic children compared to the control children. SAH and adenosine concentrations were higher in autistic children compared to control children. The SAM/SAH ratio was almost 50% lower in the autistic children than in the control children (metabolic biomarkers?) (5). In both studies, the intracellular ratio GSH/GSSH was shifted towards an oxidized state in children with autism when compared to their siblings and their age-matched control group. These findings contributed to the idea that there may be an autistic metabolic profile of increased SAH and increased oxidized glutathione, but not in 100% of autistic cases.

Conclusions

The various studies reviewed here concluded that a deficiency in the detoxification system can have an important association with autism. A decrease in enzymes such as superoxide dismutase, glutathione peroxidase, glycine cysteine ligase, and glutathione synthase appear to contribute to oxidative stress in children. This oxidative stress leads to increased levels of free radicals, which may damage DNA, leading to neuronal impairments seen in autism.

Unfortunately, these studies have shortcomings. One of the limitations of current research is that it fails to make a distinction of whether detoxification deficiency is actually contributing to the cause of autism or if it is secondary to or co-existent with the disorder itself. Another deficiency is seen in experimental data that only involve a small number of cases in the test population. Larger studies should be done in the future to address these concerns.

Along with the cause of autism, measures should be taken to evaluate treatments in cases where the detoxification system is suspected to be the culprit for the disorder. Few investigations have shown that supplementation of antioxidants may help improve the clinical manifestations of autistic children. In addition, whether early administration of antioxidants can prevent or reduce irreversible cellular damage in the autistic child remains to be tested. While there has been much research on autism to date, more has to be done in order to fully unmask this disorder.

Glossary
GCL- glycine cysteine ligase
GCLC- glutamate-cysteine ligase catalytic subunit
GCLM- glutamate-cysteine ligase modifier protein
GPx or **GSH-Px**- glutathione peroxidase
GR- gluthathione reductase
GSH- glutathione
GSSG- glutathione disulfide
GST- glutathione-S-transferase
GSTP1-glutathione-S-transferase P1
JNK- jun N-terminal kinase
MDA- malondialdehyde
SOD- superoxide dimutase

THERAPY

Chapter 9A: Diagnosis & Prevention

Gary Steinman

[While an effective treatment of autism is urgently needed, without a complete understanding of its cause, such an advance remain elusive. For the most part, many "therapies" have had little benefit for the affected children since what and how these treatments are supposed to ameliorate is still undefined. – Ed.]

Hypothesis

As reviewed in the Prologue to this book, there are three requirements to identify the cause of specific infections. In light of modern medical and molecular biological advances, as well as the specific factors characteristic of autism, these postulates can now be broadened and modified for the issue at hand as follows:

1. The suspected causal factors must be constantly associated with the disease.
2. The suspected causal dysfunction must be identified within an affected individual.
3. When a susceptible host (e.g., test animal) is genetically modified appropriately (e.g., deletion of the IGF gene), the same symptoms of the spontaneous disease must develop.

For example, in chapter 7A, it was emphasized that rigorous studies have failed to identify a cause-and-effect relationship between autism and vaccination. On the other hand, the appearance of autism-like behavior in mice bred to have the IGF gene deleted meets these standards (chapter 6D).

Observations

In dealing with any medical disorder, it is necessary to be able to comprehend the mechanism by which it originates and manifests itself in the patient. Once this is known, the next step is to deal with:

1) Routine diagnosis - to be able to identify the condition in any affected person;
2) Therapy/treatment – to manage and minimize the severity of the condition; and
3) Prevention – if possible.

Because of the large body of inadequately explored, potentially associated factors (e.g., autoimmune diseases), many medical disorders are not clearly understood. This makes effective management or prevention difficult in such cases. As a result, medical practice in general remains an art rather than a science. As the body of knowledge increases, the ability to apply new technology and insight becomes apparent in the care of individuals suffering from these conditions.

As a complete entity, each condition has its combination of symptoms and signs such a pain, body temperature, changes in nervous function, weight loss, laboratory abnormalities, and/or specific behavioral characteristics. However, the difficulty is that not every incident of a particular disorder manifests itself in the same manner with a full array of the same symptoms (the patient's subjective complaints) and signs (objective findings on physical examination) in every patient. In a number of cases, some idiosyncratic factors are not found, whereas in other cases, nonspecific changes may mask the true identity of the condition.

At present, the diagnosis of autism is complicated by the variability found between its sufferers and because of periodic modification of analytical criteria (chapter 1D). Major genetic anomalies occur in some cases, but not uniformly in most (chapter 8A). Identification of this disorder (or spectrum of disorders) currently relies mainly on psychological testing, which is largely subjective in nature. As a result, it is not clear in any given case if a particular ailment is a life-long illness (e.g., autism) or if improvement to varying degrees can be achieved. For example, when "infantile autism" became a named condition through the work of Leo Kanner in 1943 (1), he distinguished the malady from feeble-mindedness and schizophrenia. However, there remained much overlap in such conditions to make the biological basis difficult to define.

What was and still is needed is an understanding of specific biomarkers in affected people which distinguish it from other entities. These require a characterization (diagnosis) identified by a combination of biochemical, microscopic, anatomic, genetic, and/or physiologic changes specific to each condition. The thrust of current research deals extensively with this requirement, especially genetic. For example, a search is underway to identify biochemicals, not necessarily representing the primary cause of the disease, which may be characteristically abnormal in children exhibiting autistic behavior. These agents would be called biomarkers and could serve as sentinels and signs of the pathologic process underway.

Autism is commonly thought to be a combination of genetic predisposition and an environmental trigger inducing overt manifestations of the disorder. Whereas the cause of autism should be identifiable and comparable in 100% of the clearly diagnosed cases, many display such an etiologic characteristic in many, but not all, of the patients determined to have a form of autism spectrum disorder (ASD). In combination with the subjective psychological determinants qualifying a particular case as autism, some special coexistent objective attributes occur which qualify them as biomarkers. These indicators may stem from the same origin as the disease itself, making them co-morbid factors but not etiologic inducers.

A major subject of current investigation concerns dysmyelination (chapter 6A). While reduced myelin sheathing is commonly found in the brains of autistic individuals who died from other causes, it would be advantageous if such a deficiency could somehow be documented in living patients. Forms of brain imaging, such as MRI, have been reported to identify thinning myelin sheaths in babies who were diagnosed as autistic months later (chapters 3A,6A). As such methods become more refined and definitive, preventive therapy could begin at an early age, before autistic behavior became fully manifested.

Treatment

Once hearing and sight impairments have been ruled out, the major approach to treatment today centers on the control of behavioral disorders in children and adults labeled as autistic. Typically, a definitive diagnosis cannot now be made with certainty until the child reaches age 2 or 3 years. Such efforts usually attain only small overall improvement even with intensive efforts at behavioral modification and rehabilitation (chapters 2A-2C). However, one of the most gratifying advances so far deals with interpersonal communication. Initially, children labeled as autistic almost uniformly display seemingly insurmountable barriers to social interactions and communication with others in the general environment. However, through the successful use of word processors, the inner thoughts of many autistic individuals have been effectively transmitted to others and, surprisingly, identified mature, stimulating thinking where confusion seemed to be the rule before this.

As with any disorder, the ultimate objective is to understand the mechanism of the disease so that preventative measures can be instituted before irreversible pathologic damage has taken place. Although unique genetic changes, for example, can be observed in some autistic patients, none have been found in more than a few percent of affected individuals. Thus, it is difficult to ascertain if such mutations are coincidental or do, in fact, represent contributory processes in the patients. As a case in point, it is unlikely that a cause-and-effect connection between the rate of television watching and elevated rates of autism coexist, even though statistically there appears to be a correspondence (chapter 2D). Similarly, the time proximity of vaccination and the appearance of autistic behavior seemed to support a causal relationship at first, but subsequent studies showed that the connection was untenable (chapter 7A).

In chapters 4B,4C,5D, and 7, evidence was reviewed negating the claim that heavy metals generally are the cause autism and its overt manifestations. Even now, methods intended to remove such metals from the body, such as chelation, continue to be applied. Double-blind studies which would substantiate the use of such methods are lacking. The fallacious reasoning used to promote continued use of such ineffective and potentially harmful "therapy" continues to be applied. Much of this results from the frustrations of parents of autistic children who are willing to seek out even questionable means, in the hope that some improvement will be achieved (chapters 2A-2C).

Many of the proposed origins of autism reviewed in this book have, in fact, been disproven with additional research work, but the effort continues today to uncover and define its fundamental, primary cause. If a positive connection between a proposed initiation of the neural damage characteristically found in autistic children and a contributory event can be firmly identified, attention could be directed to impeding such a process in the early stages.

As a case in point, the stimulus of insulin-like growth factor (IGF) in promoting myelination of the developing nerves in the central nervous system was discussed in chapter 6E. It was proposed that an IGF deficiency identified in the baby at birth could be evidence for the need for additional growth factor, especially in the first year of life. Although this remains to be proven with convincing laboratory results, the prospect that IGF may be a key to the etiology of autism could lead to an effective preventative, if proven correct.

The beneficial effects of injected IGF for rescuing synaptic and motor neural deficits have been demonstrated with modified mouse models bearing autism-like conditions. For example, Phelan-McDermid syndrome, an uncommon disease lacking a copy of the SHANK3 gene (sometimes associated with autism), is characterized by major defects in excitatory synaptic transmission. *In vitro,* providing IGF supplement promotes restoration of mature synapses in these animals (2-4).

Rett Syndrome (RS), an X-linked mutant entity displaying neurologic abnormalities that mimic autism, is not now considered a part of the autism spectrum (chapters 1D,8A). However, genetically altered mice displaying RS-like characteristics have been studied in the laboratory. In such cases, symptoms have improved following administration of IGF-1 (5).

Plausible means for replacing the insufficient resource of IGF in the human newborn could be:

1) Parenterally supply (e.g., injection);
2) Oral supplementation in formula or bovine milk;
3) Massage therapy (6) (chapter 2D); and
4) Breastfeeding (7) .

An additional approach is the treatment of autistic children with fluoxetine, whereby the level of IGF-1 in their cerebrospinal fluid (typically lowered in affected children) was found to rise (8) (chapter 6D).

Prevention

One strategy for prevention is to identify the inherited elements leading to the overt manifestations of autism. Many attempts have been made to detect a specific early biomarker for the subsequent development of explicit autistic behavior. A number have searched for a unique genetic mutation, although essentially all those isolated so far have been found in only a small number of cases (chapter 8A). On the other hand, if IGF deficiency is at the center of autism generation (chapter 6E) for example, and is the consequence of IGF gene polymorphism, identifying the same gene in both prospective parents would warn about the potential of their conceiving affected children subsequently. Thus, this characteristic would serve both as a biomarker for the increased tendency to develop autism in the offspring and as a therapeutic target for prevention or reduction of subsequent autistic behavior.

Much like Tay-Sachs disease, couples planning a pregnancy could be pretested for the presence of abnormal genes in both adults, potentially leading to preventative methods before conception. Unaffected offspring could be achieved with a donor sperm or egg free of the defect. However, as noted in chapter 8A, some genetic modifications are unique to the autistically affected individual. Another prophylaactic approach would be to undergo preimplantation genetic diagnosis (PGD). This would be especially applicable with women who previously gave birth to an autistic children, since in such women the chance is much higher (1-in-5) of having another affected child than in the general population of mothers (1-in-88).

Fetal hypoxia in labor is implicated in affected newborn in some autism cases (chapters 3G,3H). Expeditious delivery, especially when fetal compromise is anticipated, is the preferred course of action. Furthermore, pharmaceuticals and pollutants known to increase the chance of autism in the neonate need to be avoided during gestation (chapters 4D,4E). Gravidas must avoid exposure to toxins including pesticides and gaseous pollutants, especially during the 1st trimester of pregnancy. Medical conditions such as diabetes and compromised blood flow from heart disease should be under effective control prior to initiation of pregnancy (chapter 3I); preventative vaccinations (e.g., against influenza) must be given before conception is attempted (chapter 6B).

It is worth repeating here that vaccination of young children has not been shown to be an initiator of autism (chapter 7A). In this way, the youngsters are protected against otherwise devastating viral infections such as mumps and measles. Unfortunately, of all the misconceptions about autism discussed in this book, this one persists the most widely in the general public without any substantiating evidence.

In chapters 6B-6C, the increased occurrence of autism in the offspring of women who had influenza during the first trimester of their pregnancy was discussed. Based on this, it would seem that prepregnancy influenza vaccination would reduce this risk. However, much like moderate fish eating discussed in chapter 5D, gravidas continue to be hesitant to "chance" this potential autism-reducing precaution primarily because of subjective apprehension and uncertainty.

Conclusions

Until the exact etiology of autism is ascertained, it will not be possible to effectively deal with the prevention of this condition. While many methods have been proposed to deal with the supposed cause (e.g., chelation to remove lead as a postulated cause – chapter 4C), none has reduced or totally prevented the onset of autistic behavior. The only therapeutic methods now available are aimed at making the child more productive within society (e.g., speech therapy – chapter 2C).

Autism most likely has both a genetic component, setting the possible outcomes within particular settings, and an environmental component, triggering the expression of inherent potential for flawed behavior traits. Thus, an integrated research agenda which exposes the idiosyncrasies of both areas of involvement needs to be initiated, using an open-minded approach to new ideas and perspectives. The "old school" approach of repeating previously reported experimental findings has not brought us much closer to a solution than what we had in the 1940s when Kanner first identified and described this unique condition (chapters 1A,2B). Claims of major progress and insights into new findings have little to show for real progress. Prior unsuccessful approaches need to be laid aside in favor of new thinking and an open-mindedness to fresh ideas.

Glossary
GSSG – glutathione (oxidized)
IFN - interferon
MeCP2 – methyl-binding protein
ROS - reactive oxygen species
SAM – S-adenosylmethionine
TS – tuberous sclerosis

Chapter 9B - Stem Cell Therapy

Brian Temple, Aldo Manresa

[With deficiencies noted in the nervous tissue of autistic individuals, such as dysmyelination, patch gaps, and immune dysregulation, it is plausible that implantation of unaffected stem cells may hold the key to reversing the abnormal neurologic manifestations and behavior disorders characteristic of this condition. – Ed.]

Hypothesis

The fundamental goal of science and medical research is to mold our current understanding of the universe into a knowledge core that has the ability to prevent or ameliorate illness in our fellow mankind. This optimistic and theoretical goal has led researchers to invest time and effort into the development of stem cell technologies in particular, and their therapeutic reach is intriguingly extending into autism. The objective of this chapter is to introduce the reader to the concepts of stem cells, discuss current research endeavors addressing the use of stem cells as potential biological models for autism and drug discovery, and to elaborate on this seeming panacea that could result in an alleviation of the travails of autism.

Observations

Ever since Robert Hooke discovered the cell while observing bottle cork under a compound microscope in the 1600's, scientist have whittled away at its hidden biological secrets. The term "stem cell" was proposed in the early 1900's, which theorized the existence of hematopoietic stem cells (HSC's) (1). HSC's were then discovered in 1978 in human cord blood. These blood-specific multipotent cells have since become a powerful treatment for patients suffering from numerous blood and bone marrow pathologies, such as leukemia, lymphoma, myelodysplastic syndromes, immunodeficiency syndromes and sickle cell anemia (2). The downside of using HSC's lies in their efficacy only in hematologic/oncologic disease and their strong potential for eliciting an immune response that can manifest as graft-vs-host disease. Embryonic stem cells were discovered three years later in the inner cell mass of a mouse blastocyst (3).

By unlocking the clandestine nature of these pluripotent, embryologic stem cells, scientists are able to regenerate any tissue in the body that, for some reason, has gone awry. However, in order for an embryonic stem cell to be created, a viable embryo had to be sacrificed, which met with much opposition. In 2001, the Federal Government only allowed funding for research on stem cell lines that already existed at that time. Many of these lines were found to be contaminated and unusable for research, leaving investigators without a reliable source of stem cells as well as decreased funding opportunities from the Department of Health, including the National Institute of Health. In 2009, a new executive order removed restrictions on federal funding involving embryonic stem cell research (4). However, the ethical and moral questions persist and embryonic stem cell therapy remains controversial.

In 1962, Gurdon discovered that the specialization of cells is reversible when he replaced an immature cell nucleus in an egg of a frog with a nucleus from a mature intestinal cell. This modified egg eventually became a tadpole, revolutionizing the dogma that specialized cells are irreversibly committed to a predestined fate. In 2006, Yamanaka introduced a novel stem cell type dubbed the Induced Pluripotent Stem cell (iPSC). Dr. Yamanaka's group not only found a way to reprogram terminally differentiated cells, but was able to do it using a simple, reproducible method. This technique utilizes somatic cells, such as fibroblasts, and introduces four factors [*Oct3/4, Sox2, Klf4* and *cMyc*] via retroviral vectors (5). These four genes were found to be integral in reprogramming somatic cells back into pluripotent stem cells that were proven to express the phenotype (condensed clusters of cells with low cytoplasmic to nuclear ratio) and genotype (pluripotent stem cell markers SSEA-3, SSEA-4, Tra-1 60 and Tra-1 81) of known stem cells. These pluripotent iPSC's then were able to differentiate into all three germ layers. Yamanaka and Gurdon were awarded the Nobel Prize in Medicine or Physiology in 2012 for this groundbreaking discovery.

Currently, three different methods have been developed to convert differentiated somatic cells into iPSC's:

1) The first method was demonstrated by Yamanaka's group, as described above.

2) The second method utilizes transdifferentiation to create induced neurons (iN's). "Transdifferentiation is a process by which one cell type is transformed to take on the identity of another cell type" (6). In autism, for instance, it is theorized that one could remove human fibroblasts from autistic patients, transdifferentiate them into iN's, and potentially use them for therapeutic purposes. Researchers proved that with the addition of NeuroD1, a basic transcription factor, human fibroblasts can be transdifferentiated into iN's in about 3 weeks. The transdifferentiated neurons demonstrated an ability to fire action potentials and further differentiate into multiple subtypes of neurons (7).

3) The third method takes fibroblasts and turns them directly into neuronal stem cells (NSC's). It has been proposed that if transcription factor Sox2 were introduced alone,

mouse fibroblasts would differentiate into neuronal stem cells (8). These NSC's were able to differentiate into astrocytes and oligodendrocytes. However, it is not yet known whether this process can occur using human adult fibroblasts.

With iPSC technology, researchers might be able to create patient-specific cellular models of autism spectrum disorder (ASD) directly from an autistic patient's somatic cells, allowing a better understanding of the pathophysiology of each patient with this disorder. Furthermore, with these *in vitro* ASD models, progress in drug discovery will no longer suffer from the failure of the predictive validity of animal models and the lack of access to post-mortem human brain tissue. iPSC's eliminate the ethical debate that shadows the use of embryological stem cells, and create an endless supply of pluripotent stem cells. Lastly, iPSC's may serve a role in organogenesis and cellular/tissue transplant in the future. In the next section we will take the topics we have introduced and delve deeper into current research to further discuss their implications and current applications in understanding and treating ASD.

Pathobiology in ASD

Neurons, once committed in children to a specific tract and function, cannot be repaired once damaged, at the present state of scientific progress. ASD is a complex and heterogenous, neurodevelopmental disorder characterized by social and language impairments along with repetitive behaviors (9). To truly understand any neurological disorder there needs to be a fundamental recognition of its neural development and clinical manifestations. This is why there has been a greater emphasis on developing animal and cellular models for neurological diseases including ASD. However, this has proven to be a difficult challenge due to limited access of live neuronal cells and the multitude of factors that this illness possesses. For apparent ethical reasons, biopsies of neuronal tissue from otherwise healthy patients with autism are not feasible and do not allow for *in vitro* studies of disease progression. Currently, researchers believe creation of cellular models with iPSC provides the future for the study of ASD. Hypothetically, iPSC's may be able to be mass developed for the benefit of drug development, drug screening, and drug testing, including the analysis of toxicities and efficacy (10). These advancements are key in providing patients with future pharmacological therapies which will most likely entail a multidisciplinary approach.

The putative pathobiology of ASD can be derived from multiple factors including a possible genetic component, immune dysregulation, and a complex neuronal communication disorder (11). Also, neurological patterns have showed an inability for neurons to establish proper connections (chapters 3F,6D) (12). However, autism is currently defined by subjective behavioral assessments and lacks objective biomarkers that would clarify diagnostic criteria (chapter 9A) (13). Thus, this becomes a key issue that is attempting to be answered by iPSC technology. In this respect, a clearer understanding of the genetic component of ASD needs to be addressed and considerable work has gone into this (chapter 8A).

Researchers have demonstrated that autism has a strong genetic component, as indicated by their twin studies (chapters 1C,8A) (14,15). The data resulted in a concordance of 70-90% in monozygotic twins, many times higher than for dizygotic twins. Stem cells would largely further the understanding of the complex, multifactorial genetic causes of autism. Moreover, many novel genes have already been discovered for autism-like monogenic disorders including Fragile X, Rett syndrome, and Timothy syndrome, although none have been identified in all ASD cases. These disorders provide a clearer genetic component that aids studying those diseases. Interestingly, roughly half of the 683 genes that have been found to be differentially expressed in ASD individuals have a role in the brain and about 5% have a role in fetal brain (16). On the other hand, autism studies have not been successful in clearly determining universal genetic causes. With the use of iPSC's and new genetic techniques, most would hope that a connection can be established.

A great amount of work has been dedicated in discovering what exactly is different about the brain of a patient with autism. Using magnetic resonance images (MRI), positron emission tomography (PET) scans, and post-mortem autopsies, researchers have provided some insight into the anatomical differences (chapter 3A). Moreover, researchers concluded that three main functional and anatomical differences in patients with autism exist when compared to IQ, age, and gender-matched controls. These include:

1) a lower degree of functional connectivity between the frontal and parietal areas
2) decreased sections of the corpus callosum, which are cortical areas used to communicate, and
3) an interaction exists between the size of the genu in the corpus callosum and frontal parietal functional connectivity (17,18).

These anatomical and functional differences provide for a lesser degree of integration of information across certain cortical areas thought to result in the phenotypic characteristics that we term ASD (chapters 3B-3F).

iPSC's as a model for ASD

Autism spectrum disorder has been shown to be associated with multiple, complex genetic abnormalities. Over 100 genes have been identified, making this illness a nightmare to create successful animal models to emulate its disease process (chapter 8A). However, major advancements have been made in creating animal/cellular models that will help us study its pathology. ASD is a multifactorial, complex pathologic process that an animal model seems unlikely to be developed using mice and other mammals. Although such examples may not be optimal for studying a human condition, helpful neuropathologic and behavioral information can be gleaned from such models. On the other hand, much work has been implemented into creating a cellular model that expresses what the pathophysiological deficiencies truly are. Researchers believe the key is in neuronal cells and their effects on autism's behavioral and emotional manifestations. In these regards, induced neuronal (iN) cells from patients with autism may provide a cellular framework from which further work can be undertaken (6).

The iN cells are very similar to regular neurons. They contain sodium and potassium channels, along with having the ability to fire action potentials when stimulated. This advancement may provide researchers the ability to delve into developmental deficiencies in autistic neuronal cells. Interestingly, iN cells follow normal developmental timelines which allow them to be used specifically for neurodevelopmental disorders (6). Despite this progression, many early neurological models have suffered from inadequacies including neuronal maturation, synaptic deficiencies, and failed connectivity (12).

A key challenge in developing proper cellular models is dependent on creating a parallel between what is observed *in vitro* and the disease pathology observed *in vivo* (12). In addition, the lack of a murine model and the availability of post-mortem brains are detrimental to advancement of a true causal pathological understanding (19). Consequently, iPSC technology can potentially be developed to overcome this hurdle. In theory, induced neuronal cells can be derived from fibroblasts of autistic patients and personalized studies could be performed. This, we hope, would yield a feasible and readily available model from which to perform studies. Also, murine models would have major limitation especially the lack of certain neocortical areas that are only present in humans (11).

The major benefits of using iPSC's to study autism is the ability to develop a disease-specific cellular model, potential for replacement cell therapies and the groundwork for drug screening. Thus, iPSC's provide an autologous cellular foundation from which to further our understanding of its pathobiology. These induced cells will also circumvent ethical concerns associated with human embryonic stem cells which include destroying embryos (11).

iPSCs use in pharmacological discovery/efficacy/safety in treating ASD

Ultimately, the goal of stem cells in autism includes their ability to be used in pharmacological discovery and treatment. Furthermore, key aspects of drug discovery include its ability to be tested for efficacy and most importantly safety before being used on human patients. The lack of modeling *in vivo* and *in vitro*, limited understanding of the pathophysiology and the heterogeneity of symptoms provides for much of the difficulty in developing pharmacological therapy. Currently, there is a severe deficiency in available treatments for these patients. Off-label use of anti-anxiety, anti-depressant, and anti-psychotics are all the existing weapons clinicians possess to combat ASD symptoms. Among these are two approved medications for ASD, risperidone and aripiprazole. These current therapies only address the symptoms of the patients and do not address the causality of disease. ASD is still diagnosed based solely on behavioral symptoms within a spectrum. Thus, the idea of a single therapy for the multitude of symptoms seems unfeasible. Rather, it reasons that a homogenous subgroup classification will provide for the best treatment outcomes. This should not only lead to the development of diagnostic biomarkers and treatments, but for the design of large scale clinical trials (19).

Hematopoietic stem cells as ASD treatment

Immune dysregulation and dysfunction have been observed in the brain, periphery and gastrointestinal tract in ASD individuals (20). Studies have shown elevated pro-inflammatory cytokines/interkeukins; TNF-α, IL-6, IL-8, GM-CSF, IFN-γ and MCP-1 and a concurrent decrease in anti-inflammatory cytokines; IL-10 and TGF-β in the central nervous system (CNS) of ASD individuals (21) (chapter 6C). Autoantibodies to myelin basic protein, Purkinje cells, neuron-axon filament and glial fibrilary acidic protein found in autistic individuals suggest an autoimmune mechanism (chapter 6A) (22,23). T-cell and B-cell abnormalities leading to decreased leukocyte proliferation and abnormal cytokine production have also been implicated (24).

Cortical minicolumn abnormalities are also noted in individuals with ASD (25). The abnormalities in minicolumn structure have been shown to be correlated with a disruption in reelin formation, a protein that is integral in neuronal migration and brain development (26). Researchers believe that an early immunological insult may disrupt reelin signaling in the CNS rendering the altered brain structure noted in ASD's. These findings have led researchers to propose the administration of hematopoietic stem cells (HSC) in order to repair and replace the damaged neural tissue at molecular, structural and functional levels (27). The HSC have the capability to not only differentiate into any cell type of hematopoietic lineage, but also to secrete transcription factors such as vascular endothelial growth factor (VEGF) and fibroblast growth factor (FGF) that act to repair these sites of inflammation by increasing proliferation, cellular recruitment and maturation of endogenous stem cells. The HSC has a key innate capability of traveling to sites of damaged tissue (28). This function of HSCs allows researchers to use them therapeutically as they will transfer to the affected sites appropriately. Animal and human studies are underway to determine the effectiveness, attainability, safety and suitability for the treatment of ASD with stem cell technologies (36,37,42).

An inflammatory process generated from prenatal maternal infection is a risk factor for ASD (chapter 6C) (20). After the 1964 rubella pandemic, 8-13% of children born to infected mothers were shown to develop ASD characteristics (29). Recently in a study in Denmark from 1980 to 2005, there was a significant association found between autism and maternal viral infection occurring in the first trimester of pregnancy (30). A mouse model was created to mimic this phenomenon where pregnant mice were injected with a synthetic, double stranded RNA, poly (I:C) in order to initiate a pro-inflammatory antiviral response. This maternal immune activation (MIA) model yielded offspring with the core behavioral and neuropathological symptoms of ASD (31).

Recently, by utilizing the MIA model in mice, Hsiao et al. have (32) found that regulatory T-cells in adult offspring of poly (I:C)-injected mothers were decreased when compared to controls. This would leave the prenatally infected mice with a decreased ability to suppress the innate and adaptive immune system. IL-6 and IL-17 in poly(I:C) offspring mice was also found to be increased, yielding a pro-inflammatory T-helper cell phenotype. The poly(I:C) offspring also showed increased production of Gr-1 (+) cells indicating that HSC's are being induced to become differentiated into granulocyte precursors and, thereby, driving inflammation via production of immune cells.

This group further investigated the utilization of bone marrow transplant in MIA offspring in ameliorating ASD behavior-like symptoms. Prepulse inhibition (PPI) was used to measure startle reflex, marble burying was used to assess increased repetitive behavior and duration spent, and entries into chamber housing a novel mouse versus a familiar mouse was used to assess decreased social interaction (32). The poly(I:C) offspring displayed abnormalities in all of the above characteristics which parallel ASD symptoms. The mice were then irradiated (to destroy the maleficent domestic blood cells) and transplanted with donor bone marrow (BM) harvested from unmutated adult mice. Following BM transplant, the MIA offspring no longer exhibited behavioral abnormalities in several of the tests described above. These findings suggest that correcting immune function may correct some autism-related behavioral abnormalities.

A preclinical study utilizing cord blood mononuclear cells (CBMC) transplant in brain ischemic animal models showed recovery (from hypoxic injury) by improving blood perfusion through increasing angiogenesis (33). Other data revealed that mesenchymal stem cells were shown to suppress T-cells, B-cells and Natural Killer cells while inducing regulatory T cells (34,35). With the insight from these experiments, Yong-Tao conducted a non-randomized, open-labeled, controlled, single center Phase I/II trial to examine the safety and efficacy of transplantation of a combination therapy which included CBMC's, umbilical cord mesenchymal stem cells (UCMSCs), and professional sensory integration and behavioral rehabilitation therapy (rehab) in 37 individuals with ASD (36). The childhood Autism Rating Scale (CARS), Clinical Global Impression (CGI) scale and Aberrant Behavior Checklist (ABC) were used to assess the therapeutic effect at baseline and following treatment (chapter 1D). The individuals with ASD who were treated with the combination therapy showed a greater statistically significant improvement in the tests 24 weeks after therapy, when compared to CBMC therapy with rehab and solely with rehab. The relief in autistic symptoms is hypothesized to stem from the combined ability of UCMSC's to decrease immunological inflammation and CD34+ cell population enriched in CBMC's to trigger angiogenesis in ischemic tissues through the release of VEGF, HGF and insulin-like growth factor-1 (IGF-1) (chapter 6D). This study, while imperfect in nature, gives hope to the use of stem cells in treating ASD in the future.

Another clinical study conducted by Sharma et al. aimed to improve perfusion through promoting angiogenesis and balance inflammation by immune regulation with the administration of autologous bone marrow mononuclear cell (BMMNC) transplant combined with occupational therapy regimes (37). Hypoperfusion results in hypoxia and an associated increase in toxic metabolites leading to neuronal damage. The magnitude of hypoxia has been shown to be inversely related to IQ (38). Thirty-two patients with autism were subjected to intrathecal injection of BMMNCs after procurement and isolation of these cells from the patients' anterior superior iliac spine. The patients were followed for 26 months, then assessed with standard behavioral scales, and compared to baseline performance before the treatment. Statistically significant improvements were noted in all aspects of ASD, including improvements in communication and social interaction and a decrease in repetitive behaviors. Very few side effects were also noted throughout the study. BMMNC transplant may not be a cure for autism but could offer a potential therapy to manage disease severity and improve overall quality of life.

These promising results represent another step forward for the application of stem cell therapy in autism.

In summary, HSC's have many characteristics that can prove beneficial in treating ASD. HSC's show self-renewal, mobilization, and multipotent differentiation capacity as they can become any myeloid or lymphoid cell type. HSC's are quantitatively low in peripheral blood under normal conditions, but are strongly mobilized by inflammation (39). They are able to molecularly traffic to sites of inflammation and can target pro-inflammatory molecules released in a specific location in the ASD's central nervous system. Once the HSC's are present at the site of inflammation, they mitigate the inflammatory response by down-regulating pro-inflammatory TNF-alpha, IFN-gamma and IL-1 and up-regulating anti-inflammatory cytokine IL-10 (38). In conclusion, transplanted HSCs have the potential to replace malfunctioning immune cells in the CNS, while also recruiting tissue-residing stem cells so that they can both decrease inflammation and promote CNS immunological homeostasis.

Non-hematopoietic stem cells as ASD treatment

Human stem cells have many unique features that bring forth potential therapeutic and diagnostic possibilities. Their ability of self renewal and differentiation potential provides researchers with the unique ability to attempt to "restart"or "replenish" deficiencies in a diseased state. Aside from the dysregulation and dysfunction of the immune system, which yield HSCs as good candidates for ASD treatment, there are also indications for non-hematopoietic stem cells as a therapy for ASD. iPSCs developed from human cortical interneurons are prospects for treatment of neurological and psychiatric disease as well as mesenchymal stem cell transplantation and iPSCs that have been converted to Oligodendrocytes and/or IGF-1 producing cells.

Cortical interneurons represent a minority of the neuronal cell type in the CNS. They are GABAergic and thus provide inhibitory inputs to help determine excitation responses of pyramidal cells. Decreased tonic inhibition has been implicated in psychiatric illness including ASD due to interneuron hypoplasia (40). Conceptually, iPSCs that can be differentiated into cortical interneurons can offer an unlimited supply of therapeutic transplant cells. However, little is known on how to differentiate iPSCs into distinct cortical interneuron subtypes. More research is needed in order for this therapeutic option to become a reality.

Mesenchymal stem cells (MSCs), as stated previously, have a particularly interesting potential in the treatment of ASD due to their ability to address the immune and neural dysregulation associated with this disease. MSCs have a mutilineage potential and are progenitor cells of mesodermal origin found mostly in the bone marrow of adults. Conceptually, MSCs may act through paracrine activity whereby these cells are able to secrete factors that activate endogenous restorative mechanisms within injured tissues, secrete survival promoting growth factors, and restore synaptic connections (41). MSCs are also noted to inhibit the immune system, more specifically, inhibit proliferation of CD4+, CD8+ and NK cells and inhibit the maturation of dendritic cells. Autism has been associated with dysregulation in the maturation and plasticity of dendritic spine morphology. The restoration of injured brain functioning might be established by stem cell based replacement.

Another possible mechanism of ASD therapy via iPSC technology is through the effects of IGF-1. This growth factor is secreted mainly by the liver and is the mediator of anabolic and mitogenic activity of the pituitary-released growth hormone (chapter 6D). However, it is also produced in many other tissues including brain microvascular endothelial cells (BMECs). IGF-1 has a profound influence on intrauterine growth, as demonstrated by a study measuring growth in mice with an IGF-1 knockout mutation. These mice, who were ultimately unable to produce the IGF-1 protein, were 30% smaller than matched controls (43). IGF-1 that is secreted by BMECs has also been shown in mouse models to attenuate injury caused by ischemia (middle cerebral artery occlusion) (44). A well regulated expression of IGF-1 secretion is necessary for proper function, overexpression can result in brain overgrowth while underexpression can cause brain growth retardation (45). As an embryo, IGF-1 stimulates neuronal progenitor proliferation and later is involved in neuron maintenance, outgrowth, and synaptogenesis. IGF-1 has also been shown to stimulate oligodendrocyte progenitor proliferation and stimulating myelin production.

IGF-1 production is believed to be abnormal in autistic individuals, which may hinder proper neurogenesis and myelination (46). Therefore, a therapeutic mechanism that may relieve or prevent the pathologic processes of ASD would be the preservation or administration of proper levels of IGF-1 in the fetal and infant body. One possibility of achieving this goal would be to create iPSCs from autistic patients and transform them into oligodendrocytes, replacing myelin that has been damaged and brain microvascular endothelial cells that secrete IGF-1 (47). Administration of stem cells could prove superior to synthetic IGF-1 administration because it would decrease the need for regular injections of the hormone and resulting compliance issues, and would allow for the patient's own reprogrammed cells to generate the lack of hormone.

Cellular therapy represents a new frontier in treatment of human disease. Clinical trials have already begun implementing stem cell technology into treatment regimes of all types of human illness. The world's first application of iPSCs for regenerative medicine in humans is set to take place this year. A group led by Takahashi in Japan will be surgically transplanting iPSCs that have been differentiated into retinal epithelial cells into patients with wet age-related macular degeneration. As more research is undertaken and clinical trials are set in motion we will be able to understand more about the efficacy and safety of using non-hematopoietic stem cells as a form of regenerative medicine.

Conclusions

The exact etiology of autism remains a mystery. Through this book we have examined many hypotheses related to its disease mechanism. The triggering pathophysiology and subsequent mechanisms being unclear creates a particularly difficult task of coming up with a curative solution. Presently, therapy for ASD is targeted primarily to control behavioral symptomatology without addressing the underlying disease and is palliative in nature. Through the use of iPSC technology, stem cells may be used to emulate the pathophysiology and further our understanding of autism. With further elucidation of ASD using iPSC models, a better classification of this disease will translate into improved diagnostic criteria and patient-specific care for each individual that correlates with his/her particular pathophysiology and respective location on the autism spectrum. As the models become a reality, researchers will be able to conduct *in vitro* pharmacological clinical trials with iPSCs created directly from a patient population yielding key information on efficacy, potential side effects, and overall safety of a specific treatment regime.

Stem cell therapy also reveals a promising approach in curing currently untreatable human diseases. Their ability to self-renew, give rise to terminally differentiated cells, and bring about intrinsic regulatory function allows stem cells to be considered as a possible therapeutic option for ASD. The beneficial effects of stem cells are not restricted to cellular regenerative medicine, but intriguingly seem to exert an immunomodulatory effect in the CNS of autistic individuals.

Despite the many recent advances in stem cell technology and neurobiology, more detailed investigations are needed before it can become a reality in treating ASD. Focus should not be lost on understanding the pathophysiology of the disease before clinical use of stem cell therapy becomes routine. Questions of the financial burden on research and development on patient-specific therapy, ethical issues and qualifying criteria for this treatment option may surface in the future. Further research investigation on proper stem cell dosing, site of administration, and proper therapy application must be addressed. Continued monitoring of side effects and long term safety will need to be documented. As research continues in this field and as the exciting and mysterious nature of stem cell therapy becomes revealed, the potential for a revolutionary shift in medicine remains lingering among our grasps.

CONCLUSIONS AND PROSPECTUS

Correlation versus *Causation*

As noted in the Prologue of this book, autism has recently become a central issue of concern in medical research. In part, this is the result of a reported increase in the frequency (or diagnosis) of this neuropathologic disorder (chapter 1C). Currently adjusted criteria defining this malady may account, in part, for the apparent contemporary growth in cases (chapter 1D). Increasing public awareness, especially through the media (chapter 2B), may have sensitized parents to have young children with seemingly inappropriate behavioral patterns analyzed earlier and more often than had been the case previously (chapter 1B).

Autism is clearly a condition which impinges broadly on the quality of life not only of the patient him/herself, but also of the family and educators of that child as well (chapters 2A-2C). Extensive research over many years has uncovered some hints of what may be the cause of autism. However, unless a "eureka moment" occurs in a laboratory somewhere or a serendipitous discovery is made, we seem to be years away from a convincing explanation of the etiology of this syndrome. As a consequence, preventive therapy remains a later objective.

With these prior research efforts, especially in the examination of pathologic changes in the brains of affected individuals (chapters 3B-3F), much has been learned about the central nervous system. Impairments remain difficult to remedy. However, the rapidly progressing field of stem cell investigation may hold out some hope. Early discoveries have demonstrated the ability of stem cells and stimulated oligodendrocytes to replace or repair myelin sheathing, possibly improving nerve performance in affected patients (chapters 6A,6D,9B).

Recent changes and updates in the Diagnostic and Statistical Manual of Mental Disorders (DSM) have sought, among other things, to refine the diagnosis and definition of autism (chapter 1D), althoughit is currently under review (and probable revision). A summary of the symptom domains defined by the two most recent editions would be:

DSM-IV	DSM-5
1) Social deficits	1) Social communication/interaction difficulties
2) Communication impairments	2) Fixated interests; repetitive behaviors
3) Repetitive behaviors	

Many researchers believe that the etiology of autism is linked to one or more gross mutations of genes or changes in their transcription/translation in affected patients. However, these defects are usually found in only a small percentage of such cases, leaving this enigma to be clarified in otherwise genetically normal autistic children (chapter 8A). By themselves, certain single-gene disorders such as tuberous sclerosis, neurofibromatosis type I, Fragile X syndrome, and phenylketonuria are manifested in part by autistic-like behavior (3). However, only a subset of such disorders is characterized by this abnormal behavioral quality. A direct, uniform correlation is not evident 100% of the time between such genetic abnormalities and autism, thereby putting into question the connection between these disorders. For example, as noted in chapters 1D,8A, Rett syndrome does not meet the classical definition of autism, although it has some characteristics in common with it. Similarly, 10% of Down's syndrome children are classified as "autistic", while not being the case for the other 90%.

Confounding the difficulty in studying the genetics of autism and its possible role in trait inheritance is that most autistic patients do not engage in reproductive activities. Similarly, the parents of affected children are not ovetly autistic themselves.

Profound progress made in scientific technology recently has made possible the sequencing of whole genomes expeditiously. As a result, numerous mutations have been identified in autistic patients that might not otherwise have been sought or observed. Whether these uncommon mutations, found in only a few percent of such cases, are relevant to the primary etiologic process of autism is uncertain and remains to be determined. An example of this is the PTEN (phosphatase/tensin homolog) gene, which is found together with various cancers. A total of 10 % of children with this mutation also are diagnosed as being autistic (4). What has yet to be determined is the relevance of this finding to the other 90%.

Whole-genome scans have identified recurrent abnormal sequences in a subset of autistic patients, but results so far are inconclusive and not all-encompassing (5). This has been blamed on a previously unrealized increase in perceived complexity of the disorder. Linkage scans have failed to identify genomic regions that are consistently replicated. Conclusive relationship and association results are lacking. The rationalization expressed is that previous speculations on the number of genes involved in the etiology of autism were underestimates (chapter 8A).

Based on these various hypotheses proposed to explain the etiology of autism, especially from twin studies, there is currently believed to be a need for both a ***genetic predisposition(s)*** and a corresponding ***environmental trigger(s)*** in order to generate this disease. At least four possible scenarios can be proposed to explain the relationship of this to the etiology of autism:

1) Autistic patients sometimes appear to demonstrate marked genetic changes, especially in severe cases (chapter 8A). It is possible that such individuals have a greater tendency to bear genetic aberrations than unaffected or less affected ones. ASD may be a single disease in all ailing patients, where the spectrum is characterized by a range of increasing severity. This would suggest that ASD is an ascending array of a single, all-encompassing behavioral disorder, where significant genetic anomalies appear in only the most complex;

2) ASD may be a spectrum of several neurological disorders, some of which possess identifiable genetic anomalies, but all of which display conventional "autistic" behavioral and social dysfunction in some form. The array may consist of more than one disorder generally comparable to the group overall, where each is promoted by a different genetic or environmental factor;

3) This disease may be an autosomal recessive trait. This could explain why mothers and fathers of affected children typically have no autistic behavioral characteristics

themselves (i.e., are carriers) and may yet conceive two or more impaired offspring (in addition to unaffected ones) (chapter 1C). In such circumstances, the occurrence of affected siblings in a family is 10-20 times more frequent than in a random population;

4) As noted in chapter 6D, gravidas carrying genetically female fetuses may exhibit higher levels of fetal growth hormone in their own sera, the effector of insulin-like growth factor (IGF), than those bearing males. If IGF deficiency in the fetus and/or neonate retards neural myelination, this could correlate with and follow from the gender differences noted.

Dating back to the original observations of Leo Kanner in the 1940s, an uncertainty has persisted whether or not reduced IQ is a hallmark of autism (6). A seemingly low intelligence in autistic children may, in fact, be related to an inability of professional testers to communicate effectively with such individuals, making a realistic determination of mental capacity difficult to ascertain. Modern devices, such as word processors and hearing aids, have enhanced the inherent capability of such patients to express themselves and demonstrate their true mental aptitudes in a constructive fashion.

Rather than being the primary causative agents inducing autism, many of the various associated, coexistent features discussed in this book may be co-morbidities ("PARALLEL CO-MOBIDITY") that appear in parallel in the same autistic individual ("AUTISM"), possibly resulting from the same, yet-to-be-determined, etiology ("SINGLE ETIOLOGY"). Co-morbidities may be psychological/ psychiatric (e.g., depression, obsessive-compulsive behaviors, intellectual disability, or attention deficits) or medical/genetic (e.g., Down's syndrome, mitochondrial disease, or tuberous sclerosis) disorders. As noted in chapter 5B, maladies such as GI lymphoid nodular hyperplasia may be co-morbid with autism or may be free of it. This might represent a single etiology which evokes one or both disorders independently but concurrently.

SINGLE ETIOLOGY $\nearrow$ PARALLEL CO-MORBIDITY

$\searrow$ *AUTISM*

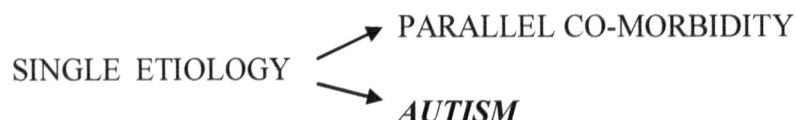

On the other hand, these associated phenomena ("CO-MORBIDITY") may be the consequence of environmental triggers ("ENVIRONMENTAL TRIGGER"), such as pollutants, hypoxia, or heavy metals, which effect the expression of promoter genes ("GENE") by epigenetic activation. In the latter case, a modified (e.g., polymorphic) gene may be more sensitive to the trigger than a normal gene.

ENVIRONMENTAL TRIGGER $\rightarrow$ CO-MORBIDITY

CO-MORBIDITY + GENE $\rightarrow$ *AUTISM*

Corrales and Herbert view the roles of genetic-environmental factors as interactions by at least four possible mechanisms to result in the appearance of autism (7):

1) Environmental factors induce neurologically relevant genetic damage;
2) Environmental factors promote epigenetic modifications of gene expression;
3) Mutant genes enhance the effects of environmental factors, which then promote genesis of autistic behavior; and
4) Genes interact in concert with environmental factors (e.g., pollutants, oxidative stress) to increase susceptibility to the latter.

Research into the cause of autism has both utilized and promoted pioneering advances in brain physiology and pathology (chapters 3A-3F). New findings in biochemical and molecular biology have laid the foundation for a broad, fresh approach to elucidate the underlying mechanism of autism. However, none has been successful so far in identifying the key, fundamental defect which is at the core of the process bringing about the aberrant behavioral patterns characteristic of this disease.

Proposal #3 above is much like the rationalization of why there are polymorphisms and mutations which each appear to increase the probability that a particular environmental factor (e.g., cigarette smoke) will promote distinct malignancies (e.g., lung cancer). Dissimilar mutations on different chromosomes may induce the same cancer (e.g., BRCA1 on #17 and BRCA2 on #13 for familial breast malignancies). In addition, not everyone with a particular cancer-promoting gene will develop the disease, possibly related to variable DNA repair mechanisms or socioeconomic conditions (7).

Conditions such as phenylketonuria (PKU) which are often (but not always) found as co-morbid with autism are frequently related to specific genetic defects. In untreated PKU patients, dysmyelination is commonly seen (8), as it is with IGF deficiency (chapter 6E). If PKU is left untreated, its coexistence with autism may be related to hyperphenylalanemia causing damage to and reduction of early myelin production. This induces a deteriorating course, resulting in irreversible autistic behavior (9). Even more inclusive is the realization that currently no diet modification, chemical/pharmaceutical therapy, or manipulative process promotes any lasting improvement in affected individuals in general (10). Until the fundamental cause and progression of autism are elucidated, no functional repair of damaged neurons can be expected. The main hope today for restitution of some "conventional" human behavior is guided educational therapy (chapter 2C). Claims of isolated cures of autism appear from time to time. In the absence of a clearcut elucidations of the mechanism of cause, effective treatment to achieve cure is ephemeral at best at the present state of knowledge.

The information presented in this book is intended to provide the reader with information based on scientific research and well-founded reasoning which give clues to the basic neuropathologic mechanism causing autism. Some of the chapters have reviewed proposals which have turned out to be baseless. They should be eliminated from consideration; however, large segments of the public continue to view them (e.g., childhood vaccinations) as credible. After numerous detailed reports to the contrary (chapters 7A-7C), it is disturbing that children are still being deprived of the protections offered by MMR. A recent rise in the number of measles cases attests to this consequential danger. Similarly, the reported correlation of first trimester maternal influenza and an increased incidence of autism in the neonates (chapter 6C) has not succeeded in promoting significantly more preconception vaccination against this virus in particular.

In the interest of possibly *reducing* the risk of autism, one of the most important conclusions presented in this book includes the need to advise pregnant or potentially pregnant women to decrease their exposure to teratogens such as alcohol, viral infections, air pollution, and smoking, especially in the early months of gestation. Also, breast-feeding following delivery for at least one year should be encouraged.

It is the hope of the authors and editors of this volume that the astute reader will evaluate each hypothesis that comes along in the future, especially in the popular press, and act according to sound, scientifically based conclusions instead of emotional misunderstanding. Disorders affecting children are especially prone to subjective misdirection when an urgency for cure is sensed. A rush to employ the latest "breakthrough" in purportedly curative therapy may lead to devastating disappointment in the end.

In short, large sums have been invested in research investigations to determine the cause of autism, with minimal tangible results realized thus far to be germane to effective therapy and prevention. For example, the employment of high tech procedures or new epigenetic, proteomic, and imprinting principles has not brought us significantly closer to a final, conclusive solution of the autism enigma (3). Frustration and the lack of meaningful discovery in these studies seem to have made the latest hypotheses more convoluted and less comprehensible.

As Albert Einstein said,

"Any intelligent fool can make things bigger and more complex; It takes a touch of genius – and a lot of courage – to move in the opposite direction."

REFERENCES

PROLOGUE

1) Brimberg, L, Sadiq, A, Gregersen, PK, Diamond, B. Brain-reactive IgG correlates with autoimmunity in mothers of a child with autism spectrum disorder. Mol Psychiatry 2013;18(11):1171-7.

2) Steinman, G. Mechanisms of Twinning: I. Effect of environmental diversity on genetic expression in monozygotic multifetal pregnancies. J Reprod Med 2001;46(5):467-72.

3) Glinianaia, SV, Rankin, J, Wright, C. Congenital anomalies in twins: a register-based study. Hum Reprod 2008;23(6):1306-11.

4) Rosenberg, RE, Law, JK, Yenokyan, G, er al. Characteristics and concordance of autism spectrum disorders among 277 twin pairs. Arch Pediatr med. 2009;163(10):907-14.

5) Muhle, R, Trentacoste, SV, Rapin, I. The genetics of autism. Pediatrics 2004;113(5): e472-86.

6) Gupta, AR, State, MW. Recent advances in the genetics of autism. Biol Psychiatry 2007;61:429-37.

7) Autism Genome Project Consortium. Mapping autism risk loci using genetic linkage and chromosomal rearrangements. Nature Genetics 2007;39:329-28.

8) Steinman, G, Mankuta, D. Insulin-like growth factor and the etiology of autism. Med Hypoth 2013;80(4):475-80.

Chapter 1A – Scientific approach

1) NYTimes, "Measles cases in US reach a 20 year high," p.A21, 5/23/14.

2) "Plagarism in scientific publishing," Acta Inform Med 2012, 20(4):208-13.

3) Shewan, LG, Coats, AJS, Ethics in the authorship and publishing of scientific articles. 2010;144(4):p.1-2.

4) NIH Funding Report, 1/14/14.

5) Brawley, OW. The study of untreated syphilis in the negro male, Int J Radiat Oncol Biol Phys 1998;40(1):5-8.

6) Berger, RL, Nazi Science – the Dachau hypothermia experiments. NEJM 1990;322(20):1435-40.

7) LATimes, "Scientist accused of manipulating data in STAP stem cell therapy. 4/1/14.

8) Fleecks, BM. Esearcher admits to HIV vaccine fraud, Liberty Voice, 6/25/14.

9) Marshall, BJ. "The pathogenesis of non-ulcer dyspepsia". Med. J. Aust. 1985;143(7): 319.

Chapter 1B – Geographic trends

1) Data Accountability Center (2012, November 5). CSV Data Part B Child Count 2010. Individuals with Disabilities Education Act (IDEA) Data, US Department of Education. Available: https://www.ideadata.org/PartBChildCount.asp

2) Howden, LM., Meyer, JA (2011, May). Age and Sex Composition: 2010. US Census Bureau, 2010 Census Briefs. http://www.census.gov/prod/cen2010/briefs/c2010br-03.pdf

3) US Census Bureau. Resident Population Data (text Version). Available: http://www.census.gov/2010census/data/apportionment-dens-text.php

4) US Census Bureau (2012). Table 233 Educational Attainment by State: 1990-2009. Available: http://www.census.gov/compendia/statab/2012/tables/12s0233.pdf

5) US Census Bureau (2012, March). Table H-8 Median Household Income by State: 1984-2011. Available:http://www.census.gov/hhes/www/income/data/historical/household/2011/H08_201 1.xls

Chapter 1C – Occurrence rate

1) Centers for Disease Control and Prevention. Prevalence of autism spectrum disorders—Autism and Developmental Disabilities Monitoring Network, 14 sites, United States, 2008. MMWR 2012;61(3):1-18

2) Fombonne, E., Epidemiology of pervasive developmental disorders. Pediatr Res. 2009;65(6):591-8.

3) Centers for Disease Control and Prevention. Prevalence of Autism Spectrum Disorder Among Children Aged 8 Years — Autism and Developmental Disabilities Monitoring Network, 11 Sites, United States, 2010. MMWR 2014;63(2): 1-21

4) Manning-Courtney, P, Murray, D, Currans, K, et al. Autism spectrum disorders. Curr Probl Pediatr Adolesc Health Care 2013;43(1):2-11.

5) Young, SK, Bennett, LL, Yun-Joo, K, et al. Prevalence of Autism Spectrum Disorders in a Total Population Sample. Am J Psychiatry 2011;168:904-912.

6) Shattuck, PT. The contribution of diagnostic substitution to the growing administrative prevalence of autism in US special education. Pediatrics 2006;117(4):1028-37.

7) Ozonoff, S, Young, GS, Carter, A, et al. Recurrence risk for autism spectrum disorders: a baby siblings research consortium study. Peds 2011;128:e488-95.

8) Rosenberg, RE, Law, JK, Yenokyan, G, et al. Characteristics and concordance of autism spectrum disorders among 277 twin pairs. Arch Pediatr Adolesc Med 2009;163(10):907-14.

9) Hallmayer, J, Cleveland, S, Torres, A, et al. Genetic Heritability and Shared Environmental Factors Among Twin Pairs With Autism. Arch Gen Psychiatry 2011;68(11):1095-1102.

10) American Psychiatric Association. Diagnostic and statistical manual of mental disorders. 4. Washington, DC: American Psychiatric Association; 2000. (Text revision)

11) Wong, VC, Hui, SL. Epidemiological study of autism spectrum disorder in China. J Child Neurol 2008;23:67–72.

12) Centers for Disease Control and Prevention. Summary of Autism Spectrum Disorder (ASD) Prevalence Studies. http://www.cdc.gov/ncbddd/autism/documents/ autism_prevalencesummarytable_2011.pdf/. 2013.

13) Kočovská, E, Biskupstø, R, Carina Gillberg, I, et al. The rising prevalence of autism: a prospective longitudinal study in the faroe islands. J Autism Dev Disord. 2012;12:1959–66.

14) Al-Farsi, YM, Al-Sharbati, MM, Al-Farsi, OA, et al. Brief report: prevalence of autistic spectrum disorders in the sultanate of Oman. J Autism Dev 2011; 41(6):821-5.

15) Posserud, M, Lundervold, AJ, Lie, SA, et al. The prevalence of autism spectrum disorders: impact of diagnostic instrument and non-response bias. Soc Psychiatr Epidemiol 2010;45:319–327.

16) Zuckerman, KE, Mattox, K, Donelan, K, et al. Disorder Pediatrician Identification of Latino Children at Risk for Autism Spectrum Disorder. Pediatrics 2013;132:445-453.

17) Keen, DV, Reid, FD, Arnone, D. Autism, ethnicity and maternal immigration. Br J Psychiatry 2010. 196: 274–281.

18) Croen, LA, Grether, JK, Hoogstrate, J, et al. The changing prevalence of autism in California. J Autism Dev Disord 2002;32: 207–15.

19) Yeargin-Allsop, A, Rice, C, Karapurkar, T, et al. Prevalence of autism in a US metropolitan area. JAMA 2003; 289: 49–55.

20) Barnevik-Olsson, M, Gillberg, C, Fernell, E. Prevalence of autism in children born to Somali parents living in Sweden: a brief report. Dev Med Child Neurol 2008; 50: 598–601.

21) Kolevzon, A, Gross, R, Reichenberg, A. Prenatal and perinatal risk factors in autism. Arch Pediatr Adolesc Med 2007; 161: 326–33.

Chapter 1D – DSM-5

1)   American Psychiatric Association 2013. Highlights of Changes from DSM-IV TR to DSM -5: 1-2.

2)   American Psychiatric Association, 1994. Desk Reference to the Diagnostic Criteria from DSM-IV: 59, 61-62.

3)   American Psychiatric Publishing, 2013. Diagnostic and Statistical Manual of Mental Disorders Fifth Edition: DSM-5: 50-59: Table-2, 52.

4)   Babsoun, P. (2012, December 3). Changes to Autism Definition Approved for Publication in DSM-V, *The Examiner.*   Retrieved August, 15, 2013, from http://www.examiner.com.

5)   The College of William and Mary (2013). Asperger's, Autism and the New DSM, *William & Mary.* Retrieved August 7, 2013 from http://www.wm.edu.

6)   Autism, Research Institute (2013). DSM-V: What Changes May Mean: Updates to the APA in DSM-V – What do the changes mean to families living with Autism? *Autism.com.* Retrieved August 7, 2013 from http://autism.com.

7)   Duffy FH, Shankardass, A, McAnulty, G.B, Als, H. A Stable Pattern Of EEG Spectral Coherence Distinguishes Children With Autism From Neuro-Typical Controls — A Large Case Control Study. *BMC Medicine.* 2013.

8)   The Economist. (2013, May 18). DSM-5 By the Book: The American Psychiatric Association's latest diagnostic manual remains a flawed attempt to categorize mental illness. *The Economist.* Retrieved June 12, 2013 from http://www.economist.com.

9)   Kaplan, B, Sadock, H, J, Grebb. Synopsis of Psychiatry: Behavioral Sciences Clinical Psychiatry 1994:1060.

10) Mientka, M. (2013, August 5). Asperger's Syndrome and Autism Are Biologically Distinct According To New Brain Study. *Medical daily.com.* Retrieved August 7, 2013 from http://www.medicaldaily.com.

11) Robison, J.E. (2013, August 25). My Life with Asperger's. Autism and Asperger's: Two Separate Conditions, Or Not [Web log post]? *Psychologytoday.com.* Retrieved September 18, 2013 from http://www.psychologytoday.com.

12) Willingham, E. (2012, December 4). Just In: Asperger's Prevalence Predicted to Fall to Zero. *Forbes.* Retrieved August 7, 2013 from http://www.forbes.com.

13) DeChello, P. 2013. The DSM-5, The Next Generation: 5.

Additional Sources

1)   Autism Society, http://www.autism-society.org.

2)   Morrison, J. DSM-IV Made Easy: The Clinician's Guide to Diagnosis. Guilford Press, 1994.

3)   The Johnson Center for Child and Health Development http://www.johnson-center.org

4)   Geshwind, D, Levitt, P (2007). Autism, Spectrum Disorders: Developmental Disconnection Syndromes. *Current Opinion in Neurobiology*, 17:103-111.

Chapter 2A – Family dynamics

1)   Gray, D.E., Coping over time: the parents of children with autism. Journal of Intellectual Disability Research 2006; 50: 970-976.

2)   American Psychiatric Association. Diagnostic and Statistical Manual of Mental Disorders, 5th Edition, 2013.

3)   Jabr,F., Redefining Autism: Will New DSM-5 Criteria for ASD Exclude Some People? ScientificAmerican.com, Jan 30, 2012.

4)   Blumberg, S.J., Bramlett, M.D., Kogan, M.D., et al. Changes in Prevalence of Parent-reported Autism Spectrum Disorder in School-aged U.S. Children: 2007 to 2011–2012. National Health Statistics Report, 65, March 20, 2013.

5) Zahorodny, W., Shenouda, J., Howell, S., et al. Increasing autism prevalence in metropolitan New Jersey. Online:Autism, 2012.

6) Wakefield,AJ, Murch, S, Anthony, A,et al. Ileal-lymphoid-nodular hyperplasia, non-specific colitis, and pervasive developmental disorder in children. Lancet 1998;351:637-41,1998.

7) Taylor, B.,Miller,E.,Farrignton, G.,et al. Autism and measles, mumps, and rubella vaccine: no epidemiological evidence for a causal association. Lancet 1999;353:2026-29.

8) Deer, B., How the case against the MMR vaccine was fixed. British Medical Journal 2011;342:c5347.

9) Deer, B., Revealed: MMR research scandal. The Sunday Times (London). February, 2004.

10) Mckee, M., Controversial MMR and autism study retracted. New Scientist. March 2004.

11) BBC News, MMR doctor to face GMC charges. June 2006.

12) Boseley, S., Andrew Wakefield found 'irresponsible' by GMC over MMR vaccine scare. The Guardian (London). January, 2010.

13) The Editors Of The Lancet . "Retraction – Ileal-lymphoid-nodular hyperplasia, non-specific colitis, and pervasive developmental disorder in children". The Lancet 2010;375 (9713):445.

14) The Editorial Board, Aftermath of an Unfounded Vaccine Scare. The New York Times, May 22, 2013.

15) Kirby, D., Vaccine Court Awards Millions to Two Children with Autism. The Blog, Huffington Post, January, 2013.

16) Callaway, E., Fathers bequeath more mutations as they age. Online: Nature 2010;488:439.

17) Kong, A., Frigge, M.L., Masson, G., Rate of de novo mutations and the importance of father's age to disease risk. Nature 2012;488:471-457.

18) Moisse, K.,StudyConfirms Link between Older Maternal Age and Autism. Scientificamerican.com, Feb 11, 2010.

19) Roberts, A., Lyall, K., Rich-Edwards, J., et al. Association of Maternal Exposure to Childhood Abuse with Elevated Risk for Autism in Offspring. JAMA Psychiatry 2013;70(5):508-515.

20) Dumas, J. E., Wolf, L. C., Fisman, S. N., et al. Parenting stress, child behavior problems, and dysphoria in parents of children with autism, Down syndrome, behavior disorders, and normal development. Exceptionality 1991;2: 97-110.

21) Kennedy Krieger Institute, 80 percent autism-divorce rate debunked in first-of-its kind scientific study. Science Daily, May 19, 2010.

22) Dickler, J. The financial toll of autism. @CNNMoney April 2, 2012.

23) Weiss, T. Autism and the Affordable Care Act. Disabled World. Nov 08, 2013.

24) Bristol, M. M. (1984). Family resources and successful adaptation to autistic children. in
E. Schopler & G. B. Mesibov (Eds), The effects of autism on the family. New York: Plenum Press, 1984, pp. 289-310

25) Hastings, R., Kovshoff, H., Ward, N., et. al. Systems analysis of stress and positive perceptions in mothers and fathers of pre-school children with autism. Journal of Autism and Developmental Disorders, 2005;35(5):635–44.

26) Tuteur, A. Autism and maternal self-blame. www.skepticalob.com. October 28, 2013.

27) Boyd, B. Examining the Relationship Between Stress and Lack of Social Support in Mothers of children with Autism. Focus Autism Other Dev Disablties, 2002; 17: 208.

28) Baker, D., Drapela, L. Mostly the mother: Concentration of adverse employment effects on mothers of children with autism. The Social Science Journal, doi:10.1016/k/spscok/2010/01.013.

29) Sabih, F., Sajid, W. There is Significant Stress among Parents Having Children with Autism. Rawal Medical Journal. 2008; 33(2): 214-216

30) Vogel, D., Wester, S., Heesacker, M., et al. Confirming Gender Stereotypes: A Social Role Perspective. Sex Roles, 2003; 48(11/12):519-27.

31) DeMyer, M. K. Parents and children in autism. Washington, DC: V. H. Winston. 1979.

32) Altiere, M. Family Functioning and Coping Behaviors in Parents of Children with Autism Master's Theses and Doctoral Dissertations. Paper 54. 2006

33) Muhl, K., Eisenbeis, H. Lotton, A. The Four Key Dads You Need to Know Now www.iconoculture.com, August 2013

34) Bågenholm, A., Gillberg, C. Psychosocial effects on siblings of children with autism and mental retardation: a population-based study. Journal of Mental Deficiency Research. 1991;35(4):291-307.

35) Wheeler, M. Siblings perspectives: Some guidelines for parents. Reporter 2006;11(2)13-15.

36) Glicksman, E., Catching autism earlier. American Psychological Association 2012;43(9):56.

37) Office of Special Education, Early Intervention Program for Infants and Toddlers with Disabilities, U.S. Department of Education, 2004

38) Karoly, L., Killburn, M., Cannon, J. Proven Benefits of Early Childhood Interventions. RAND Corporation. Web Only. RB-9145-PNC, 2005

39) Brauser, D., New Practice Guidelines for Autism. Online, Medscape Medical News. January 29, 2014.

Chapter 2B – Societal implications

1) Rhoades, R. A., Scarpa, A., & Salley, B. The importance of physician knowledge of autism spectrum disorder: Results of a parent survey. BMC Pediatric 2007;7(1):37.

2) Harrington, J. W., Patrick, P. A., Edwards, K. S., & Brand, D. A. Parental beliefs about autism implications for the treating physician. Autism, 2006;10(5):452-462.

3) Freedman, B. H., Kalb, L. G., Zablotsky, B., & Stuart, E. A. Relationship status among parents of children with autism spectrum disorders: A population-based study. Journal of Autism and Developmental Disorders, 2012;42(4): 539-548.

4) Hartley, S. L., Barker, E. T., Seltzer, M. M., Floyd, F., Greenberg, J., Orsmond, G., & Bolt, D. (2010). The relative risk and timing of divorce in families of children with an autism spectrum disorder. Journal of Family Psychology, 2010;24(4):449.

5) Krauss, MW, Orsmond, GI, Vestal, C, et al. Families of adolescents and adults with autism: Uncharted territory, International Review of Research in Mental Retardation, 2001;23:267-

6) Kogan, MD., Strickland, BB, Blumberg, SJ, et al. A national profile of the health care experiences and family impact of autism spectrum disorder among children in the united states, 2005–2006. Pediatrics, 2008;122(6): e1149-e1158. doi:10.1542/peds.2008-1057

7) Smith, L. E., Hong, J., Seltzer, M. M.,et al. Daily experiences among mothers of adolescents and adults with autism spectrum disorder. Journal of Autism and Developmental Disorders,2010: 40(2):167-178.

8) American psychiatric association: DSM-5 development. (2012). Retrieved September 5, 2013 from http://www.dsm5.org/Documents/changes from dsm-iv-tr to dsm-5.pdf

9) American psychiatric association: DSM. (2013). Retrieved September 5, 2013 from http://www.psychiatry.org/practice/dsm.

10) Mandell, D. S., Ittenbach, R. F., Levy, S. E., & Pinto-Martin, J. Disparities in diagnoses received prior to a diagnosis of autism spectrum disorder. Journal of Autism & Developmental Disorders,2007; 37(9): 1795-1802.

11) U.S. Department of Health and Human Services. Patient centered medical home resource center. Retrieved September 5, 2013 from http://www.pcmh.ahrq.gov/portal/server.pt/community/pcmh__home/1483/pcmh_home_v2

12) Thomas, K. C., Ellis, A. R., McLaurin, C., et al. Access to care for autism-related services. Journal of Autism & Developmental Disorders, 2007;37(10): 1902-12.

Chapter 2C – Therapy difficulties

1) http://www.asha.org/div40/definitions.htm. Accessed 3/12/14.
2) http://www.asha.org/public/speech/disorders/Autism.htm. Accessed 3/12/14.
3) http://www.asha.org/uploadedFiles/public/TESAutisticSpectrum.pdf. Accessed 3/12/14.
4) http://nichcy.org/schoolage/accommodations. Accessed 3/12/14.
5) Bzech, K, League, R. Receptive-Expressive Emergent Language Scale (REEL Scale). The Tree of Life Press, First addition, 1971.
6) http://www.asha.org/public/speech/disorders/AAC/ . Accessed 3/12/14.

Chapter 2D – Refrigerator mom

1) Refrigerator Mothers. Dir. David Simpson. Kartemquin Films, 2003. DVD.
2) Rodriguez, A. Autism and Asperger Syndrome. Minneapolis: Lerner Publishing Group, Inc., 2009: 59.
3) Silverman, C. Understanding Autism: Parents, Doctors, and the History of a Disorder. Princeton: Princeton University Press, 2012: 32.
4) Vicedo, M. The Social Nature of the Mother's Tie to Her Child: John Bowlby's Theory of Attachment in Post-War America. British Journal for the History of Science 2011; 44 (3): 404
5) Bernier, R, Gerdts, J. Autism Spectrum Disorders: A Reference Handbook. Santa Barbara: ABC CLIO, 2010: 47-148.
6) Severson, K, Aune, J, Jodlowski, D. Bruno Bettelheim, Autism, and the Rhetoric of Scientific
7) Authority. Autism and Representation. Ed. Mark Osteen. New York: Routledge, 2007: 65.
8) Feinstein, A. A History of Autism: Conversations with the Pioneers. West Sussex, UK: John Wiley Sons, 2011: 5-6, 48-75.
9) Kanner, L. Autistic Disturbances of Affective Contact. Nervous Child 1943; 2: 248-250.
10) Kanner, L. Problems of Nosology and Psychodynamics of Early Infantile Autism. The American Journal of Orthopsychiatry 1949; 19(3): 425.
9) Nadesan, MH. Constructing Autism: Unravelling the 'Truth' and Understanding the Social. New York: Routledge, 2005: 82-97.
11) Bowlby, J. Maternal Care and Infant Health. World Health Organization, 1952: 11-55.
12) Bowlby, J. The Nature of the Child's Tie to His Mother. International Journal of Psycho-Analysis 1958; 39: 350.
14) Bretherton, I. The Origins of Attachment Theory: John Bowlby and Mary Ainsworth. Developmental Psychology 1992; 28: 764-765.
15) Medicine: The Child Is Father. Time 1960; 76(4)
http://www.time.com/time/magazine/0,9263,7601600725,00.html
16) Bettelheim, B. The Empty Fortress: Infantile Autism and the Birth of the Self. New York: The Free Press, 1967: 7-392.
17) Holder, A. Anna Freud, Melanie Klein, and the Psychoanalysis of Children and Adolescents. London: H. Karnac Ltd, 2005: 39.
18) Berzoff, J, Flanagan, L, Hertz, P. Inside Out and Outside In: Psychodynamic Clinical Theory and
19) Psychopathology in Contemporary Multicultural Contexts. Plymouth, UK: Rowman & Littlefield Publishers, 2011: 118.
20) Rimland, B. Infantile Autism: The Syndrome and Its Implications for a Neural Theory of Behavior. Englewood Cliffs, NJ: Prentice-Hall, Inc, 1964.
21) Venables, S. Bernard Rimland: Psychologist researcher into autism who overturned the theory that it was a reaction to bad parenting. The Independent. 28 Nov 2006. http://www.independent.co.uk/news/obituaries/bernard-rimland-426132.html

20)   Davis, A, ed. Psychopathology of Childhood and Adolescence, a Neuropsychological Approach. New York: Springer Publishing Company, LLC, 2013: 52-53.

21)   Carey, B."Bernard Rimland, 78, Scientist Who Revised View of Autism, Dies. The New York Times. 28 Nov. 2006. http://www.nytimes.com/2006/11/28/obituaries/28rimland.html

22)   Bird, D. Dr. Leo Kanner, 86, Child Psychologist. The New York Times. 7 Apr. 1981. http://www.nytimes.com/1981/04/07/obituaries/dr-leo-kanner-86-child-psychologist.html

23)   Kanner, L. In Defense of Mothers: How to Bring Up Children in Spite of More Zealous Pyschologists. Dodd, Mead & Company, 1949.

24)   Eyal, Gil, Hart, B. Onculer, E, Oren, N, et al. The Autism Matrix. Malden, MA: Polity Press, 2010: 144-145.

25)   Park, C. The Siege: A Family's Journey into the World of an Autistic Child. Little, Brown and Company, 1982.

26)   Hevesi, D. Clara Claiborne Park, 86, Dies; Wrote about Autistic Child. The New York Times. 13 July 2010. <http://www.nytimes.com/2010/07/13/health/13park.html>

27)   Folstein, S, Rutter, M. Infantile Autism: A Genetic Study of 21 Twin Pairs. Journal of Child Psychology and Psychiatry 1977; 18(4): 297-321.

28)   National Vaccine Information Center. Autism & Vaccines: A New Look At An Old Story. <http://www.nvic.org/nvic-archives/newsletter/autismandvaccines.aspx>.

29)   DeMyer, M, Barton, S, DeMyer, W et al. Prognosis in Autism: A Follow-Up Study. Journal of Autism and Childhood Schizophrenia 1973; 3(3): 199-246.

30)   Autism Spectrum Disorder: Data and Statistics. Centers for Disease Control and Prevention. March 2014. <http://www.cdc.gov/ncbddd/autism/data.html>

31)   Kwang Hwang, S, Charnley, H. Making the familiar strange and making the strange familiar: Understanding Korean children's experiences of living with an autistic sibling. Disability and Society 2010; 25(5): 579-592.

32)   Grinker, R. Unstrange Minds Remapping the World of Autism. Philadelphia: Perseus Books Group, 2007: 91-93.

33)   Field, T, Diego, M, Hernandez-Reif, M et al. Insulin and Insulin-Like Growth Factor 1 (IGF-1) Increased in Preterm Neonates. Journal of Developmental & Behavioral Pediatrics 2008; 29(6): 463-466.

Chapter 3A – Brain imaging

1)   Acosta, MT, Pearl, PL. Imaging data in autism: from structure to malfunction. Semin Pediatr Neuro 2004; 11(3):205-213.

2)   Nordahl, CW, Scholz, R, Yang, X, et al. Increased rate of amygdale growth in children aged 2 to 4 years with autism spectrum disorders: a longitudinal study. Arch Gen Psychiatry 2012;69(1):53-3)Courchesne, E, Karns, CM, Davis, HR, et al. Unusual brain growth patterns in early life in patients with autistic disorder. Neuro 2001; 57(2):245-254.

3)   .

4)

5)   Akshoomoff, N, Lord, C, Lincoln, AJ, et al. Outcome classification of preschool children with autism spectrum disorders using MRI brain measures. J Am Acad Child Adolesc Psych 2004; 43:349–357.

6)   Amaral, DG, Schumann, CM, Nordahl, CW. Neuroanatomy of autism. Trends Neurosci 2008; 31(3):137-45.

7)   Bolton, PF, Roobol, M, Allsopp, L, et al. Association between idiopathic infantile macrocephaly and autism spectrum disorders. Lancet 2001; 358:726–727.

8) Courchesne, E, Pierce, K, Schumann, CM, et al. Mapping early brain development in autism. Neuron 2007; 56(2):399-413.

9) Critchley, HD, Daly, EM, Bullmore, ET, et al. The functional neuroanatomy of social behaviour: changes in cerebral blood flow when people with autistic disorder process facial expressions. Brain 2000; 123:2203– 2212.

10) Cui, R, Cunnington, R, Beisteiner, R, et al. Effects of force-load on cortical activity preceding voluntary finger movement. Neuro Psych Brain Res 2012;18(3):97-104.

11) Dawson, G, Finley, C, Phillips, S, et al. Hemispheric specialization and the language abilities of autistic children. Cild Development. 1986;57:1440-53.

12) Edgar, JC, Keller, J, Heller, W, et al. Psychophysiology in research on Psychopathology. Cambridge Univ. Press, New YHork, 2007.

13) Toal, F, Murphy, DGM, Murphy, KC. Autistic spectrum disorders: lessons from neuroimaging. Brit J Psych 2005;187:395-7.

14) Hamalainen, M, Hari, R. Magnetoencephalography – theory, instrumentation, and applications to noninvasive studies of the working uman brain. Rev Mod Phys 1993;65:413-97.

15) Hadjikhani, N, Joseph, RM, Snyder, J, et al. Activation of the fusiform gyrus when individuals with autism spectrum disorder view faces. Neuroimage 2004;22:1141-50.

16) Hirano, Y, Hirano, S, Maekawa, T, et al. Auditory gating deficit to human voices in schizophrenia: a MEG study. Schizophr Res 2010;117:61-67.

17) Jacobson, GP, Magnetoencephalogaphic studies of auditory system function. J Clin Neurophysiol 1994;11(3):343-64.

18) Kanner, L. Autistic disturbances of affective contact. Nervous Child 1943;2:217-50.

19) Lainhart, JE, Lazar, M, Bigler, ED, et al. The brain during life in autism: Advances in neuroimaging research. Nova Science Press, New YHork, 2005.

20) McAlonan, GM, Cheung, V, Cheung, C, et al. Mapping the brain in autism. A voxel-based MRI study of volumetric differences and intercorrelations in autism. Brain 2005;128:268-76.

21) Nordahl, CW, Simon, TJ, Zierhut, C, et al. Brief report: methods for acquiring structural MRI data in very young children without the use of sedation. J Autism Dev Disord 2008; 38(8): 1581-1590.

22) Oram Cardy, JE, Ferrari ,P, Flagg, EJ, et al. Prominence of M50 auditory evoked response over M100 in childhood and autism. Neuroreport 2004; 15:1867–1870.

23) Pierce K. Early functional brain development in autism and the promise of sleep fMRI. Brain Res. 2011; 1380:162–74.

24) Pierce, K, Haist, F, Sedaghat, F, et al. The brain response to personally familiar faces in autism: findings of fusiform activity and beyond. Brain 2004; 127:2703– 2716.

25) Roberts, TP, Khan, SY, Rey, M, et al. MEG detection of delayed auditory evoked responses in autism spectrum disorders: towards an imaging biomarker for autism. Autism Res. 2010; 3(1):8-18.

26) Scherg, M. Fundamentals of dipole source potential analysis. In: Gandori MHGLR, editor. Auditory evoked magnetic fields and electric potentials. Advances in audiology. 6th ed. S Karger publishing, Switzerland, 1990, 40–69.

27) Sparks, BF, Friedman, SD, Shaw, DW, et al. Brain structural abnormalities in young children with autism spectrum disorder. Neuro 2002; 59(2):184-192.

28) Yamada, T, Nakamura, A, Horibe, K, et al. Asymmetrical enhancement of middle-latency auditory evoked fields with aging. Neurosci Lett. 2003; 337(1): 21-4.

29) Pelphrey, K. A., Morris, J. P., & McCarthy, G. (2005). Neural basis of eye-gaze processing deficits in autism. Brain, 128, 1038-1048.

30) Chandana SR, Behen ME, Juhasz Cet al. (2005). Significance of abnormalities in develop-

mental trajectory and asymmetry of cortical serotonin synthesis in autism. Int J Dev Neurosci 23:171–182.

31) Boddaert, N., Barthelemy, C., Poline, J.-B., et al (2005) Autism: functional brain mapping of exceptional calendar capacity. British Journal of Psychiatry, 187, 83-86.

32) Kliemann, D, Dziobek I, Hatri A, et al (2012). The role of the amygdala in atypical gaze on emotional faces in autism spectrum disorders. J Neuroscience.11;32(28):9469-76

33) Luders, C., Gaser, L., and Schlaug 2004. A voxel-based approach to gray matter asymmetries. Neuroimage. 22(2):656-64

34) Radua, E. Via, M. Catani and D. Mataix-Cols (2011). Voxel-based meta-analysis of regional white-matter volume differences in autism spectrum disorder versus healthy controls. Psychological Medicine, 41, pp 1539-1550.

35) Cauda, E. Geda, K. Sacco, F. D'Agata,(2011). Grey matter abnormality in autism spectrum disorder: an activation likelihood estimation meta-analysis study. Journal of Neurology, Neurosurgery, and Psychiatry, 82 (2011), pp. 1304–1313

36) Abell F, Krams M, Ashburner J, Passingham R, Friston K, Frackowiak R, Happe F, Frith C, Frith U (1999). The neuroanatomy of autism: a voxel-based whole brain analysis of structural scans. Neuroreport 10, 1647-1651.

37) Heilman KM, Scholes R, Watson RT (1975). Auditory affective agnosia. Disturbed comprehension of affective speech. Journal of Neurology, Neurosurgery, and Psychiatry38, 69–72

38) Schmahmann JD, Pandya DN, Wang R, Dai G, D'Arceuil HE, de Crespigny AJ, Wedeen VJ(2007). Association fibre pathways of the brain : parallel observations from diffusion spectrum imaging and autoradiography. Brain 130, 630–653.

39) Damasio AR, Maurer RG (1978). A neurological model for childhood autism. Archives of Neurology 35, 777–786.

Chapter 3B – Brain macropathology

1) American Psychiatric Association (2013). Diagnostic and statistical manual of mental disorders (5th ed.). Arlington, VA: American Psychiatric Publishing.

2) Akshoomoff, N, Lord,C, Lincoln, AJ, et al. Outcome Classification of Preschool Children With Autism Spectrum Disorders Using MRI Brain Measures. Journal of the American Academy of Child & Adolescent Psychiatry 2002;43.3:349-57.

3) Schumann CM, Bloss CS, Barnes CC, et al. Longitudinal magnetic resonance imaging study of cortical development through early childhood in autism. J Neurosci. 2010;30:4419-4427.

4) Courchesne E, Mouton PR, Calhoun ME, et al. Neuron number and size in prefrontal cortex of children with autism. JAMA. 2011; 306:2001-10.

5) Nordahl, CW,Lange,N, Li,DD, et al. Amaral Brain enlargement is associated with regression in preschool-age boys with autism spectrum disorders 2011, doi:10.1073/pnas.1107560108.

6) Hardan, A. Y., Jou, R. J., Keshavan, M. S., et al. Increased frontal cortical folding in autism: A preliminary MRI study. Psychiatry Research, 2004;131:263–68.

7) Wallace, GL,Robustelli,B, Dankner, N, et al. Increased gyrification, but comparable surface area in adolescents with autism spectrum disorders. Brain first published online May 28, 2013 doi:10.1093/brain/awt106

8) Cheung, C, McAlonan, GM, Fung,YY, et al. MRI Study of Minor Physical Anomaly in Childhood Autism Implicates Aberrant Neurodevelopment in Infancy. Plos One 2011;6(4):e18914.

9) Thomas, D,Krissy, AR, Duerden, EG. Effects of Age and Symptomatology on Cortical Thickness in Autism Spectrum Disorders. Research in Autism Spectrum Disorders, 2013;7(1):141-50.

10) Hua, X, Paul, MT, Leow, AD, et al. Brain Growth Rate Abnormalities Visualized in Adolescents with Autism. Human Brain Mapping (2011).

11) Mak-FanMargot, KM, Taylor, M J, Roberts, W,et al. Measures of Cortical Grey Matter Structure and Development in Children with Autism Spectrum Disorder. Journal of Autism and Developmental Disorders. doi:10.1007/s10803-011-1261-6

12) Dickstein,P, Pescosolido,MF, B.A., Reidy,BL. Developmental Meta-Analysis of the Functional Neural Correlates of Autism Spectrum Disorders. Journal of the American Academy of Child & Adolescent Psychiatry 2013;52(3):279-89.

13) Clarke, JM, Zaidel, E. Anatomical–behavioral relationships: corpus callosum morphometry and hemispheric specialization. Behavioral Brain Research 1994; 64,185–202.

14) He, Q., Ye, D., Karsch, K,et al. Detecting Corpus Callosum Abnormalities in Autism Based on Anatomical Landmarks. Psychiatry Research: Neuroimaging 2010;183(2):126-32.

15) Hardan, AY, Muddasani, SR, Vemulapalli, M. An MRI Study of Increased Cortical Thickness in Autism. American Journal of Psychiatry 2006:1290-92..

16) Salmond, CH, Vargha-Khadem, F, Gadian, DG, et al. Heterogeneity in the patterns of neural abnormality in autistic spectrum disorders: evidence from ERP and MRI. Cortex, 2007;43: 686–699.

17) Ashburner, J. Voxel-Based Morphometry—The Methods. NeuroImage 2000;11(6): 805-21.

18) Schumann CM, Hamstra J, Goodlin-Jones BL, et al. The amygdala 48 is enlarged in children but not adolescents with autism; the hippocampus is enlarged at all ages. J Neurosci. 2004;24:6392-6401.

19) Klin A, Jones W. Attributing social and physical meaning to ambiguous visual displays in individuals with higher-functioning 49. autism spectrum disorders. Brain Cogn. 2006;61:40-53.

20) Bookheimer SY, Wang AT, Scott A, et al. Frontal 50 contributions to face processing differences in autism: evidence from fMRI of inverted face processing. J Int Neuropsychol Soc. 2008;14:922-932.

21) Conturo TE, Williams DL, Smith CD,et al. Neuronal fiber pathway abnormalities in autism: an initial MRI diffusion tensor tracking study of hippocampo- fusiform and amygdalo-fusiform pathways. J Int Neuropsychol Soc. 2008;14:933-946.

22) Maltbie E, Bhatt K, Paniagua B, et al. Asymmetric bias in user guided segmentations of brain structures. Neuroimage. 2012;59:1315-23.

23) Minshew NJ, Williams DL. The new neurobiology of autism: cortex, connectivity, and neuronal organization. Arch Neurol. 2007;64:945-50.

24) Via E, Radua J, Cardoner N, et al. Meta-analysis of gray matter abnormalities in autism spectrum disorder: should Asperger disorder be subsumed under a broader umbrella of autistic spectrum disorder? Arch Gen Psychiatry. 2011;68:409-418.

25) Duerdon, EC, Mak-Fam,KM,Taylor,MJ,et al. Regional Differences in Grey and White Matter in Children and Adults with Autism Spectrum Disorders: An Activation Likelihood Estimate (ALE) Meta-analysis. Autism Research, 2012, 5: 49-66

26) Cotugno, A.J. Social competence and social skills training and intervention for children with Autism Spectrum Disorders. Journal of Autism and Developmental Disorders, 2009;39:1268–77.

27) Klein, S.B., Cosmides, L., Gangi, et al. Evolution and episodic memory: an analysis and demonstration of a social function of episodic recollection. Social Cognition,2009; 27, 283–319.

Chapter 3C – Brain pathology and behavior

1) Devinsky O, Morrell MJ, Vogt BA. Contributions of anterior cingulate cortex to behavior. Brain. 1995; 118:279–306.

2) Taylor SF, Stern ER, Gehring WJ. Neural systems for error monitoring: recent findings and theoretical perspectives. Neuroscientist 2007;13:160-72.

3) Kesong Hu, Srikanth Padmala, Luiz Pessoa, Interactions between reward and threat during visual processing, Neuropsychologia,2013; 51(9): 1763-72.

4) Dawson G, Webb SJ, McPartland J. Understanding the nature of face processing impairment in autism: insights from behavioral and electrophysiological studies. Developmental Neuropsychology. 2005; 27: 403-24.

5) Thakkar KN, Polli FE, Joseph RM, et al. Response monitoring, repetitive behaviour and anterior cingulate abnormalities in autism spectrum disorders (ASD). Brain. 2008;131(9):2464-78.

6) Doyle-Thomas KA, Kushki A, Duerden EG, et al. The effect of diagnosis, age, and symptom severity on cortical surface area in the cingulate cortex and insula in autism spectrum disorders. J Child Neurol. 2013;28(6):729-36.

7) Thomas C., Humphreys K., Jung K.-J., et al. The anatomy of the callosal and visual-association pathways in high-functioning autism: A DTI tractography study, Cortex,2011; 47(7): 863-73.

8) T. Nakao, T. Takezawa, M. Miyatani, et al. Medial prefrontal cortex and cognitive regulation. Psychologia, 2009;52:93–109

9) Chevallier, C, Kohls, G, Troiani,V, et al. The social motivation theory of autism, Trends in Cognitive Sciences, 2012;16(4):231-9.

10) Kiernan JA. Barr's The Human Nervous System. Philadelphia, PA: Lippincott, Williams and Wilkins; 2009.

11) J. Morris, C. Frith, D. Perrett, D. et al. A differential neural response in the human amygdala to fearful and happy facial expressions. Nature. 1997;383:812–5.

12) E. Bonda, M. Petrides, D. Ostry, A. Evans. Specific involvement of human parietal systems and the amygdala in the perception of biological motion, Journal of Neuroscience, 1996;15:3737–37.

13) Munson J, Dawson G, Abbott R, et al. Amygdalar volume and behavioral development in autism. Arch Gen Psychiatry 2006; 63: 686–693.

14) Nacewicz BM, Dalton KM, Johnstone T, et al. Amygdala volume and nonverbal social impairment in adolescent and adult males with autism. Arch Gen Psychiatry 2006; 63:1417–1428.

15) Adolphs R, Sears L, Piven J. Abnormal Processing of Social Information from Faces in Autism. Journal Of Cognitive Neuroscience .2001;13(2): 232.

16) Hadjikhani, N., Joseph, R.M., Manoach, D.S., et al. Body expressions of emotion do not trigger fear contagion in autism spectrum disorder, Social Cognitive and Affective Neuroscience, 2009;4(1):70-78.

17) Kleinhans NM, Johnson LC, Richards T, et al. Reduced neural habituation in the amygdala and social impairments in autism spectrum disorders. Am J Psychiatry. 2009;166:467–75.

18) Critchley HD, Daly EM, Bullmore ET, et al. The functional neuroanatomy of social behaviour: changes in cerebral blood flow when people with autistic disorder process facial expressions. Brain 2000; 123:2203–12.

19) Ashwin C, Baron-Cohen S, Wheelwright S, et al. Differential activation of the amygdala and the "social brain" during fearful face-processing in Asperger syndrome. Neuropsychologia 2007; 45:2–14.

20) Baron-Cohen S, Ring HA, Wheelwright S, et al. Social intelligence in the normal and autistic brain: an fMRI study. Eur J Neurosci 1999; 11:1891–98.

21) Dalton KM, Nacewicz BM, Johnstone T, et al. Gaze fixation and the neural circuitry of face processing in autism. Nat Neurosci 2005; 8:519–26.

22) Monk CS, Weng SJ, Wiggins JL, et al. Neural circuitry of emotional face processing in autism spectrum disorders. J Psychiatry Neurosci. 2010 Mar; 35(2): 105-14.

23) Strick PL, Dum RP, Fiez, JA. Cerebellum and nonmotor function. Annu Rev Neurosci. 2009; 32: 413-34.

24) Martin, JH. Neuroanatomy Text and Atlas. New York, NY: McGraw-Hill; 2012.

25) Polsek D, Jagatic T, Cepanec M, et al. Recent developments in neuropathology of autism spectrum disorders. Transl Neurosci. 2011; 2(3): 256-64.

26) Fatemi SH, Aldinger KA, Ashwood P, et al. Consensus paper: pathological role of the cerebellum in autism. Cerebellum. 2012; 11(3): 777-807.

27) Bauman ML, Kemper TL. Neuroanatomic observations of the brain in autism: a review and future directions. Int J Devl Neuroscience. 2005; 23: 183-87.

28) Arin DM, Bauman ML, Kemper TL. The distribution of Purkinje cell loss in the cerebellum in autism [abstract]. Neurology. 1991; 41 (Suppl.): 307.

29) Pickett J, London E. The neuropathology of autism: a review. J Neuropathol Exp Neurol. 2005; 64(11): 925-35.

30) Gowen E, Hamilton A. Motor abilities in autism: a review using a computational context. J of Autism Dev Disord. 2013; 43(2): 323-44.

31) Perez-Pouchoulen M, Miquel M, Saft P, et al. The cerebellum in autism. Neurobiologia. 2012; 3(5): 1-11.

32) Horwitz B. The elusive concept of brain connectivity. NeuroImage. 2003; 19: 466-70.

33) Horwitz B, Braun AR. Brain network interactions in auditory, visual and linguistic processing. Brain and Language. 2004; 89: 377-84.

34) Booth R, Wallace GL, Happe F. Connectivity and the corpus callosum in autism spectrum conditions: Insights from comparison of autism and callosal agenesis. 2011; 189: 303-17.

35) Just MA, Cherkassky VL, Keller TA, et al. Functional and anatomical cortical underconnectivity in autism: Evidence from an fMRI study of an executive function task and corpus callosum morphometry. Cerebral Cortex. 2007; 17: 951-61.

36) Wicker B, Fonlupt P, Hubert B, et al. Abnormal cerebral effective connectivity during explicit emotional processing in adults with autism spectrum disorder. Scan. 2008; 3: 135-43.

37) Poustka L, Jennen-Steinmetz C, Henzie R, et al. Fronto-temporal disconnectivity and symptom severity in children with autism spectrum disorder. World J Biol Psychiat. 2012; 13: 269-80.

38) Bellani M, Calderoni S, Branbilla P. Brain anatomy of autism spectrum disorders I. focus on corpus callosum. Epidemiology and Psychiatric Sciences. 2013; 22: 217-21.
Lau YC, Hinckley LBN, Bukshpun P, et al. Autism traits in individuals with agenesis of the corpus callosum. J Autism Dev Disord. 2013; 43: 1106-111

Chapter 3D – Brain micropathology

1) Wegiel, J, Kuchna, I, Nowicki, K, Imaki, H, et al. The neuropathology of autism: defects of neurogenesis and neuronal migration, and dysplastic changes. Acta Neuropathol 2010;119:755-770.

2) Casanova, MF. The Neuropathology of Autism. Brain Pathology 2007;17:422-433.

3) Rutter, M. Changing concepts and findings on Autism. J Autism Dev Disorder 2012:1-9.

4) Bauman, ML. Microscopic Neuroanatomic abnormalities in Autism. Pediatrics 1991;87(5):791-796.

5) Tang, G, Rios, PG, Kuo, SH, et al. Mitochondrial abnormalities in temporal lobe of autistic brain. Neurobiology of Disease 2013;54:349-361.

6) Palmen, SJMC, Van Engeland, H, Hof, PR, et al. Review article: Neuropathological findings in Autism. Brain 2004;127:2572-83.

7) Tetreault, NA, Hakeem, AY, Jiang, S, et al. Microglia in cerebral cortex in Autism. J Autism Dev Disord 2012;42:2569-84.

8) Suzuki, K, Sugihara, G, Ouchi, Y, et al. Microglial activation in young adults with Autism Spectrum Disorder. JAMA Psychiatry 2013;70(1):49-58.

9) Morgan, JT, Chana, G, Pardo, CA, et al. Microglial activation and increased microglial density observed in the dorsolateral prefrontal cortex in Autism. Biological Psychiatry 2010;68:368-376.

10) Casanova, MF, Buxhoeveden, DP, Switala, AD, et al. Neuronal density and architecture (Gray Level Index) in the brains of Autistic patients. Journal of Child Neurol 2002;17:515-21.

11) Oblak, AL, Rosene, DL, Kemper, TL, et al. Altered posterior cingulate cortical cytoarchitecture, but normal density of neurons and interneurons in the posterior cingulate cortex and fusiform gyrus in autism. Autism Research 2011;4(3):200-11

12) Casanova, M, Trippe, J. Radial cytoarchitecture and patterns of cortical connectivity in Autism. Phil. Trans. R. Soc. B 2009;364:1433-36.

13) Buxhoeveden, DP, Semendeferi, K, Buckwalter, J, et al. Reduced minicolumns in the frontal cortex of patients with autism. Neuropathol and Appl Neurobiol 2006;32:483-91.

14) Casanova, MF, El-Baz, A, Vanbogaert, E, et al. A topographic study of minicolumnar core width by lamina comparison between Autistic subject and controls: possible minicolumnar disruption due to an anatomical element in-common to multiple laminae. Brain Pathology 2010;20: 451-58.

15) Pearson, BL, Corley, MJ, Vasconcellos, A, et al. Heparan sulfate deficiency in Autistic postmortem brain tissue from the subventricular zone of the lateral ventricles. Behav Brain Res 2013;243:138-45.

16) Simms, ML, Kemper, TL, Timbie, CM, et al. The anterior cingulate cortex in autism: heterogeneity of qualitative and quantitative cytoarchitectonic features suggests possible subgroups. Acta Neuropathologica 2009; 118(5):673–84.

17) Zikopoulos B., Barbas H. Changes in prefrontal axons may disrupt the network in autism. J. Neurosci. 2010;30,14595–609.10.1523/jneurosci.2257-10.2010

Related Sources:

1) Schumann, CM, Hamstra, J, Goodlin-Jones, BL, et al. The Amygdala is enlarged in children but not adolescents with Autism; the Hippocampus is enlarged at all ages. J Neurosci 2004;24(28):6392-6401.

2) Korkmaz, B, Benbir, G, Demirbilek, V. Migration abnormality in the left cingulate gyrus presenting with Autistic Disorder. J Child Neurol 2006;21:600-604.

3) Schumann, CM, Amaral, DG. Stereological analysis of amygdala neuron number in Autism. J Neurosci 2006;26(29):7674-7679.

4) Jacot-Descombes, S, Uppal, N, Wicinski, B, et al. Decreased pyramidal neuron size in Brodmann Areas 44 and 45 in patients with Autism. Acta Neuropathol 2012;124:67-79.

5) Ecker, C, Ginestet, C, Feng, Yue, et al. Brain surface anatomy in adults with Autism. JAMA Psychiatry 2013;70(1):59-70

6) Rogers, T, McKimm, E, Dickson, P, et al. Is Autism a disease of the cerebellum? An integration of clinical and pre-clinical research. Front Syst Neurosci 2013:1-11.

7) Deoni, SCI, Mercure, E, Blasi, A, et al. Mapping infant brain myelinations withm magnetic resonance imaging. J Neurosci 2011;31(2):784-791.

Chapter 3E – Neurotransmitter imbalance

1) R. Luján, R. Shigemoto, G. López-Bendito, Glutamate and GABA receptor signaling in the developing brain, Neuroscience, 2005;130(3):567-80.

2) Rubenstein, J. L. R., Merzenich, M. M. Model of autism: increased ratio of excitation/inhibition in key neural systems. Genes, Brain and Behavior, 2003;2(5):255-67.

3) Haijun Tu, Chanjuan Xu, Wenhua Zhang, et al. GABAb Receptor Activation Protects Neurons from Apoptosis via IGF-1 Receptor Transactivation. The Journal of Neuroscience, 2010; 30(2):749-59

4) Chebib, M, Johnston, GAR. The 'ABC' of GABA receptors: a brief review. Clinical and Experimental Pharmacology and Physiology, (1999), 26: 937–940. doi: 10.1046/j.1440-1681.1999.03151.x

5) Oblak, AL,Gibbs, TT, Blatt,GJ . Reduced GABAa receptors and benzodiazepine binding sites in the posterior cingulate cortex and fusiform gyrus in autism. Brain Research, 2011;1380:218–28

6) Doris D. Wang and Arnold R. Kriegstein. GABA Regulates Excitatory Synapse Formation in the Neocortex via NMDA Receptor Activation. The Journal of Neuroscience, 2008; 28(21):5547-58.

7) Nick Medford, Hugo D. Critchley. Conjoint activity of anterior insular and anterior cingulate cortex: awareness and response. Brain Struct Funct. 2010;214(5-6):535–549.

8) Allman, J. M., Hakeem, A., Erwin, J. M., et al., The Anterior Cingulate Cortex. Annals of the New York Academy of Sciences, 2001:935:107–117. doi: 10.1111/j.1749-6632.2001.tb03476.x

9) Miles JH. Autism spectrum disorders--a genetics review. Genet Med. 2011);13(4):278-94. doi: 10.1097/GIM.0b013e3181ff67ba. Review.

10)Fahim C, Yoon U, Sandor P, et al. Thinning of the motor-cingulate–insular cortices in siblings concordant for Tourette syndrome. Brain Topogr. 2009;22:176–84.

11) Oblak A, Gibbs TT, Blatt GJ. Decreased GABAa receptors and benzodiazepine binding sites in the anterior cingulate cortex in autism. Autism Res. 2009;2(4):205-19. doi: 10.1002/aur.88. Erratum in: Autism Res. 2009;2(4):237.

12) Dichter, G. S., Richey, J. A., Rittenberg, A. M., et al. Reward circuitry function in autism during face anticipation and outcomes. J. Autism Dev. Disord. 2012;42:147–60.

13) Chan, A.S., Han, Y. M. Y., Leung, W.W., et al. Abnormalities in the anterior cingulate cortex associated with attentional and inhibitory control deficits: A neurophysiological study on children wit h autism spectrum disorders. Research in Autism Spectrum Disorders. 2011;5(1): 254–66.

14) Baron-Cohen, S, Ring, H.A., Bullmore, E.T., et al. The amygdala theory of autism. Neuroscience and Behavioral Reviews. 2000;24:355-64.

15) Wiggins, J, Swartz, J, Martin, D, et al. Serotonin transporter genotype impacts amygdala habituation in youth with autism spectrum disorders. Social Cognitive and Affective Neuroscience Advance Access 2013.

16) Kandel ER. The molecular biology of memory storage: a dialogue between genes and synapses. Science. 2001;294(5544):1030–8.

17) Saxe MD et al. Ablation of hippocampal neurogenesis impairs contextual fear conditioning and synaptic plasticity in the dentate gyrus. Proc Natl Acad Sci USA 2006;103(46):17501–6.

18) Davis CD, Jones FL, Derrick BE. Novel environments enhance the induction and maintenance of long-term potentiation in the dentate gyrus. J Neurosci 2004;24(29): 6497–506.

19) Levitt P, Eagleson KL, Powell EM. Regulation of neocortical interneuron development and the implications for neuro- developmental disorders. Trends Neurosci 2004;27(7): 400–6.

20) Mercadante, M, Cysneiros,, R, Schwartzman, J, et al. Neurogenesis in the amygdala: A new etiologic hypothesis of autism? Medical Hypotheses 2008;70: 352-347.

21) Sweeten, T, Posey, D, Shekhar, A, et al. The amygdala and related structures in the pathophysiology of autism. Pharmacology Biochemisty and Behavior 2002;71: 449-55.

22)   Costanzo, Linda S. Physiology. Philadelphia, PA: Saunders/Elsevier, 2010. Pp. 30-31.

Chapter 3F – Synaptic pathology

1) Morrow E, Walsh C, Rubenstein J. Autism and brain development. Cell 2008; 135(3):396-400.

2) Bourgeron T, Persico A. Searching for ways out of the autism maze, epigenetic and environmental cluses. Trends Neurosci 2006; 29(7):349-68

3) Pardo, C, Vargas, DL. Zimmerman, AW, at al. Immunity, neuroglia and neuroinflammation in autism. International Review of Psychiatry 2005;17:485-495.

4) Imbrici P, Camerino D, Tricarico D. Major channels involved in neuropsychiatric disorders and therapeutic perspectives. Front Genet 2013;(7):4-76

5) Eagleson K, Judson M, Levitt P. Evidence of cell-nonautonomous changes in dendrite and dendritic spine morphology in the MET signaling deficient mouse forebrain. Vanderbilt University Medical Center 2010; 518(21):4463-78

6) Katz D, Shephard G. Synaptic microcircuit dysfunction in genetic models of neurodevelopmental disorders: focus on Mecp2 and Met. Curr Opin Neurobiol 2011; (6):827-33.3

7) Anderson C, Levitt P, Shephard G, et al. Circuit-specific intracortical hyperconnectivity in mice with deletion of the autism-associated MET receptor tyrosine kinase. J. Neurosci 2011; 31(15):5855-5a864

8) Eagleson K, Judson M, Levitt P. A new synaptic player leading to autism risk: Met receptor tyrosine kinase. J. Neurodev Disord 2011;3(3):282-2928b:

9) Rudie J, Hernandez L, Brown J, et al. Autism-Associated Promoter Variant in MET Impacts Functional and Structural Brain Networks. Neuron 2012; 75(5):904-15.

10) Patel S, Tyndall S, Walikonis R. Hepatocyte growth factor reduced enhancement of dendritic branching is blocked by inhibitors of N-methyl-D-aspartate receptors and calcium/calmodulin-dependent kinases. J Neurosci Res 2007; 11(2343-51)

11) Campbell D, Levitt P. The genetic and neurobiologic compass points toward common signaling dysfunctions in autism spectrum disorders. J Clin Invest 2009; 119(4):747-54

12) Gan W, Gooden F, Ross M, et al. Lis1 controls dynamics of neuronal filopedia and spines to impact synaptogenesis and social behavior. EMBO Mol Med 2013; 5(4):591-607

13) Gizatullin R, Imreh S, Kashuba V, et al. Assignment of the ARHA and GPX1 genes to human chromosome bands 3p21.3 by in situ hybridization and with somatic cell hybrids. Cytogenet Cell Genet 1997; 79(3-4):228-30

14) Wang L, Li J, Jia, M, et al. No association of polymorphisms in the CDK5, NDEL1, and LIS1with autism in Chinese Han population. Psychiatry Research 2011; 190(2-3):369-71

15) Spooren W, Lindemann, L, Ghosh, A, et al. Synapse dysfunction in autism: a molecular medicine approach to drug discovery in neurodevelopmental disorders. Trends in Pharamcological Sciences. 2012;33(12): 669-684.

16) Sandeep S, Eroglu C., Neuroligins Provide Molecular Links Between Syndromic and Nonsyndromic Autism 2013; 9;6(283)

17) Alarcon, M, Abrahmans, BS, Stone, JL, et al. Linkage, Association, and Gene-expression Analyses identify CNTNAP2 as an Autism-Susceptibility Gene. American Journal of Human Genetics 2008;82:150-159.

18) Strauss, K et al. Recessive symptomatic focal epilepsy and mutant contactin-associated protein-like 2. New England Journal of Medicine 2006;354:1370-1377

19) vanSpronsen, M, Hoogenraad, CC. Synapse Pathology in Psychiatric and Neurologic Disease. Curr Neurol Neurosci Reports 2010; 10(3):207-214.

20) Sudhof, T. Neuroligins and neurexins link synaptic function to cognitive disease. Nature 2008;455(7215):903-911.

21) Moessner R, Marshall C, Sutclifffe, JS, et al. Contribution of SHANK 3 mutations to Autism spectrum disorder. American Journal of Human Genetics. 2007;81 (6): 1289-1297.

22) Pizzarelli R, Cherubini E. Developmental regulation of GABAergic signalling in the hippocampus of neuroligin 3R451C knock-in mice: an animal model of Autism. Front Cell Neurosci. 2013; 7: 85.

23) Tabuchi K, Blundell J, Etherton M, et al. (2007). A neuroligin-3 mutation implicated in autism increases inhibitory synaptic transmission in mice Science 318, 71–76. doi: 0.1126/science.1146221.

24) Auerbach B, Bear M, Chattarji S, et al. Correction of fragile X syndrome in mice. Neuron 2007;56(6):955-62

25) Gauthier J, Bonnel A, St-Onge J, et al. NLGN 3/NLGN 4 gene mutations are not responsible for autism in the Quebec population. American Journal of Medical Genetics B Neuropsychiatric Genetics. 2005;132B(1):74-5.

26) Elmer, B, Garay, P, Glynn,M, et al. MHC Class I negatively regulates synapse density during the establishment of cortical connections. Nat Neurosci. 2011;14 (4): 442-451

27) Morgan, J, Chana, G, Pardo, CA, et al. Microglial activation and increased microglial density observed in the dorsolateral prefrontal cortex in autism. Biological Psychiatry 2010;68:368-376.

28) Gesundheit ,B, Rosenzweig, J, Naor, D, et al. Immunological and autoimmune considerations of Autism spectrum disorders. Journal of Autoimmunity 2013;44:1-7

29) Wei, H, Chadman, KK, McCloskey, DP, et al. Brain IL-6 elevation causes neuronal circuitry imbalances and mediates autism-like behaviors. BBA 2012:831-842.

30) Canitano, R. Epilepsy in autism spectrum disorders. Eur. Child Adolesc. Psychiatry 2007;16:61-66.

31) Braunschweig D, Krakowiak P, Duncanson P,et al. Insulin-like growth factor and the etiology of autism. Medical Hypotheses 2013 Apr;80(4):475-80.

32) Steinman, G, Mankuta, D, Insulin-like growth factor and etiology of autism, Med Hypotheses 2013;80(4):475-80.

33) Aldinger K, Levitt P, Qui S. Modeling of autism genetic variations in mice: focusing on synaptic and microcircuit dysfunctions. Dev Neurosci 2012;34:2-3.

34) Levy, S. Autism. The Lancet 2009;374:1627-38.

Chapter 3G - Hypoxia

1) Rees, S, Harding, R. Brain development during fetal life: influences of the intra-uterine environment. Neuroscience Letters 2004; 361(1-3):111-114.

2) Pittman RN. "Oxygen Transport in Normal and Pathological Situations: Defects and Compensations". Regulation of Tissue Oxygenation. San Rafael: Morgan & Claypool Life Sciences, 2011. 7 Sep, 2013.

3) Leach, RM, Treacher, DF. Oxygen transport – 2. Tissue hypoxia. BMJ 1998; 317:1370-1373.

4) Dugan, LL, Choi, DW. "Hypoxia-Ischemia and Brain infarction". Basic Neurochemistry: Molecular, Cellular and Medical Aspects (6th ed.). Siegel, GJ, Agranoff, BW, Albers, RW, et al. eds. Philadelphia: Lippincott-Raven, 1999. Accessed 25 Sep 2013.

5) Thong, YH. Reptilian behavioural patterns in childhood autism. Medical Hypotheses 1984; 13(4):399-405.

6) Zikopoulos, B, Barbas, H. Changes in prefrontal axons may disrupt the network in autism. J Neuroscience 2010; 30(44):14595-609.

7) Kemper, TL, Bauman, ML. Neuropathology of infantile autism. Molecular Psychiatry 2002;7:S12-S13.

8) Kiernan, JA. Barr's The Human Nervous System: An Anatomical Viewpoint (9th ed). Baltimore: Lippincott Williams & Wilkins, 2009.

9) Kier, EL, Kim, JH, Fulbright, RK, et al. Embryology of the human fetal hippocampus: MR imaging, anatomy, and histology. Am J Neuroradiol 1997;18:525-32.

10) Farovik, A, Dupont, LM, Eichenbaum, H. Distinct roles for dorsal CA3 and CA1 in memory for sequential nonspatial events. Learning & Memory 2010;17:12-17.

11) Daumas, S, Halley, H, Francés, B, et al. Encoding, consolidation, and retrieval of contextual memory: Differential involvement of dorsal CA3 and CA1 hippocampal subregions. Learning & Memory 2005; 12:375-82.

12) Ji, J, Maren, S. Differential roles for hippocampal areas CA1 and CA3 in the contextual encoding and retrieval of extinguished fear. Learning & Memory 2008;15:244-51.

13) Ishikawa, A, Nakamura, S. Ventral hippocampal neurons project axons simultaneously to the medial prefrontal cortex and amygdala in the rat. J Neurophysiol 2006; 96:2134-38.

14) Purves, D, Augustine, GJ, Fitzpatrick, D, et al. (Eds.). "Emotions". Neuroscience (2nd ed). Sunderland: Sinauer Associates, Inc., 2001:625-44.

15) Snider, RS, Maiti, A. Cerebellar contributions to the papez circuit. J Neuroscience Research 1976; 2(2):133-46.

16) Tanimura, Y, Vaziri, S, Lewis, MH. Indirect basal ganglia pathway mediation of repetitive behavior: Attenuation by adenosine receptor agonists. Behav Brain Res 2010; 210(1): 116-122.

17) Kemper, TL, Bauman, ML. Neuropathology of infantile autism. Molecular Psychiatry 2002; 7:S12-S13.

18) Bauman, ML, Kemper, TL. Neuroanatomic observations of the brain in autism: a review and future directions. Int J Devl Neuroscience 2005; 23:183-187.

19) Centers for Disease Control. Tobacco Use and Pregnancy. Pregnancy Risk Assessment and Monitoring System (PRAMS) and Smoking, Data from 2000-2008. 7 Sep 2013. http://www.cdc.gov/reproductivehealth/tobaccousepregnancy/

20) Abbott, LC, Winzer-Serhan UH. Smoking during pregnancy: lessons learned from epidemiological studies and experimental studies using animal models. Crit Rev Toxicol 2012; 42(4): 279-303.

21) Bureau, MA, Monette, J, Shapcott, D, et al. Carboxyhemoglobin concentration in fetal cord blood and in blood of mothers who smoked during labor. Pediatrics 1981; 69(3):371-373.

22) "High Blood Pressure in Pregnancy". National Institute of Health. 9 Sep 2013. http://www.nhlbi.nih.gov/health/public/heart/hbp/hbp_preg.htm

23) "Gestational Hypertension". University of Rochester Medical Center. 9 Sep 2013. http://www.urmc.rochester.edu/Encyclopedia/Content.aspx?ContentTypeID=90&ContentID=P02484

24) Letourneur, A, Freret, T, Roussel, S, et al. Maternal hypertension during pregnancy modifies the response of the immature brain to hypoxia-ischemia: Sequential MRI and behavioral investigations. Experimental Neurology 2012; 233:264-272.

25) Harvey, R, Ferrier, D. "Chronic Effects and Prevention of Diabetes" Biochemistry (5th ed). Baltimore: Lippincott, Williams and Wilkins, 2010.

26) Goldin, A, Beckman, J, Schmidt, AM, et al. "Basic Science for Clinicians: Advanced Glycation End Products". American Heart Association. Web. 22 Sep 2013. http://circ.ahajournals.org/content/114/6/597.

27) Daskalakis, G, Marinopoulos, S, Krielesi, V, et al. Placental pathology in women with gestational diabetes. Acta Obstetrica et Gynecologica 2008; 87:403-407

28) Taricco, E, Radaelli, T, Rossi, G, et al. Effects of gestational diabetes on fetal oxygen and glucose levels in vivo. BGOJ 2009; 116:1729-1735.

29) Martin, RJ, Fanaroff, AA, Walsh, MC. Fanaroff & Martin's Neonatal-Perinatal Medicine: Disease of the Fetus and Infant (8th ed.) St. Louis: Mosby, 2006.

30) Bush, M, Eddleman, K, Belogolovkin, V, et al. In: UpToDate, Basow, DS (Ed), UpToDate, Waltham, MA, 2013.

31) Cleveland Clinic. Uterine Cord Prolapse – Complications. 9 Nov 2013. http://my.clevelandclinic.org/healthy_living/pregnancy/hic_umbilical_cord_prolapse.aspx

32) Gregory, SG, Anthopolos, R, Osgood, CE, et al. Association of autism with induced or augmented childbirth in North Carolina birth record (1990-1998) and education research (1997-2007) databases. JAMA Pediatrics 2013;167(10):1-11.

33) Modahl, C, Green, LA, Fein, D, et al. Plasma oxytocin levels in autistic children. Biol Psychiatry 1998;43:270-77.

Chapter 3H – Perinatal complications

1) Gillberg C, Gillberg IC. Infantile autism: a total population study of reduced optimality in the pre-, peri-, and neonatal period. *Journal of autism and developmental disorders.* Jun 1983;13(2):153-166.

2) Gardener H, Spiegelman D, Buka SL. Perinatal and neonatal risk factors for autism: a comprehensive meta-analysis. *Pediatrics.* Aug 2011;128(2):344-355.

3) Lyall K, Pauls DL, Spiegelman D, et al. Pregnancy complications and obstetric suboptimality in association with autism spectrum disorders in children of the Nurses' Health Study II. *Autism research : official journal of the International Society for Autism Research.* Feb 2012;5(1):21-30.

4) Juul-Dam N, Townsend J, Courchesne E. Prenatal, perinatal, and neonatal factors in autism, pervasive developmental disorder-not otherwise specified, and the general population. *Pediatrics.* Apr 2001;107(4):E63.

5) Steffenburg S, Gillberg C, Hellgren L, et al. A twin study of autism in Denmark, Finland, Iceland, Norway and Sweden. *Journal of child psychology and psychiatry, and allied disciplines.* May 1989;30(3):405-416.

6) Brimacombe M, Ming X, Lamendola M. Prenatal and birth complications in autism. *Maternal and child health journal.* Jan 2007;11(1):73-79.

7) Burd L, Severud R, Kerbeshian J, Klug MG. Prenatal and perinatal risk factors for autism. *Journal of perinatal medicine.* 1999;27(6):441-450.

8) Lord C, Mulloy C, Wendelboe M, Schopler E. Pre- and perinatal factors in high-functioning females and males with autism. *Journal of autism and developmental disorders.* Jun 1991;21(2):197-209.

9) Piven J, Simon J, Chase GA, et al. The etiology of autism: pre-, peri- and neonatal factors. *Journal of the American Academy of Child and Adolescent Psychiatry.* Nov 1993;32(6):1256-1263.

10) Hultman CM, Sparen P, Cnattingius S. Perinatal risk factors for infantile autism. *Epidemiology.* Jul 2002;13(4):417-423.

11) Glasson EJ, Bower C, Petterson B, et al. Perinatal factors and the development of autism: a population study. *Archives of general psychiatry.* Jun 2004;61(6):618-627.

12) Larsson HJ, Eaton WW, Madsen KM, et al. Risk factors for autism: perinatal factors, parental psychiatric history, and socioeconomic status. *American journal of epidemiology.* May 15 2005;161(10):916-925; discussion 926-918.

13) Maimburg RD, Vaeth M. Perinatal risk factors and infantile autism. *Acta psychiatrica Scandinavica.* Oct 2006;114(4):257-264.

14) Croen LA, Grether JK, Selvin S. Descriptive epidemiology of autism in a California population: who is at risk? *Journal of autism and developmental disorders.* Jun 2002;32(3):217-224.

15) Wier ML, Yoshida CK, Odouli R, et al. Congenital anomalies associated with autism spectrum disorders. *Developmental medicine and child neurology.* Jun 2006;48(6):500-507.

16) Williams K, Helmer M, Duncan GW, et al. Perinatal and maternal risk factors for autism spectrum disorders in New South Wales, Australia. *Child: care, health and development.* Mar 2008;34(2):249-256.

17) Qazi G. Obstetric and perinatal outcome of multiple pregnancy. *Journal of the College of Physicians and Surgeons--Pakistan : JCPSP.* Mar 2011;21(3):142-145.

18) Hack M, Taylor HG, Drotar D, et al. Chronic conditions, functional limitations, and special health care needs of school-aged children born with extremely low-birth-weight in the 1990s. *JAMA : the journal of the American Medical Association.* Jul 20 2005;294(3):318-325.

19) Kolevzon A, Gross R, Reichenberg A. Prenatal and perinatal risk factors for autism: a review and integration of findings. *Archives of pediatrics & adolescent medicine.* Apr 2007;161(4):326-333.

20) Moster D, Lie RT, Markestad T. Long-term medical and social consequences of preterm birth. *The New England journal of medicine.* Jul 17 2008;359(3):262-273.

21) Schothorst PF, van Engeland H. Long-term behavioral sequelae of prematurity. *Journal of the American Academy of Child and Adolescent Psychiatry.* Feb 1996;35(2):175-183.

22) Wood NS, Marlow N, Costeloe K, et al. Neurologic and developmental disability after extremely preterm birth. EPICure Study Group. *The New England journal of medicine.* Aug 10 2000;343(6):378-384.

23) Buchmayer S, Johansson S, Johansson A, et al. Can association between preterm birth and autism be explained by maternal or neonatal morbidity? *Pediatrics.* Nov 2009;124(5):e817-825.

24) Sandin S KA, Levine SZ, Hultman CM, Reichenberg A. Parental and Perinatal Risk Factors for Autism: Epidemiological Findings and Potential Mechanisms In: Buxbaum J, ed. *The Neuroscience of Autism Spectrum Disorders*: Elsevier Science; 2013.

25) Eaton WW, Mortensen PB, Thomsen PH, Frydenberg M. Obstetric complications and risk for severe psychopathology in childhood. *Journal of autism and developmental disorders.* Jun 2001;31(3):279-285.

26) Stein D, Weizman A, Ring A, Barak Y. Obstetric complications in individuals diagnosed with autism and in healthy controls. *Comprehensive psychiatry.* Jan-Feb 2006;47(1):69-75.

27) Mason-Brothers A, Ritvo ER, Pingree C, et al. The UCLA-University of Utah epidemiologic survey of autism: prenatal, perinatal, and postnatal factors. *Pediatrics.* Oct 1990;86(4):514-519.

28) Dodds L, Fell DB, Shea S, et al. The role of prenatal, obstetric and neonatal factors in the development of autism. *Journal of autism and developmental disorders.* Jul 2011;41(7):891-902.

29) Krakowiak P, Walker CK, Bremer AA, et al. Maternal metabolic conditions and risk for autism and other neurodevelopmental disorders. *Pediatrics.* May 2012;129(5):e1121-1128.

30) Baron-Cohen S LSKR. *Prenatal testosterone in mind.* Cambridge, MA: MIT Press; 2004.

31) Eidelman AI, Samueloff A. The pathophysiology of the fetus of the diabetic mother. *Seminars in perinatology.* Jun 2002;26(3):232-236.

32) Mann JR, McDermott S, Bao H, et al. Pre-eclampsia, birth weight, and autism spectrum disorders. *Journal of autism and developmental disorders.* May 2010;40(5):548-554.

33) Grether JK, Li SX, Yoshida CK, Croen LA. Antenatal ultrasound and risk of autism spectrum disorders. *Journal of autism and developmental disorders.* Feb 2010;40(2):238-245.

34) Bolton PF, Murphy M, Macdonald H, et al. Obstetric complications in autism: consequences or causes of the condition? *Journal of the American Academy of Child and Adolescent Psychiatry.* Feb 1997;36(2):272-281.

35) Zwaigenbaum L, Szatmari P, Jones MB, et al. Pregnancy and birth complications in autism and liability to the broader autism phenotype. *Journal of the American Academy of Child and Adolescent Psychiatry.* May 2002;41(5):572-579.

Chapter 3I - Diabetes; obesity

1) Gardener H, Spiegelman D, Buka SL. Prenatal risk factors for autism: comprehensive meta-analysis. Br J psychiatry. 2009; 195(1): 7-14.

2) Krakowiak, P, Walker, CK, Bremer, A, et al. Maternal Metabolic Conditions and Risk for Autism and Other Neurodevelopmental Disorders. Pediatrics 2012;129(5):Q1121-8.

3) FG Cunningham, et al., eds. Williams Obstetrics, McGraw-Hill, New York, 2001, Diabetes. pp.1359-84.

4) Kumar, V, Fauston, Abbas, A. Robbins and Cortan Pathologic Basis of Disease, 7th edition, Elsevier, New York, 2004, pp. 1197-98.

5) RS Gibbs, et al. eds. Danforth Obstetrics and Gynecology. 10th edition: Diabetes Mellitus and Pregnancy, pp.246-56.

6) Eidelman Al, Samueloff A. The Pathophysiology of the Fetus of the Diabetic Mother. Semin Perinatal 2002;26(3):232-236

7) Georgieff MK. The role of Iron in Neurodevelopment: Fetal Iron Deficiency and the Developing Hippocampus. Biochem Soc Trans. 2008;36(6):1267-71.

8) Georgieff MK. The Effect of Maternal Diabetes During Pregnancy on the Development of Offspring. Minn Med 2006; 89 (3):44-47

9) Lozoff B Georgieff MK. Iron Deficiency and Brain Development. Semin Pediatric Neurology. 2006; 13(3)158-165.

10) Zinkhan E, Fu Q, Wang Y. Maternal Hyperglycemia Disrupts Histone 3 Lysine 36 Trimethylation of the IGF-1. Gene 2012.

11) Steinman G, Mankuta D. Insulin Like Growth Factor and the Etiology of Autism. Medical Hypotheses 2013; 475(2) 21-33.

12) Wuarin, L, Guertin, DM, Ishii, DN. Early reduction in insulin-like growth factor gene expression in diabetic nerve. Exp Neurol 1994;130:106-14.

Chapter 4A – Heavy metals

1) Grandjean P, Landrigan PJ. Developmental Neurotoxicity of Industrial Chemicals. The Lancet 2006;368:2167-78.

2) Caserta, D., Graziano, A., Monte Lo G., et al. Heavy Metals and placental fetal- maternal barrier: a mini- review on the major concerns. European Review for Medical and Pharmacological Sciences 2013;17:2198-2206.

3) Lathe, R. (2006). Autism, brain, and environment. Jessica Kingsley Publishers.

4) Yasuda, H., Kobayashi, M., Yasuda, Y & Tsutsui, T. Estimation of autistic children by metallomics analysis. Sci Rep. 3, 1199; DOI 10.1038/srep01199 (2013).

5) Tomljenovic, L., Shaw, C. A. Do aluminum vaccine adjuvants contribute to the rising prevalence of autism?. Journal of Inorganic Biochemistry, 2011;105(11) 1489-1499.

6) Bishop, N.J. Morley, R., Day, J.P. et al. The New England Journal of Medicine 1997;336: 1557-1561

7) Baylor, N.W., Egan, W., Richman, P. Vaccine 2002;20(Suppl. 3): S18-S23.

8) Yokel, R. A., Hicks, C. L., & Florence, R. L. Aluminum bioavailability from basic sodium aluminum phosphate, an approved food additive emulsifying agent, incorporated in cheese. Food and chemical toxicology, 2008;46(6);2261-66.

9) Ellingson R.J., Peters, J.F. Electroencephalography and Clinical Nuerophysiology 1980;49:112-124.

10) Vergani, L., Lanza, C., Rivaro, P. Metals, metallothioneins and oxidative stress in blood of autistic children. Elsevier Research in Autism Spectrum Disorders 2010;5:286-83.

11) Obrenovich E. M., Shamberger J. R., Lonsdale D. Altered Heavy Metals and Transketalase Found in Autistic Spectrum Disorder. Biol Trace Elem Res 2010;144:475-86.

12) Blaucok-Busch, E., Amin, O. R., Dessoki, H. H., Rabah, T. Toxic Metals and Essential Elements in Hair and Severity of Symptoms among Children with Autism. Mædica, 2012;7(1):38-48.

13) Blaucok-Busch, E., Amin, O. R., Rabah, T. Heavy Metals and Trace Elements in Hair and Urine of a Sample of Arab Children with Autistic Spectrum Disorder. Mædica,2011; 6(4):247-57.

14) Bhatty, Javed I. (1995). "Role of Minor lements in Cement anufacture and Use."

15) Ogunbileje, J. O., et al. (2012) "Lead, mercury, cadmium, chromium, nickel, copper, zinc, calcium, iron, manganese and chromium (VI) levels in Nigeria and United States of America cement dust." Chemosphere.

16) Baranowska-Dutkiewicz, B. Absorption of hexavalent chromium by skin in man. Archives of Toxicology, 1981;47(1): 47-50.

17) Malarveni D. L. P., Arumigam G. Level of Trace Elements (Copper, Zinc, Magnesium and Selenium) and Toxic Elements (Lead and Mercury) in Hair and Nail of Children with Autism. Biol Trace Elem Res 2011;142:148-158.

18) Dietary Supplement Fact Sheet: Selenium,http://ods.od.nih.gov/factsheets/Selenium-HealthProfessional.

19) American Psychiatric Association, & American Psychiatric Association. Task Force on DSM-IV. (1994). Diagnostic and statistical manual of mental disorders: DSM-IV. Amer Psychiatric Pub Inc.

20) Adams, J. B., et al. "Analyses of toxic metals and essential minerals in the hair of Arizona children with autism and associated conditions, and their mothers." Biological trace element research 2006;110.3:193-209.

21) Adams, J. B., Romdalvik, J., Ramanujam, V. S., & Legator, M. S. Mercury, lead, and zinc in baby teeth of children with autism versus controls. Journal of Toxicology and Environmental Health, Part A, 2007;70(12):1046-1051.

22) Green, V. A., Pituch, K. A., Itchon, J., et al,. Internet survey of treatments used by parents of children with autism. Research in Developmental Disabilities,2006; 27(1): 70-84.

23) Golnik, A. E., & Ireland, M. Complementary alternative medicine for children with autism: A physician survey. Journal of Autism and Developmental Disorders, 2009;39(7),996-1005.

Chapter 4B - Lead

1) Hernberg S. Lead poisoning in a historical perspective. Am J Ind Med. 2000;38:244–54. doi: 10.1002/1097-0274(200009)38:3<244::AID-AJIM3>3.0.CO;2-F.

2) Lidsky TI, Schneider JS. Lead neurotoxicity in children: basic mechanisms and clinical correlates. Brain. 2003;12:5–19. doi: 10.1093/brain/awg014.

3) Cohen DJ, Johnson WT, Caparulo BK. Pica and elevated blood lead level in autistic and atypical children. Am J Dis Child. 1976;130:47–8.

4) Kinnell HG. Pica as a feature of Autism. Br J Psychiatry. 1985;147:80–2.

5) Cohen DJ, Paul R, Anderson GM, et al. Bloodlead in autistic children. Lancet. 1982;2:94–5.

6) Goldstein, G. W. (1990). Lead Poisoning and Brain Cell Function. Environmental Health perspective, 1990;89: 91-94.

7) Lidsky, T. I., Schneider, J. S. Lead neurotoxicity in children: basic mechanisms and clinical correlates. brain, a journal of neurology, 2003;126(1):5-19. Retrieved from http://brain.oxfordjournals.org.lb-proxy13.touro.edu/content/126/1/5.long

8) Anderson AC, Pueschel SM, Linakis JG. Pathophysiology of lead poisoning. In: Pueschel SM, Linakis JG, Anderson AC, editors. Lead poisoning in children. Baltimore (MD): P.H. Brookes; 1996.pp. 75-96.

9) El-Ansary, A. K., Bacha, A. B., Al- Ayahdi, L. Y. Relationship between chronic lead toxicity and plasma neurotransmitters in autistic patients from Saudi Arabia.Elsevier, 2011;44(13): 1116–1120

10) Bressler JP, Goldstein GW. Mechanisms of lead neurotoxicity. [Review]. Biochem Pharmacol 1991; 41: 479-84.

11) Nihei MK, McGlothan JL, Toscano CD, Guilarte TR. Low level Pb2+ exposure affects hippocampal protein kinase CaÄ gene and protein expression in rats. Neurosci Lett 2001; 298: 212-6.

12) Young JG, Kavanagh ME, Anderson GM, et al. Clinical neurochemistry of autism and associated disorders. J Autism Dev Disord 1982;12:147–65.

13) Stone JM, Morrison PD, Pilowsky LS. Glutamate and dopamine dysregulation in schizophrenia—a synthesis and selective review. J Psychopharmacol 2007;21: 440–52.

14) Tsai G, Coyle JT. Glutamatergic mechanisms in schizophrenia. Annu Rev Pharmacol Toxicol 2002; 42:165–79.

15) American board of family medicine, . N.p.. Web. 25 Sep 2013. http://www.medscape.com/viewarticle/405804_3.

16) Shannon M, Graef JW. Lead intoxication in children with pervasive developmental disorders. J Toxicol Clin Toxicol. 1996;34:177–81.

17) Clark B, Vandermeer B, Simonetti A, Buka I. Is lead a concern in Canadian autistic children?. Paediatr Child Health. 2010;15(1):17-22.

18) Grabrucker AM. Environmental factors in Autism. Front Psychiatry. 2012;3:118.

19) Bedrosian, Katie, Jonathan Charest, Victoria DeVault, and Emily Lumley. "Neurotoxic Chemicals in the Environment." (2008): n.pag. Web. 24 Sep 2013.

20) Lidsky TI, Schneider JS. Autism and autistic symptoms associated with childhood lead poisoning. J Appl Res. 2005;5:80–4.

21) 29 Sep 2013. http://www.poison.org/current/chelationtherapy.htm

22) Lowry, Jennifer. "Oral Chelation Therapy For Patients With Lead Poisoning" (2010): n.pag. Web. 27 Sep 2013. http://www.who.int/selection_medicines/committees/expert/18/applications/4_2_LeadOral Chelators.pdf

23) Davis,TN, O'Reilly, M, Kang, S, et al. Chelation treatment for Autism spectrum disorders: A systematic review, Research in Autism Spectrum Disorders, 2013;7(1):49-55, http://dx.doi.org/10.1016/j.rasd.2012.06.005. (http://www.sciencedirect.com/science/article/pii/S1750946712000724)

24) Lofthouse N, Hendren R, Hurt E, et al. A review of complementary and alternative treatments for Autism spectrum disorders. Autism Res Treat. 2012;2012:870391.

25) Rossignol DA. Novel and emerging treatments for Autism spectrum disorders: a systematic review. Ann Clin Psychiatry. 2009;21(4):213-36.

26) Accardo P, Whitman B, Caul J, Rolfe U. Autism and plumbism, a possible association. Clin Pediatrics. 1988;27:41–4.

27) Dietrich KN, Ware JH, Salganik M, et al. Effect of chelation therapy on the neuropsychological and behavioral development of lead-exposed children after school entry. Pediatrics. 2004;114(1):19-26.

28) Stangle DE, Smith DR, Beaudin SA, et al. Succimer chelation improves learning, attention, and arousal regulation in lead-exposed rats but produces lasting cognitive impairment in the absence of lead exposure. Environ Health Perspect. 2007;115(2):201-9.

29) Mitka , M. "Chelation Therapy Trials Halted." 300(19).2236 (2008): JAMA. Database. 25 Sep 2013.

30) Baxter AJ, Krenzelok EP. Pediatric fatality secondary to EDTA chelation. Clin Toxicol (Phila). 2008;46(10):1083-4.

Chapter 4C – Teratogenic classification

1) Food and Drug Administration, HHS, (2008). Content and format of labeling for human prescription drug and biological products; requirements for pregnancy and lactation labeling. Federal Register.

2) Sannerstedt, R., Lundborg, P., Danielsson, B., et al. Drugs during pregnancy: an issue of risk classification and information to prescribers. Drug Safety 1996; 2: 69-77.

3) Addis, A., Sharabi, S., & Bonati, M. Risk classification systems for drug use during pregnancy: Drug Safety 2000;3: 245-53.

4) Sachdeva, P., Patel, B., & Patel, B. Drug use in pregnancy; a point to ponder!. Indian Journal of Pharmaceutical Sciences 2009;71:1-7.

5) Draper, J, K Cox, and K Matthews Jr. Teratology and Drug Use During Pregnancy. Medscape Reference, 2013.

6) Roullet, F., Wollaston, L., deCatanzaro, D., & Foster, J. Behavioral and molecular changes in the mouse in response to prenatal exposure to the anti-epileptic drug valproic acid. Cellular and Molecular Neuroscience 2010;170(2): 514-522.

7) Kim, J., & Scialli, A. Thalidomide: The tragedy of birth defects and the effective treatment of disease. Toxicological Sciences 2011;122(1):1-6.

Chapter 4D – Autism-promoting drugs

1) Miller, M. T., Stromland, K., Ventura, L., et al. Autism with ophthalmologic malformations: The plot thickens. Transactions of the American Ophthalmological Society 2004; 102, 107–122.

2) Dufour-Rainfray, D., Vourc'h, P., Tourlet, S., et al. Fetal exposure to teratogens: Evidence of genes involved in autism. Neuroscience & Biobehavioral Reviews 2011;35(5), 1254–1265. doi:10.1016/j.neubiorev.2010.12.013

3) Ema, M., Ise, R., Kato, H., et al. Fetal malformations and early embryonic gene expression response in cynomolgus monkeys maternally exposed to thalidomide. Reproductive Toxicology 2010;29(1), 49–56. doi:10.1016/j.reprotox.2009.09.003

4) Rinaldi, T., Silberberg, G., & Markram, H. Hyperconnectivity of Local Neocortical Microcircuitry Induced by Prenatal Exposure to Valproic Acid. Cerebral Cortex 2008; 18(4), 763–770. doi:10.1093/cercor/bhm117

5) Narita, N., Kato, M., Tazoe, M., et al. Increased Monoamine Concentration in the Brain and Blood of Fetal Thalidomide- and Valproic Acid–Exposed Rat: Putative Animal Models for Autism. Pediatric Research 2002;52(4), 576–579. doi:10.1203/00006450-200210000-00018

6) Therapontos, C., Erskine, L, Gardner, et al. Thalidomide induces limb defects by preventing angiogenic outgrowth during early limb formation. PNAS 2009;106 (21) 8573-8578; doi:10.1073/pnas.0901505106

7) Bandim, José Marcelino, Ventura, et al. Autism and Möbius sequence: an exploratory study of children in northeastern Brazil. Arquivos de Neuro-Psiquiatria 2003;61(2A), 181-185

8) Hsieh, C.-L., Wang, H.-E., Tsai, W.-J., et al. Multiple point action mechanism of valproic acid-teratogenicity alleviated by folic acid, vitamin C, And N-acetylcysteine in chicken embryo model. Toxicology 2012;291(1–3), 32–42. doi:10.1016/j.tox.2011.10.015

9) Tamiji, J., & Crawford, D. A. Prostaglandin E(2) and misoprostol induce neurite retraction in Neuro-2a cells. Biochemical and biophysical research communications 2010;398(3), 450–456. doi:10.1016/j.bbrc.2010.06.098

Chapter 4E – Pesticides, pollutants

1) Becerra, TA, et al. "Ambient Air Pollution and Autism in Los Angeles County, California." Environmental health perspectives 2013; 121.3: 380.

2)   Roberts, JR., Reigart, JR. "Organophosphate Insecticides." Recognition and Management of Pesticide Poisonings. 6th ed., 2013. 43-55.

3)   Stamou, M, et al. "Neuronal connectivity as a convergent target of gene-environment interactions that confer risk for Autism Spectrum Disorders." Neurotoxicology and teratology (2012).

4)   Sheng, L, et al. "Prenatal polycyclic aromatic hydrocarbon exposure leads to behavioral deficits and downregulation of receptor tyrosine kinase, MET." Toxicological Sciences 2010;118.2: 625-634.

5)   Volk, E., et al. "Residential proximity to freeways and autism in the CHARGE study." Environmental health perspectives 2011;119.6: 873.

6)   Casida, JE. Pest Toxicology: the Primary Mechanisms of Pesticide Action. Chem Res Toxicol 2009;22(4):609-619

7)   Belmonte MK, Bourgeron T. Fragile X syndrome and autism at the intersection of genetic and neural networks. Nat Neurosci 2006; 9(10):1221–25.

8)   Varju P, Katarova Z, Madarasz E, Szabo G. 2001. GABA signalling during development: new data and old questions. Cell Tissue Res 2001;305(2):239–246.

9)   Brannen KC, Devaud LL, Liu J, Lauder JM. 1998. Prenatal expo- sure to neurotoxicants dieldrin or lindane alters tert-butyl- bicyclophosphorothionate binding to GABAA receptors in fetal rat brainstem. Dev Neurosci 1998;20(1):34–41.

10)   Liu J, Brannen KC, Grayson DR, et al. Prenatal exposure to the pesticide dieldrin or the GABAA receptor antagonist bicuculline differentially alters expression of GABAA receptor subunit mRNAs in fetal rat brainstem. Dev Neurosci 1998;20(1):83–92.

11)   Ming X, Brimacombe M, Wagner GC. Prevalence of motor impairment in autism spectrum disorders. Brain Dev 2007;29(9):565–570.

12)   Bolton PF, Carcani-Rathwell I, Hutton J,. Epilepsy in autism: features and correlates. The Br J Psychiatry 2011;198(4):289–294.

13)   Rossignol, DA, Frye, RE. Mitochondrial dysfunction in autism spectrum disorders: a systematic review and meta- analysis. Mol Psychiatry 2012;17(3):290–314.

14)   Shi, X, Gu, A, Ji, G, et al. Developmental toxicity of cypermethrin in embryo–larval stages of zebrafish. Chemosphere 2011;85(6):1010–16.

15)   Shelton, JF., Hertz-Picciotto, I, Pessah, IN. Tipping the Balance of Autism Risk: Potential Mechanisms Linking Pesticides and Autism. Environmental Health Perspectives 2012;120.7: 944-51.

16)   Brown, B La'Nissa, A., et al. "Down-regulation of early ionotrophic glutamate receptor subunit developmental expression as a mechanism for observed plasticity deficits following gestational exposure to benzo(a) pyrene." Neurotoxicology 2007;28.5: 965-978.

17)   Judson, MC., et al. "Dynamic gene and protein expression patterns of the autism-associated met receptor tyrosine kinase in the developing mouse forebrain." Journal of Comparative Neurology 2009;513.5: 511-531.

18)   Campbell, DB., et al. "Association of MET with social and communication phenotypes in individuals with autism spectrum disorder." American Journal of Medical Genetics Part B: Neuropsychiatric Genetics 2010;153.2: 438-446.

19)   Roberts, EM, English, PB, Grether, JK, et al. Maternal residence near agricultural pesti- cide applications and autism spectrum disorders among children in the California Central Valley. Environ Health Perspect 2007;115:1482–1489.

20)   Canfield, MA, Ramadhani, TA, Langlois, PH, Waller, DK. Residential mobility patterns and exposure misclassification in epidemiological studies of birth defects. J Expo Sci Environ Epidermiol 2006;16(6):53-543.

21) London, Eric, Etzel, RA. "The Environment as an Etiologic Factor in Autism: A New Direction for Research." Environmental Health Perspectives 2000;108.3: 401-04.

22) Aluigi, MG, Angelini, C, Falugi, C, et al. Interaction between organophosphate compounds and cholinergic functions during development. Chem Biol Interact 2005;157–158:305–316.

23) Zerbo, O, Iosif, AM, Delwiche, L, et al. "Month of Conception and Risk of Autism." Epidemiology 2011;22.4: 469-75.

24) Volk, HE., et al. "Traffic-Related Air Pollution, Particulate Matter, and Autism." JAMA psychiatry 2013;70.1: 71-77.

Chapter 4F - Television

1) American Academy of Pediatrics Committee on Public Education. Children, Adolescents, and Television. Pediatrics 2001; 107(2): 423.

2) Centers for Disease Control and Prevention. Autism Spectrum Disorders (ASDs): Data & Statistics. 27 June 2013. <http://www.cdc.gov/ncbddd/autism/data.html>.

3) Waldman, M, Nicholson, S, Adilov, N. Does Television Cause Autism? Cambridge: National Bureau of Economic Research 2006; Working Paper No. 12632:11-43©.

4) Christakis, D, Zimmerman, F, DiGiuseppe, D. Early Television Exposure and Subsequent Attentional Problems in Children. Pediatrics 2004; 113(4): 708-711.

5) Zwaigenbaum, L, Bryson, S, Rogers, T. Behavioral Manifestations of Autism in the First Year of Life. International Journal of Developmental Neuroscience 2005; 23: 146-148.

6) Whitehouse, M. Is An Economist Qualified To Solve Puzzle of Autism? The Wall Street Journal. 27 February 2007. <http://online.wsj.com/article/SB117131554110006323.html>.

7) Braun, J, Kalkbrenner, A. Autism Prevalence and Precipitation: The Potential for Cross-Level Bias. JAMA Pediatrics 2009; 163 (5): 492.

8) Campbell, D, Sutcliffe, J, Levitt, P. A Genetic Variant that Disrupts MET Transcription is Associated with Autism. Proceedings of the National Academy of Sciences of the United States of America 2006; 103 (43): 16834-16839.

9) Wells, C. Does Watching TV Cause Autism? TIME. 20 October 2006. <http://content.time.com/time/health/article/0,8599,1548682,00.html>.

10) American Academy of Pediatrics. Media and Children. <http://www.aap.org/en-us/advocacy-and-policy/aap-health-initiatives/Pages/Media-and-Children.aspx>

Chapter 5A – Folic acid

1) Scholl TO, Johnson WG. Folic acid: influence on the outcome of pregnancy. Am J Clin Nutr 2000;71(5 Suppl): 1295S-1303S.

2) Daly LE, Kirke PN, Molloy A, Weir DG, Scott JM. Folate levels and neural tube defects: implications for prevention. JAMA. 1995;274(21):1698-1702.

3) Surén P, Roth C, Bresnahan M, Haugen M, et al. Association between maternal use of folic acid supplements and risk of autism spectrum disorders in children. JAMA. 2013; 309:570-77.

4) Roth,C, Magnus,P, Schjolberg,S, et al.Folic acid supplements in pregnancy and severe language delay in children JAMA, 2011;306 : pp. 1566–1573

5) Christian, P, Murray-Kolb, LE, Khatry, SK,et al. Prenatal micronutrient supplementation and intellectual and motor function in early school-aged children in Nepal. JAMA,2010; 304:2716–2723

6) Schmidt RJ, Hansen RL, Hartiala J, et al. Prenatal vitamins, one-carbon metabolism gene variants, and risk for autism. Epidemiology. 2011; 22(4):476- 485.

7) Schmidt, RJ, Tancredi DJ, Ozonoff S, et al. Maternal periconceptional folic acid intake and risk of autism spectrum disorders and developmental delay in the CHARGE (CHildhood Autism Risks from Genetics and Environment) case-control study. Am J Clin Nutr. 2012; 96(1):80-89.

8) Czeizel, AE, Duda´s, I. Prevention of the first occurrence of neural-tube defects by periconceptional vitamin supplementation. N Engl J Med. 1992;327(26):1832-1835.

9) Werler, MM, Shapiro, S, Mitchell, AA. Periconceptional folic acid exposure and risk of occurrent neural tube defects. JAMA. 1993;269(10):1257-61.

10) Daly, LE, Kirke, PN, Molloy, A, et al. Folate levels and neural tube defects: implications for prevention.JAMA. 1995;274(21):1698-1702.

11) Shaw, GM, Schaffer, D, Velie, EM, et al. Periconceptional vitamin use, dietary folate, and the occurrence of neural tube defects. Epidemiology. 1995;6(3):219-226.

12) Schmidt, RJ, Hansen, RL, Hartiala, J, et al., Prenatal vitamins, one-carbon metabolism gene variants, and risk for autism. 2011;22(4):476-85. doi: 10.1097/EDE.0b013e31821d0e30.

13) Födinger, M, Hörl, WH, Sunder-Plassmann, G.. Molecular biology of 5,10-methylenetetrahydrofolate reductase. J Nephrol. 2000 Jan-Feb;13(1):20-33.

14) Nozaki, T, Shigeta, Y, Saito-Nakano, Y, et al. (March 2001). "Characterization of transsulfuration and cysteine biosynthetic pathways in the protozoan hemoflagellate, Trypanosoma cruzi. Isolation and molecular characterization of cystathionine beta-synthase and serine acetyltransferase from Trypanosoma". The Journal of Biological Chemistry 276 (9): 6516–23. doi:10.1074/jbc.M009774200.

15) Kałużna-Czaplińska, J, Żurawicz, E, Michalska, M, Rynkowski, J. A focus on homocysteine in autism. Acta Biochim Pol. 2013;60(2):137-42.

16) Pasca, S, Nemes, B, Vlase, L, et al., High levels of homocysteine and low serum paraoxonase 1 arylesterase activity in children with autism," Life Sciences, November 16, 2005

17) Adams, M, Lucock, M, Stuart, J, et al. Preliminary evidence for involvement of the folate gene polymorphism 19-bp deletion-DHFR in occurrence of autism. Neurosci Lett 2007;422:24–9

18) Grossman, MH, Emanuel, BS, Budarf, ML. Chromosomal mapping of the human catechol-O-methyltransferase gene to 22q11.1-q11.2. Genomics 1992;12 (4): 822–5.

19) Lotta, T, Vidgren J, Tilgmann, C, et al. Kinetics of human soluble and membrane-bound catechol O-methyltransferase: a revised mechanism and description of the thermolabile variant of the enzyme. Biochemistry 34 (13): 4202–10.

20) Lachman, HM, Morrow, B, Shprintzen, R, et al. Association of codon 108/158 catechol-o-methyltransferase gene polymorphism with the psychiatric manifestations of velo-cardio-facial syndrome. Am J Med Genet 67 (5): 468–72.

21) Bruder, GE, Keilp, JG, Xu, H, et al. Catechol-O-methyltransferase (COMT) genotypes and working memory: associations with differing cognitive operations. Biol. Psychiatry 58 (11): 901–7.

22) Sharp, WG, Berry, RC, McCracken, C, et al.. Feeding problems and nutrient intake in children with autism spectrum disorders: a meta-analysis and comprehensive review of the literature. J Autism Dev Disord. 2013 Sep; 43(9):2159-73.

Chapter 5B – Leaky gut (gluten/opiates)

1) Brewster, G, RD. CPE Article: Review of the Literature Regarding the Gut-brain Connection in Autism Spectrum Disorders and Associated Special Diet Therapies. The Integrative RD 2013. 62(4).

2) Mahikoa, K. Gastrointestinal Illness in Autism: An Interview with Tim Buie, M.D. Autism Advocate Fifth Ed. 2006.

3) Liu Z, Li N, Neu J. Tight Junctions, Leaky intestines and pediatric diseases. Acta Pediatrica April 2005;94(4):386-93.

4) Reichelt K.L. and A.M. Knivsberg. The Possibility and Probablity of a gut-to-brain connection in Autism. Annals of Clinical Psychiatry 2009;41(4):205-11.

5) Brantl, W. and Teschemacher, H. A matrial opioid activity in bovine milk and milk products. Naunyn Schmiedebergs Archivder Pharmacology. 1929; 306:301–304.

6) Fukudome, S.I. Yoshikawa, M. Opioid peptides derived from wheat gluten: their isolation and characterization. FEBS Letters. 1992; 296: 107–111.

7) De Magistris, L, Familiari, V, Pascotto, A, et al. Alterations of the Intestinal Barrier in Patients with Autism Spectrum Disorders and in their First Degree Relatives. Journal of Pediatric Gastroenterology and Nutrition October 2010: 51(4): 418-424.

8) Wakefield, AJ. The Gut-Brain Axis in Childhood Developmental Disorders. Journal of Pediatric Gastroenterology and Nutrition 2002;Supp 1:S14-7.

9) D'Eufemia, P, Celli, M, Finnochiaro, R, et al. Abnormal intestinal permeability in children with autism. Acta Pediatrica 1996; 85:1076-9

10) Christison, GW, Ivany, K. Journal of Developmental and Behavioral Pediatrics 2006; 27(2):S162-S171.

11) Reichelt, KL, Tveiten, D, Knivsberg, A, et al. Peptides' role in autism with emphasis on exorphins. Microbial Ecology in Health & Disease 2012;Aug:23.

12) Knivsberg, A, Reichelt, K, Hoien, T, et al. A Randomised, Controlled Study of Dietary Intervention in Autistic Syndromes. Nutritional Neuroscience 2002;5(4):251-61.

13) Elder, J, Shankar, M, Shuster, J, et al. The Gluten-Free, Casein-Free Diet in Autism: Results of a Preliminary Double Blind Clinical Trial. Journal of Autism and Developmental Disorders April 2006;36(3):413-20.

14) Hyman, S, Stewart, P, Smith, T, et al.: The Gluten Free and Casein Free Diet in Young Children with Autism. Brown University Child and Adolescent Behavior Letter. August 2, 2010.

Chapter 5C – Vitamin D

1) Lippincott's Illustrated Reviews: Biochemistry, Fifth Edition. Harvey, RA, Ferrier, DR, Karandish, S. Lippincott Williams & Wilkins, 2012.

2) Kocovska, E., Fernell, E., Billstedt, E., et al. Vitamin D and autism: Clinical Review. Research in Developmental Disabilities 2012; 33(5):1541-50.

3) Gentile, I., Zappulo, E., Militerni, R., et al. Etiopathogenesis of autism spectrum disorders: Fitting the pieces of the puzzle together. Medical Hypotheses 2013;81(1):26-35.

4) Cannell, JJ. Autism and vitamin D. Medical Hypotheses 2008;70(4):750-9.

5) Humble, MB. Vitamin D, light and mental health. Journal of Photochemistry and Photobiology. B; Biology 2010;101(2):142-9.

6) Almeras, L., Eyles, D., Benech, P., et al. Developmental vitamin D deficiency alters brain protein expression in the adult rat: Implications for neuropsychiatric disorders. Proteomics 2007; 7(5):769-80.

7) Eyles, DW, Smith, S., Kinobe, R., et al. Distribution of the vitamin D receptor and 1-a-hydrolyase in human brain. Journal of Chemical Neuroanatomy 2005;29(1):21-30.

8) Eyles, DW, Burne, TH, McGrath, JJ. Vitamin D in fetal brain development. Seminars in Cell and Developmental Biology 2011;22(6):629-36.

9) Feron, F., Burne, TH, Brown, J., et al. Developmental vitamin D3 deficiency alters the adult rat brain. Brain Research Bulletin 2005;65(2):141-8.

10) Eyles, DW, Burne, TH, McGrath, JJ. Vitamin D, effects on brain development, adult brain function and the links between low levels of vitamin D and neuropsychiatric disease. Frontiers in Neuroendocrinology 2013;34(1):47-64.

11) Veenstra, TD, Prufer, K., Koenigsberger, C., et al. 1,25-Dihydroxyvitamin D3 receptors in the central nervous system of the rat embryo. Brain Research 1998;804(2):193-205.

12) Harms, LR, Burne, TH, Eyles, DW, et al. Vitamin D and the Brain. Best Practice & Research Clinical Endocrinology & Metabolism 2011;25(4):657-69.

13) Burkert, R., McGrath, JJ, Eyles, DW. Vitamin D receptor expression in the embryonic rat brain. Neuroscience Research Communications 2003;33(1):63-71.

14) Meguid, NA, Hashish, AF, Amwar, M., et al. Reduced serum levels of 25-hydroxy and 1,25-dihydroxy vitamin D in Egyptian children with autism. The Journal of Alternative and Complementary Medicine 2010;16(6):641-5.

15) Mostafa, GA, Al-Ayadhi, LY. Reduced serum concentrations of 25-hydroxy vitamin D in children with autism: Relation to autoimmunity. Journal of Neuroinflammation 2012;9:201.

16) Herndon, AC, DiGuiseppi, C., Johnson, SL, et al. Does nutritional intake differ between children and Autism Spectrum Disorders and children with typical development? Journal of Autism and Developmental Disorders 2009;39(2):212-22.

17) Molloy, CA, Kalkwarf, HJ, Manning-Courtney, P., et al. Plasma 25(OH)D concentration in children with autism spectrum disorder. Developmental Medicine and Child Neurology 2010;52(10):969-71.

18) Humble, MB, Gustafsson, S., Bejerot, S. Low serum levels of 25-hydroxyvitamin D (25-OHD) among psychiatric out-patients in Sweden: Relations with season, age, ethic origin and psychiatric diagnosis. Journal of Steroid Biochemistry and Molecular Biology 2010;121(1-2):467-70.

19) Dealberto, MJ. Prevalence of autism according to maternal immigrant status and ethnic origin. Acta Psychiatrica Scandinavica 2011;123(5):339-48.

20) EPA website. http://www.epa.gov/sunwise/doc/uvradiation.html. Visited 09/19/13.

21) Fernell, E., Barnevik-Olsson, M., Bagenholm, G. Serum levels of 25-hydroxyvitamin D in mothers of Swedish and of Somali origin who have children with and without autism. Acta Paediatrica 2010;99(5):743-7.

22) Whitehouse, AJ, Holt BJ, Serralha M. Maternal Vitamin D Levels and the Autism Phenotype Among Offspring. Journal of Autism and Developmental Disorders 2013;43(7):1495-504.

23) Committee Opinion No.495. Screening and Supplementation During Pregnancy. American College of Obstetricians and Gynecologists. Obstet Gynecol 2011;118:197-8.

Chapter 5D-I – Mercury pollution of fish

1) Chisso, Corp. (2011). Historical Overview of the Company. Retrieved from http://www.chisso.co.jp/english/company/time_line.html

2) Toshihide, T. Takashi Y, Soshi T, et al. Minamata disease: Catastrophic poisoning due to a failed public health response. 2009 Palgrave Macmillan 0197-5897 Journal of Public Health Policy 2009;30(1):54–67

3) Ekino S, Susa M, Ninomiya T,et al. Minamata disease revisited: an update on the acute and chronic manifestations of methyl mercury poisoning. J Neurol Sci. 2007;262(1-2):131-44.

4) Komyo, E. Masumi, M. and Motohiro, T. The pathology of methylmercury poisoning (Minamata disease). Neuropathology 2010;30:471–479.

5) Ministry of the Environment. (2002). Minamata disease the history and measures. Retrieved from http://www.env.go.jp/en/chemi/hs/minamata2002/ch3.html

6) Eto, K. Minamata Disease. Neuropathology. 2000 Sep;20 Suppl:S14-9.

7) Harada M. Global lessons of Minamata disease—a man's worth. Nihon Hansenbyo Gakkai Zasshi. 2009;78(1):55-60.

8) Jenks, J. L. The Minamata Disaster and the True Costs of Japanese Industrialization. In A. Andrea (Ed.), Perils of Progress: Environmental Disasters in the 20th Century. Upper Saddle River, NJ: Pearson, 2010.

9) Dales L, Kahn E, Wei E. Methylmercury poisoning. An assessment of the sportfish hazard in California. Calif Med. 1971;114(3):13-5.

10) Wing L, Potter D. The epidemiology of autistic spectrum disorders: is the prevalence rising? Ment Retard Dev Disabil Res Rev. 2002;8:151-161

11) Nelson KB, Bauman ML. Thimerosal and autism? Pediatrics. 2003;111(3):674–679.

12) Baker JP. Mercury, vaccines, and autism: One controversy, Three histories. American Journal of Public Health. 2008;98:244-53.

13) Southcott, RV. The neurological effects of noxious marine creatures. Contemporary Neurological Series. 1975;12:165-258.

14) Clarkson TW, Magos L. The toxicology of mercury and its chemical compounds. Crit Rev Toxicol. 2006;36(8):609-62.

15) Davidson PW, Myers GJ, Cox C, et al. Effects of prenatal and postnatal methylmercury exposure from fish consumption on neurodevelopment: outcomes at 66 months of age in the Seychelles Child Development Study. JAMA. 1998;280(8):701-7.

16) Davidson PW, Myers GJ, Weiss B, et al. Prenatal methyl mercury exposure from fish consumption and child development: a review of evidence and perspectives from the Seychelles Child Development Study. Neurotoxicology. 2006;27(6):1106-9.

17) Lyketsos CG. Should pregnant women avoid eating fish? Lessons from the Seychelles. Lancet. 2003;361(9370):1667-8.

18) Weihe P, Joensen HD. Dietary recommendations regarding pilot whale meat and blubber in the Faroe Islands. Int J Circumpolar Health. 2012;10;71:18594. doi: 10.3402/ijch.v71i0.18594.

19) Evaluation of certain food additives and contaminants (Sixty-first report of the

Chapter 5D-II – Mechanism of mercury pollution

1) Sakamoto M, Yasutake A, Domingo JL, et al. (2013). Relationship between trace element concentrations in chorionic tissue of placenta and umbilical cord tissue: Potential use as indicators for prenatal exposure. *Environ Int*60: 106-11.

2) Marques RC, Bernardi JV, Dórea JG, et al.(2013). Mercury transfer during pregnancy and breastfeeding: hair mercury concentrations as a biomarker. *Biol Trace Elem Res* 154(3): 1733-8.

3) Carrier G, Bouchard M, Brunet RC, Caza M. (2001). A toxicokinetic model for predicting the tissue distribution and elimination of organic and inorganicmercury following exposure to methyl mercury in animals and humans. II. Application and validation of the model in humans.*ToxicolApplPharmacol*171(1): 50-60.

4) Steinman G, Mankuta D. (2013). Insulin-like growth factor and the etiology of autism. *Med Hypoth*80: 475-80.

5) Onuma TA, Ding Y, Abraham E, et al. (2011). Regulation of temporation and spatial organization of newborn GnRH neurons by IGF signaling in zebrafish. *J Neurosci*31(33): 11814-24.

6) Beck KD, Powell-Braxton L, Widmer HR, et al. (1995). IGF1 gene disruption results in reduced brain size, CNS hypomyelination, and loss of hippocampal granule and striatal parvalbumin-containing neurons. *Neuron* 14: 717-30.

7) Tropea D, Giacometti E, Wilson NR, et al. (2009). Partial reversal of Rett Syndrome-like symptoms in MeCP2 mutant mice. *ProcNatlAcadSci*109106(6): 2029-34.

8) Sara VR, Carlsson-Skwirut C. (1988). The role of insulin-like factors in the regulation of brain development. *Prog Brain Res* 73: 87-99.

9) Waly M, Olteanu H, Banerjee R, et al. Activation of methionine synthase by insulin-like growth factor-1 and dopamine: a target for neurodevelopmental toxins and thimerosal.*Mol Psychiatry* 9(4): 358-70.

10) Fahrion JK, Komuro Y, Li Y, et al. (2012). Rescue of neuronal migration deficits in a mouse model of fetal Minamata disease by increasing neuronal Ca2+ spike frequency. *ProcNatlAcadSci*109(13): 5057-62.

11) Zikopolous B, Barbas H. (2010). Changes in prefrontal axons may disrupts the network in autism. *J Neurosci*30(44): 14595-609.

12) Damarla SR, Keller TA, Kana RK, et al. (2010). Cortical underocnnectivity coupled with preserved visuospatial cognition in autism: Evidence from an fMRI study of an embedded figures task. *Autism Res*3(5): 273-9.

13) Deoni SC, Mercure E, Blasi A, et al. (2011). Mapping infant brain myelination with magnetic resonance imaging. *J Neurosci*31(2): 784-91.

14) Wass S. (2011). Distortions and disconnections: disrupted brain connectivity in autism. *Brain Cogn*75(1): 18-28.

15) Windebank AJ. (1986). Specific inhibition of myelination by lead in vitro: comparison with arsenic, thallium, and mercury. *ExpNeurol*94(1): 203-12.

16) Stankovic R. (2006). Atrophy of large myelinated motor axons and declining muscle grip strength following mercury vapor inhalation in mice. *InhalToxicol*18(1): 57-69.

17) Vargas DL, Nascimbene C, Krishnan et al. (2005). Neuroglial activation and neuroinflammation in the brain of patients with autism. *Ann Neurol*57(1): 67-81.

18) Lee RH, Mills EA, Schwartz N, et al. (2010). Neurodevelopmental effects of chronic exposure to elevated levels of pro-inflammatory cytokines in a developing visual system. *Neural Dev*5(2): 1749-8104.

19) Gardner RM, Nyland JF, Silbergeld EK. (2010). Differential immunotoxic effects of inorganic and organic mercury species in vitro. *ToxicolLett*198(2): 182-90.

20) Gardner RM, Nyland JF, Silva IA, et al. (2010). Mercury exposure, serum antinuclear/antinucleolar antibodies, and serum cytokine levels in mining population in Amazonian Brazil: a cross-sectional study. *Environ Res* 110(4): 345-54.

21) Ni M, Li X, Yin Z, et al. (2011). Comparative study on the response of rat primary astrocytes and microglia to methylmercury toxicity. *Glia* 59(5): 810-20.

22) Itoh K, Korogi Y, Tomiguchi S, et al. (2001). Cerebellar blood flow in methylmercury poisoning (Minamata disease). *Neuroradiology* 43(4): 279-84.

23) Williams CA, Dagli A, Battaglia A. (2008). Genetic disorders associated with macrocephaly. *Am J Med Genet A* 146A(15): 2023-37.

24) Peltz A, Sherwani SI, Kotha SR, et al. Calcium and calmodulin regulate mercury-induced phospholipase D activation in vascular endothelial cells. *Int J Toxicol*28(3): 190-206.

25) Yao Y, Walsh WJ, McGinnis WR, Pratico D. (2006). Altered vascular phenotype in autism: correlation with oxidative stress. *Arch Neurol*63(8): 1161-4.

26) Sakamoto M, Yasutake A, Domingo JL, Chan HM, Kubota M, Murata K. (2013). Relationship between trace element concentrations in chorionic tissue of placenta and umbilical cord tissue: Potential use as indicators for prenatal exposure. *Environ Int*60: 106-11.

27) Marques RC, Bernardi JV, Dórea JG, et al. (2013). Mercury transfer during pregnancy and breastfeeding: hair mercury concentrations as a biomarker. *Biol Trace Elem Res* 154(3): 1733-8.

28) Carrier G, Bouchard M, Brunet RC, Caza M. (2001). A toxicokinetic model for predicting the tissue distribution and elimination of organic and inorganicmercury following exposure to methyl mercury in animals and humans. II. Application and validation of the model in humans.*ToxicolApplPharmacol*171(1): 50-60.

29) Steinman G, Mankuta D. (2013). Insulin-like growth factor and the etiology of autism. *Med Hypoth*80: 475-80.

30) Onuma TA, Ding Y, Abraham E, et al. (2011). Regulation of temporation and spatial organization of newborn GnRH neurons by IGF signaling in zebrafish. *J Neurosci*31(33): 11814-24.

31) Beck KD, Powell-Braxton L, Widmer HR, et al. (1995). IGF1 gene disruption results in reduced brain size, CNS hypomyelination, and loss of hippocampal granule and striatal parvalbumin-containing neurons. *Neuron* 14: 717-30.

32) Tropea D, Giacometti E, Wilson NR, et al. (2009). Partial reversal of Rett Syndrome-like symptoms in MeCP2 mutant mice. *ProcNatlAcadSci*109106(6): 2029-34.

33) Sara VR, Carlsson-Skwirut C. (1988). The role of insulin-like factors in the regulation of brain development. *Prog Brain Res* 73: 87-99.

34) Waly M, Olteanu H, Banerjee R, et al. (2004). Activation of methionine synthase by insulin-like growth factor-1 and dopamine: a target for neurodevelopmental toxins and thimerosal.*Mol Psychiatry* 9(4): 358-70.

35) Fahrion JK, Komuro Y, Li Y, et al. (2012). Rescue of neuronal migration deficits in a mouse model of fetal Minamata disease by increasing neuronal Ca2+ spike frequency. *ProcNatlAcadSci*109(13): 5057-62.

36) Zikopolous B, Barbas H. (2010). Changes in prefrontal axons may disrupts the network in autism. *J Neurosci*30(44): 14595-609.

37) Damarla SR, Keller TA, Kana RK, et al. (2010). Cortical underconnectivity coupled with preserved visuospatial cognition in autism: Evidence from an fMRI study of an embedded figures task. *Autism Res*3(5): 273-9.

38) Deoni SC, Mercure E, Blasi A, et al. (2011). Mapping infant brain myelination with magnetic resonance imaging. *J Neurosci*31(2): 784-91.

39) Wass S. (2011). Distortions and disconnections: disrupted brain connectivity in autism. *Brain Cogn*75(1): 18-28.

40) Windebank AJ. (1986). Specific inhibition of myelination by lead in vitro: comparison with arsenic, thallium, and mercury. *ExpNeurol*94(1): 203-12.

41) Stankovic R. (2006). Atrophy of large myelinated motor axons and declining muscle grip strength following mercury vapor inhalation in mice. *InhalToxicol*18(1): 57-69.

42) Vargas DL, Nascimbene C, Krishnan C, et al. (2005). Neuroglial activation and neuroinflammation in the brain of patients with autism. *Ann Neurol*57(1): 67-81.

43) Lee RH, Mills EA, Schwartz N, et al. (2010). Neurodevelopmental effects of chronic exposure to elevated levels of pro-inflammatory cytokines in a developing visual system. *Neural Dev*5(2): 1749-8104.

44) Gardner RM, Nyland JF, Silbergeld EK. (2010). Differential immunotoxic effects of inorganic and organic mercury species in vitro. *ToxicolLett*198(2): 182-90.

45) Gardner RM, Nyland JF, Silva IA, et al. (2010). Mercury exposure, serum antinuclear/antinucleolar antibodies, and serum cytokine levels in mining population in Amazonian Brazil: a cross-sectional study. *Environ Res* 110(4): 345-54.

46) Ni M, Li X, Yin Z, S, et al. (2011). Comparative study on the response of rat primary astrocytes and microglia to methylmercury toxicity. *Glia* 59(5): 810-20.

47) Itoh K, Korogi Y, Tomiguchi S, et al. (2001). Cerebellar blood flow in methylmercury poisoning (Minamata disease). *Neuroradiology* 43(4): 279-84.

48) Williams CA, Dagli A, Battaglia A. (2008). Genetic disorders associated with macrocephaly. *Am J Med Genet A* 146A(15): 2023-37.

49) Peltz A, Sherwani SI, Kotha SR, Mazerik JN, et al. (2009). Calcium and calmodulin regulate mercury-induced phospholipase D activation in vascular endothelial cells. *Int J Toxicol*28(3): 190-206.

Chapter 5D-III – Mercury vs. omega-3 fats

1) Garrecht,M, Austin DW. The plausibility of a role for mercury in the etiology of autism: a cellular perspective. *Toxicology Environ Chem.* 2011; 93(5-6):1251-73.

2) Hites R, Foran J. Global Assessment of Organic Contaminants in Farmed Salmon. Science 2004; 6: 226-29.

3) Innis, SM. Dietary omega 3 fatty acids and the developing brain. Brain Res. 2008;1237:35-43.

4) Burger J, Jeitner C. Mercury and selenium levels, and selenium: mercury molar ratios of brain, muscle and other tissues in bluefish (Pomatomus saltatrix) from New Jersey, USA. Science of the Total Environment 2013;443;278–86.

5) Smith, KL, Guentzel,JL. Mercury concentrations and omega-3 fatty acids in fish and shrimp: Preferential consumption for maximum health benefits. Marine Pollution Bulletin 2010;60:1615–18.

6) Kelly B, Ikonomou M, Higgs D, et al. Mercury and Other Trace Elements in Farmed and Wild Salmon From British Columbia, Canada. Environmental Toxicology and Chemistry . 2008;27(6):1361-70.

7) Marsh DO, Clarkson TW. The Seychelles study of fetal methylmercury exposure and child development. Neurotoxicology. 1995;16(4):583-96.

8) Mozaffarian D, Rimm EB. Fish intake, contaminants, and human health: evaluating the risks and benefits. JAMA 2006; 296(15):1885-99.

9) Ouedraogo O, Amyot M. Effect of various cooking methods and food components on bioaccessibility of mercury from fish. Environmental Research 2009;111:1064-69.

10) Politi P, Cena H, Cornelli M, et al. Behavioral effects of omega-3 Fatty acid supplementation in young adults with severe autism: an open label study. Arch Med Res. 2008;39(7):682-5.

11) Rodrigues MV, Yamatogi RS, Sudano MJ, et al. Mercury concentrations in South Atlantic swordfish, Xiphias gladius, caught off the coast of Brazil. Bull Environ Contam Toxicology 2013;90(6):697-701.

12) Sapkota A, Sapkota AR, Kucharski M, et al. Aquaculture practices and potential human health risks: Current knowledge and future priorities. Environmental International 2008;34:1215-26.

13) United States Environmental Protection Agency (EPA). Consumption advice: joint federal advisory for mercury in fish; backgrounder for the 2004 FDA/EPA consumer advisory: what you need to know about mercury in fish and shellfish. Washington (DC). http://water.epa.gov/scitech/swguidance/fishshellfish/outreach/factsheet.cfm 2013, Dec. 2.

14) United States Environmental Protection Agency (EPA). Trends in blood mercury concentrations and fish consumption among U.S. women of childbearing age NHANES, 1999- 2010. Final Report July 2013. Washington (DC): Report No.: EPA-823-R-13-022. http://water.epa.gov/scitech/swguidance/fishshellfish/fishadvisories/upload/Trends-in-Blood-Mercury-Concentrations-and-Fish-Consumption-Among-U-S-Women-of-Childbearing-Age-NHANES-1999-2010.pdf 2013, Dec. 2.

15) Wijngaarden EV, Davidson PW, Smith TH et al. Autism spectrum disorder phenotypes and prenatal exposure to methylmercury. Epidemiology 2013;24(5):651-59.

16) National Health and Nutrition Examination Survey [internet]. 2013. Washington (DC): National Center for Health Statistics. Available from: http://www.cdc.gov/nchs/nhanes.htm (accessed 2014, Jan. 11).

Chapter 6A - Myelination

1) A. J. Barkovich. Magnetic resonance techniques in the assessment of myelin and myelination. Journal of Inherited Metabolic Disease. 2005;28(3):311-43.

2) Courchesne E, Karns CM, Davis HR, et al. Unusual brain growth patterns in early life in patients with autistic disorder: an MRI study. Neurology 2001;57(2):245-54.

3) Aylward EH, Minshew NJ, Field K, et al. Effects of age on brain volume and head circumference e in autism. Neurology 2002;59(2):175-83.

4) Aoki ,Y, Abe ,O, Nippashi ,Y, et al. Comparison of white matter integrity between autism spectrum disorder subjects and typically developing individuals: a meta analysis of diffusion tensor imaging tractography studies. Molecular Autism 2013; 4:25.

5) Courchesne E, Pierce K. Why the frontal cortex in autism might be talking only to itself: local over-connectivity but long-distance disconnection. Curr Opin Neurobiol. 2005;15: 225-30.

6) Zikopoulos B, Barbas H. Changes in Prefrontal Axons May Disrupt the network in Autism. Journal of Neuroscience. 30(44): 14595-609.

7) Rasband MN, Macklin WB. Myelin structure and biochemistry. in: Brady ST, Siegel GJ, Albers RW, Price DL, editors. Basic Neurochemistry: Principles of Molecular, Cellular, and Medical Neurobiology. Oxford: Elsevier, 2012. p. 180-197.

8) Nelson CA, Luciana M. Handbook of Developmental Cognitive Neuroscience. MIT Press, 2008.

9) Paul LK, Brown WS, Adolphs R, et al. Agenesis of the corpus callosum: genetic, development and functional aspects of connectivity. Nature Reviews Neuroscience.2007; 8: 287-99.

10) Krestel H, Annoni J-M, Jagella. White matter in aphasia: A historical review of the Dejerine's Studies. Brain and Language. Online publication 26 July 2013.

11) Mostafa GA, El-Sayed ZA, El-Aziz MMA, et al. Serum Anti-Myelin—Associated Glycoprotein Antibodies in Egyptian Autistic Children. J Child Neurol. 2008, 23:1413-8.

12) Vojdani A, Campbell AW, Anyanwu E, et al. Antibodies to neuron-pecific antigen in children with autism: possible cross reaction with encephalitogenic proteins from milk, Chlamydia pneumonia and Streptococcus Group A. Journal of Neuroimmunology 2002; 129:168-77.

13) Whitaker-Azmitia PM. Serotonin and brain development: Role in human developmental diseases. Brain Research Bulletin. 2001;5: 479-85.

14) Mostafa GA, Al-Ayadhi LY. A lack of association between hyperseronemia and the increased frequency of serum anti-myelin basic protein auto-antibodies in autistic children. Journal of Neuroinflammation 2011;8:71.

15) Steinman G, Mankuta, D. Insulin-like growth factor and the etiology of autism. Medical Hypotheses 2013;80:475-80.

16) Steinman, G, Mankuta, D. Predicting autism at birth. Medical Hypotheses 2013;81:21-25.

17) Stoner, R, Chow, M, Boyle, MP, et al. Patches of disorganization in the neocortex of children with autism. NEJM 2014;370(13):1209-19.

Chapter 6B - Infection

1) Adams Waldorf, K.M. and R.M. McAdams, Influence of infection during pregnancy on fetal development. Reproduction, 2013;146(5):R151-62.

2) Libbey, J.E., et al., Autistic disorder and viral infections. J Neurovirol, 2005; 11(1): 1-10.

3) Zhao, J., et al., Effect of intrauterine infection on brain development and injury. Int J Dev Neurosci, 2013;31(7):543-49.

4) Depino, A.M., Peripheral and central inflammation in autism spectrum disorders. Mol Cell Neurosci, 2013; 53: 69-76.

5) Atladottir, H.O., et al., Autism after infection, febrile episodes, and antibiotic use during pregnancy: an exploratory study. Pediatrics, 2012. 130(6): e1447-54.

6) Atladottir, HO, Thorsin, P, Ostergaard, L, et al., Maternal infection requiring hospitalization during pregnancy and autism spectrum disorders. J Autism Dev Disord, 2010;40(12):1423-30.

7) Garay, PA, Hsaio, EY, Patterson, PH, et al., Maternal immune activation causes age- and region-specific changes in brain cytokines in offspring throughout development. Brain Behav Immun, 2013;31:54-68.

8) Patterson, P.H., Maternal infection and immune involvement in autism. Trends Mol Med, 2011;17(7):389-94.

9) David, J, Mortari,F, Chemokine receptors: A brief overview. Clinical and Applied Immunology Reviews, 2000;1(2): 105-25.

10) Oskvig, D.B., Elkahloun, AG, Johnson, KR, et al., Maternal immune activation by LPS selectively alters specific gene expression profiles of interneuron migration and oxidative stress in the fetus without triggering a fetal immune response. Brain Behav Immun, 2012;26(4):623-34.

11) Parker-Athill, E.C., Tan, J. Maternal immune activation and autism spectrum disorder: interleukin-6 signaling as a key mechanistic pathway. Neurosignals, 2010; 18(2): 113-28.

12) Paintlia, M.K., et al., N-acetylcysteine prevents endotoxin-induced degeneration of oligodendrocyte progenitors and hypomyelination in developing rat brain. J Neurosci Res, 2004; 78(3): 347-61.

13) Rezai-Zadeh, K, Ehrhart, J, Bai, Y, et al., Apigenin and luteolin modulate microglial activation via inhibition of STAT1-induced CD40 expression. J Neuroinflammation, 2008;5: 41.

14) Parker-Athill, E, Luo, d, Baiey, A, et al., Flavonoids, a prenatal prophylaxis via targeting JAK2/STAT3 signaling to oppose IL-6/MIA associated autism. J Neuroimmunol, 2009;217(1-2): 20-7.

Chapter 6C - Inflammation

1) Theoharides TC, Angelidou A, Alysandratos KD, et al. Mast cell activation and autism, Biochimica et Biophysica Acta (BBA) - Molecular Basis of Disease,2012;1822(1):34-41.

2) Theoharides TC, Asadi S, Patel AB. Focal brain inflammation and autism. J Neuroinflammation. 2013;10:46.

3) Roberts AL, Lyall K, Hart JE, et al. Perinatal Air Pollutant Exposures and Autism Spectrum Disorder in the Children of Nurses' Health Study II Participants. Environ Health Perspect. 2013;121(8):978-84.

4) Theoharides TC. Is a subtype of autism an allergy of the brain? Clinical Therapeutics. 2013;35(5):584-91.

5) Kempuraj D, Asadi S, Zhang B, et al. Mercury induces inflammatory mediator release from human mast cells. J Neuroinflammation. 2010;7:20.

6) Steinman G, Mankuta D. Insulin-like growth factor and the etiology of autism. Med Hypotheses. 2013;80(4):475-80.

7) Rodriguez JI, Kern JK. Evidence of microglial activation in autism and its possible role in brain underconnectivity. Neuron Glia Biol. 2011;7(2-4):205-13.

8) Kettenmann H, Kirchhoff F, Verkhratsky A. Microglia: new roles for the synaptic stripper. Neuron. 2013;77(1):10-8.

9) Tetreault NA, Hakeem AY, Jiang S, et al. Microglia in the cerebral cortex in autism. J Autism Dev Disord. 2012;42(12):2569-84.

10) Beck KF, Eberhardt W, Frank S, et al. Inducible NO synthase: role in cellular signalling. J Exp Biol. 1999;202(Pt 6):645-53.

11) Tostes MH, Teixeira HC, Gattaz WF, et al. Altered neurotrophin, neuropeptide, cytokines and nitric oxide levels in autism. Pharmacopsychiatry. 2012;45(6):241-3.

12) Sweeten TL, Posey DJ, Shankar S, et al. High nitric oxide production in autistic disorder: a possible role for interferon-gamma. Biol Psychiatry. 2004;55(4):434-7.

13) Ebisch SJ, Gallese V, Willems RM, et al. Altered intrinsic functional connectivity of anterior and posterior insula regions in high-functioning participants with autism spectrum disorder. Hum Brain Mapp. 2011;32(7):1013-28.

14) Brown CM, Mulcahey TA, Filipek NC, et al. Production of proinflammatory cytokines and chemokines during neuroinflammation: novel roles for estrogen receptors alpha and beta. Endocrinology. 2010;151(10):4916-25.

15) Theoharides TC, Zhang B. Neuro-inflammation, blood-brain barrier, seizures and autism. J Neuroinflammation. 2011;8:168.

16) Hsiao EY, McBride SW, Chow J, et al. Modeling an autism risk factor in mice leads to permanent immune dysregulation. Proc Natl Acad Sci U S A. 2012;109(31):12776-81.

17) Buehler MR. A proposed mechanism for autism: an aberrant neuroimmune response manifested as a psychiatric disorder. Med Hypotheses. 2011;76(6):863-70.

18) Stolp HB, Dziegielewska KM. Review: Role of developmental inflammation and blood-brain barrier dysfunction in neurodevelopmental and neurodegenerative diseases. Neuropathol Appl Neurobiol. 2009;35(2):132-46.

19) Depino AM. Peripheral and central inflammation in autism spectrum disorders. Mol Cell Neurosci. 2013;53:69-76.

20) Zorzella-Pezavento SF, Chiuso-Minicucci F, França TG, et al. Persistent Inflammation in the CNS during Chronic EAE Despite Local Absence of IL-17 Production. Mediators Inflamm. 2013;2013:519-27.

21) Beeton C, Garcia A, Chandy KG. Induction and clinical scoring of chronic-relapsing experimental autoimmune encephalomyelitis. J Vis Exp. 2007;(5):224.

22) Egwuagu CE, Larkin Iii J. Therapeutic targeting of STAT pathways in CNS autoimmune diseases. JAKSTAT. 2013 Jan 1;2(1):e24134 Review.

23) Lavrnja I, Savic D, Bjelobaba I, et al. The effect of ribavirin on reactive astrogliosis in experimental autoimmune encephalomyelitis. J Pharmacol Sci. 2012;119(3):221-32.

24) Kreutzberg GW. Microglia: a sensor for pathological events in the CNS. Trends Neurosci. 1996 Aug;19(8):312-8. Review.

25) Centonze D, Muzio L, Rossi S, et al. Inflammation triggers synaptic alteration and degeneration in experimental autoimmune encephalomyelitis. J Neurosci. 2009;29(11):3442-52.

26) van Horssen J, Witte ME, Schreibelt G, et al. Radical changes in multiple sclerosis pathogenesis. Biochim Biophys Acta. 2011;1812(2):141-50.

27) Sospedra M, Martin R. Immunology of multiple sclerosis. Annu Rev Immunol. 2005;23:683-747. Review.

28) Shindler KS, Guan Y, Ventura E, et al. Retinal ganglion cell loss induced by acute optic neuritis in a relapsing model of multiple sclerosis. Mult Scler. 2006;12(5):526-32.

29) Baruth JM, Wall CA, Patterson MC, et al. Proton magnetic resonance spectroscopy as a probe into the pathophysiology of autism spectrum disorders (ASD): a review. Autism Res. 2013;6(2):119-33.

30) Bejjani A, O'Neill J, Kim JA, et al. Elevated glutamatergic compounds in pregenual anterior cingulate in pediatric autism spectrum disorder demonstrated by 1H MRS and 1H MRSI. PLoS One. 2012;7(7):e38786.

31) Brown MS, Singel D, Hepburn S, et al. Increased glutamate concentration in the auditory cortex of persons with autism and first-degree relatives: a (1)H-MRS study. Autism Res. 2013;6(1):1-10.

32) Horder J, Lavender T, Mendez MA, et al. Reduced subcortical glutamate/glutamine in adults with autism spectrum disorders: a [¹H]MRS study. Transl Psychiatry. 2013 Jul 9;3:e279.

33) Shinohe A, Hashimoto K, Nakamura K, et al. Increased serum levels of glutamate in adult patients with autism. Prog Neuropsychopharmacol Biol Psychiatry. 2006;30(8):1472-7.

34) Li X, Chauhan A, Sheikh AM, et al. Elevated immune response in the brain of autistic patients. J Neuroimmunol. 2009;207(1-2):111-6.

35) Dutt M, Tabuena P, Ventura E, et al. Timing of corticosteroid therapy is critical to prevent retinal ganglion cell loss in experimental optic neuritis. Invest Ophthalmol Vis Sci. 2010;51(3):1439-45.

36) Arnold AC. Evolving management of optic neuritis and multiple sclerosis. Am J Ophthalmol. 2005;139(6):1101-8. Review.

37) Trip SA, Schlottmann PG, Jones SJ, et al. Retinal nerve fiber layer axonal loss and visual dysfunction in optic neuritis. Ann Neurol. 2005;58(3):383-91.

38) Ecker C, Ronan L, Feng Y, et al. Intrinsic gray-matter connectivity of the brain in adults with autism spectrum disorder. Proc Natl Acad Sci U S A. 2013;110(32):13222-7.

39) Hendry J, DeVito T, Gelman N, et al. White matter abnormalities in autism detected through transverse relaxation time imaging. Neuroimage. 2006;29(4):1049-57.

40) Palmer AM. The role of the blood brain barrier in neurodegenerative disorders and their treatment. J Alzheimers Dis. 2011;24(4):643-56.

41) Goines PE, Croen LA, Braunschweig D, et al. Increased midgestational IFN-γ, IL-4 and IL-5 in women bearing a child with autism: A case-control study. Mol Autism. 2011;2:13.

42) Ponzio NM, Servatius R, Beck K, et al. Cytokine levels during pregnancy influence immunological profiles and neurobehavioral patterns of the offspring. Ann N Y Acad Sci. 2007;1107:118-28.

43) Molloy CA, Morrow AL, Meinzen-Derr J, et al. Elevated cytokine levels in children with autism spectrum disorder. J Neuroimmunol. 2006;172(1-2):198-205.

44) Singh VK. Plasma increase of interleukin-12 and interferon-gamma. Pathological significance in autism. J Neuroimmunol. 1996;66(1-2):143-5.

45) Croonenberghs J, Bosmans E, Deboutte D, et al. Activation of the inflammatory response system in autism.Neuropsychobiology. 2002;45(1):1-6.

46) Gupta S, Aggarwal S, Rashanravan B, et al. Th1- and Th2-like cytokines in CD4+ and CD8+ T cells in autism. J Neuroimmunol. 1998;85(1):106-9.

47) Gupta S, Aggarwal S, Heads C. Dysregulated immune system in children with autism: beneficial effects of intravenous immune globulin on autistic characteristics. J Autism Dev Disord. 1996;26(4):439-52.

48) Croonenberghs J, Wauters A, Devreese K, et al. Increased serum albumin, gamma globulin, immunoglobulin IgG, and IgG2 and IgG4 in autism. Psychol Med. 2002;32(8):1457-63

49) Al-Ayadhi LY, Mostafa GA. Elevated serum levels of interleukin-17A in children with autism. J Neuroinflammation. 2012;9:158.

50) Banks WA, Kastin AJ, Gutierrez EG. Penetration of interleukin-6 across the murine blood-brain barrier. Neurosci Lett. 1994;179(1-2):53-6.

51) Arima Y, Kamimura D, Sabharwal L, et al. Regulation of immune cell infiltration into the CNS by regional neural inputs explained by the gate theory. Mediators Inflamm. 2013;2013:898165.

52) Nishioku T, Matsumoto J, Dohgu S, et al. Tumor necrosis factor-alpha mediates the blood-brain barrier dysfunction induced by activated microglia in mouse brain microvascular endothelial cells. J Pharmacol Sci. 2010;112(2):251-4.

53) Mazur-Kolecka B, Cohen IL, Gonzalez M, et al. Autoantibodies against neuronal progenitors in sera from children with autism. Brain Dev. 2013,Jul 6.pii:50387-7604.

54) Colton CA, Gilbert DL. Production of superoxide anions by a CNS macrophage, the microglia. FEBS Lett. 1987;223(2):284-8.

55) Bennett J, Basivireddy J, Kollar A, et al. Blood-brain barrier disruption and enhanced vascular permeability in the multiple sclerosis model EAE. J Neuroimmunol. 2010;229(1-2):180-91.

56) Ignarro RS, Vieira AS, Sartori CR, et al. JAK2 inhibition is neuroprotective and reduces astrogliosis after quinolinic acid striatal lesion in adult mice. J Chem Neuroanat. 2013;48-49:14-22.

57) Hariri RJ, Chang VA, Barie PS, et al. Traumatic injury induces interleukin-6 production by human astrocytes. Brain Res. 1994;636(1):139-42.

58) Okada S, Nakamura M, Mikami Y, et al. Blockade of interleukin-6 receptor suppresses reactive astrogliosis and ameliorates functional recovery in experimental spinal cord injury. J Neurosci Res. 2004;76(2):265-76.

59) McCoy MK, Tansey MG. TNF signaling inhibition in the CNS: implications for normal brain function and neurodegenerative disease. J Neuroinflammation. 2008;5:45.

60) Carpentier PA, Dingman AL, Palmer TD. Placental TNF-α signaling in illness-induced complications of pregnancy. Am J Pathol. 2011;178(6):2802-10.

61) Rossignol DA, Frye RE. Mitochondrial dysfunction in autism spectrum disorders: a systematic review and meta-analysis. Mol Psychiatry. 2012;17(3):290-314.

62) Honorat JA, Kinoshita M, Okuno T, et al. Xanthine oxidase mediates axonal and myelin loss in a murine model of multiple sclerosis. PLoS One. 2013;8(8):e71329.

63) Das UN. Autism as a disorder of deficiency of brain-derived neurotrophic factor and altered metabolism of polyunsaturated fatty acids.Nutrition. 2013;29(10):1175-85.

64) Perry EK, Lee ML, Martin-Ruiz CM, et al. Cholinergic activity in autism: abnormalities in the cerebral cortex and basal forebrain. Am J Psychiatry. 2001;158(7):1058-66.

65) Das UN. Can vagus nerve stimulation halt or ameliorate rheumatoid arthritis and lupus? Lipids Health Dis. 2011;10:19.

66) Deutsch SI, Urbano MR, Burket JA, et al.Pharmacotherapeutic implications of the association between genomic instability at chromosome 15q13.3 and autism spectrum disorders. Clin Neuropharmacol. 2011;34(6):203-5.

67) Yao X, Huang J, Zhong H, et al. Targeting Interleukin-6 in Inflammatory Autoimmune Diseases and Cancers. Pharmacol Ther. 2014;141(2):125-39.

68) Naugler WE, Karin M. The wolf in sheep's clothing: the role of interleukin-6 in immunity, inflammation and cancer. Trends Mol Med. 2008 Mar;14(3):109-19.

69) Tanabe K, Matsushima-Nishiwaki R, Yamaguchi S, et al. Mechanisms of tumor necrosis factor-alpha-induced interleukin-6 synthesis in glioma cells. J Neuroinflammation. 2010;7:16.

70) Heinrich PC, Behrmann I, Haan S, et al. Principles of interleukin (IL)-6-type cytokine signalling and its regulation. Biochem J. 2003;374(Pt 1):1-20. Review.

71) Deng MY, Lam S, Meyer U, et al. Frontal-subcortical protein expression following prenatal exposure to maternal inflammation. PLoS One. 2011;6(2):e16638.

72) Fahmi A, Smart N, Punn A, et al. p42/p44-MAPK and PI3K are sufficient for IL-6 family cytokines/gp130 to signal to hypertrophy and survival in cardiomyocytes in the absence of JAK/STAT activation. Cell Signal. 2013;25(4):898-909.

73) Aida Y, Honda K, Tanigawa S, et al. IL-6 and soluble IL-6 receptor stimulate the production of MMPs and their inhibitors via JAK-STAT and ERK-MAPK signalling in human chondrocytes. Cell Biol Int. 2012;36(4):367-76.

74) Akira S. IL-6-regulated transcription factors. Int J Biochem Cell Biol. 1997;29(12):1401-18. Review.

75) Rébé C, Végran F, Berger H, et al. STAT3 activation: A key factor in tumor immunoescape. JAKSTAT. 2013;2(1):e23010. Review.

76) Swiatek-Machado K, Kaminska B. STAT signaling in glioma cells. Adv Exp Med Biol. 2013;986:189-208. Review.

77) Zhang S, Morrison JL, Gill A, et al. Maternal dietary restriction during the periconceptional period in normal weight or obese ewes results in adrenocortical hypertrophy, an upregulation of

the JAK/STAT and downregulation of the IGF1R signalling pathways in the adrenal of the postnatal lamb. Endocrinology. 2013;154(12):4650-62.

78) Zong CS, Chan J, Levy DE, et al. Mechanism of STAT3 activation by insulin-like growth factor I receptor. J Biol Chem. 2000;275(20):15099-105.

79) Inaba M, Saito H, Fujimoto M, et al. Suppressor of cytokine signaling 1 suppresses muscle differentiation through modulation of IGF-I receptor signal transduction. Biochem Biophys Res Commun. 2005;328(4):953-61

80) Shalita-Chesner M, Glaser T, Werner H. Signal transducer and activator of transcription-1 (STAT1), but not STAT5b, regulates IGF-I receptor gene expression in an osteosarcoma cell line. J Pediatr Endocrinol Metab. 2004;17(2):211-8.

81) Parker-Athill E, Luo D, Bailey A, et al. Flavonoids, a prenatal prophylaxis via targeting JAK2/STAT3 signaling to oppose IL-6/MIA associated autism. J Neuroimmunol. 2009;217(1-2):20-7.

82) He F, Ge W, Martinowich K, et al. A positive autoregulatory loop of Jak-STAT signaling controls the onset of astrogliogenesis. Nat Neurosci. 2005;8(5):616-25.

83) Oskvig DB, Elkahloun AG, Johnson KR, et al. Maternal immune activation by LPS selectively alters specific gene expression profiles of interneuron migration and oxidative stress in the fetus without triggering a fetal immune response. Brain Behav Immun. 2012;26(4):623-34.

84) Hsiao EY, Patterson PH. Activation of the maternal immune system induces endocrine changes in the placenta via IL-6.Brain Behav Immun. 2011;25(4):604-15.

85) Park SY, Baik YH, Cho JH, et al. Inhibition of lipopolysaccharide-induced nitric oxide synthesis by nicotine through S6K1-p42/44 MAPK pathway and STAT3 (Ser 727) phosphorylation in Raw 264.7 cells. Cytokine. 2008;44(1):126-34.

86) Yamashita T, Sawamoto K, Suzuki S, et al. Blockade of interleukin-6 signaling aggravates ischemic cerebral damage in mice: possible involvement of Stat3 activation in the protection of neurons. J Neurochem. 2005;94(2):459-68.

87) Planas AM, Gorina R, Chamorro A. Signalling pathways mediating inflammatory responses in brain ischaemia.Biochem Soc Trans. 2006;34(Pt 6):1267-70. Review.

88) Bellik L, Vinci MC, Filippi S, et al. Intracellular pathways triggered by the selective FLT-1-agonist placental growth factor in vascular smooth muscle cells exposed to hypoxia. Br J Pharmacol. 2005;146(4):568-75.

89) Arrode-Brusés G, Brusés JL. Maternal immune activation by poly I:C induces expression of cytokines IL-1β and IL-13, chemokine MCP-1 and colony stimulating factor VEGF in fetal mouse brain. J Neuroinflammation. 2012;9:83.

90) Kim do Y, Hao J, Liu R, et al. Inflammation-mediated memory dysfunction and effects of a ketogenic diet in a murine model of multiple sclerosis. PLoS One. 2012;7(5):e35476.

91) Ruskin DN, Svedova J, Cote JL, et al. Ketogenic diet improves core symptoms of autism in BTBR mice. PLoS One. 2013;8(6):e65021

92) McFarlane HG, Kusek GK, Yang M, et al. Autism-like behavioral phenotypes in BTBR T+tf/J mice. Genes Brain Behav. 2008;7(2):152-63.

93) Moy SS, Nadler JJ, Perez A, et al. Sociability and preference for social novelty in five inbred strains: an approach to assess autistic-like behavior in mice. Genes Brain Behav. 2004;3(5):287-302.

94) Herbert MR, Buckley JA. Autism and dietary therapy: case report and review of the literature. J Child Neurol. 2013;28(8):975-82.

95) Cunningham AB, Schreibman L. Stereotypy in Autism: The Importance of Function. Res Autism Spectr Disord. 2008;2(3):469-479.

96) Ramaekers VT, Sequeira JM, Blau N, et al. A milk-free diet downregulates folate receptor autoimmunity in cerebral folate deficiency syndrome. Dev Med Child Neurol. 2008;50(5):346-52.

97) Sussman D, Ellegood J, Henkelman M. A gestational ketogenic diet alters maternal metabolic status as well as offspring physiological growth and brain structure in the neonatal mouse. BMC Pregnancy Childbirth. 2013 Oct;13(1):198.

98) Yoon JR, Kim HD, Kang HC. Lower fat and better quality diet therapy for children with pharmacoresistant epilepsy. Korean J Pediatr. 2013;56(8):327-331.

99) Kim JT, Kang HC, Song JE, et al. Catch-up growth after long-term implementation and weaning from ketogenic diet in pediatric epileptic patients. Clin Nutr. 2013;32(1):98-103.

100) Mobbs CV, Mastaitis J, Isoda F, et al. Treatment of diabetes and diabetic complications with a ketogenic diet. J Child Neurol. 2013;28(8):1009-14.

101) Liu YM, Lowe H, Zak MM, et al. Can children with hyperlipidemia receive ketogenic diet for medication-resistant epilepsy? J Child Neurol. 2013;28(4):479-83.

102) Jones ML, Mark PJ, Keelan JA, et al. Maternal dietary omega-3 fatty acid intake increases resolvin and protectin levels in the rat placenta. J Lipid Res. 2013;54(8):2247-54.

103) Serhan CN, Petasis NA. Resolvins and protectins in inflammation resolution. Chem Rev. 2011;111(10):5922-43.

104) Weylandt KH, Chiu CY, Gomolka B, et al. Omega-3 fatty acids and their lipid mediators: towards an understanding of resolvin and protectin formation.Prostaglandins Other Lipid Mediat. 2012;97(3-4):73-82

105) Lu Y, Zhao LX, Cao DL, et al. Spinal injection of docosahexaenoic acid attenuates carrageenan-induced inflammatory pain through inhibition of microglia-mediated neuroinflammation in the spinal cord. Neuroscience. 2013;241:22-31.

106) Ramirez-Ramirez V, Macias-Islas MA, Ortiz GG, et al. Efficacy of fish oil on serum of TNF α, IL-1 β, and IL-6 oxidative stress markers in multiple sclerosis treated with interferon beta-1b. Oxid Med Cell Longev. 2013;2013:709493.

107) Wang TM, Hsieh SC, Chen JW, et al. Docosahexaenoic acid and eicosapentaenoic acid reduce C-reactive protein expression and STAT3 activation in IL-6-treated HepG2 cells. Mol Cell Biochem. 2013;377(1-2):97-106.

108) Yang K, Cao F, Sheikh AM, et al. Up-regulation of Ras/Raf/ERK1/2 signaling impairs cultured neuronal cell migration, neurogenesis, synapse formation, and dendritic spine development. Brain Struct Funct. 2013;218(3):669-82.

109) Kiecolt-Glaser JK, Belury MA, Andridge R, et al. Omega-3 supplementation lowers inflammation and anxiety in medical students: a randomized controlled trial.Brain Behav Immun. 2011;25(8):1725-34.

110) Cordain L, Eaton SB, Sebastian A, et al. Origins and evolution of the Western diet: health implications for the 21st century.Am J Clin Nutr. 2005;81(2):341-54. Review.

111) Burdge GC, Calder PC. Conversion of alpha-linolenic acid to longer-chain polyunsaturated fatty acids in human adults.Reprod Nutr Dev. 2005;45(5):581-97. Review.

112) Rees D, Miles EA, Banerjee T, et al. Dose-related effects of eicosapentaenoic acid on innate immune function in healthy humans: a comparison of young and older men. Am J Clin Nutr. 2006;83(2):331-42.

113) Kris-Etherton PM, Harris WS, Appel LJ; American Heart Association. Nutrition Committee. Fish consumption, fish oil, omega-3 fatty acids, and cardiovascular disease. Circulation. 2002;106(21):2747-57. Erratum in: Circulation. 2003;107(3):512..

114) Cunningham E. Are krill oil supplements a better source of n-3 fatty acids than fish oil supplements? J Acad Nutr Diet. 2012;112(2):344.

115) Tur JA, Bibiloni MM, Sureda A, et al. Dietary sources of omega 3 fatty acids: public health risks and benefits. Br J Nutr. 2012;107 Suppl 2:S23-52.

116) Vigerust NF, Bjørndal B, Bohov P, et al. Krill oil versus fish oil in modulation of inflammation and lipid metabolism in mice transgenic for TNF-α. Eur J Nutr. 2013;52(4):1315-25.

117) James S, Montgomery P, Williams K. Omega-3 fatty acids supplementation for autism spectrum disorders (ASD).Cochrane Database Syst Rev. 2011;(11):CD007992.

118) Bent S, Bertoglio K, Hendren RL. Omega-3 fatty acids for autistic spectrum disorder: a systematic review. J Autism Dev Disord. 2009;39(8):1145-54.

119) Yang CY, Leung PS, Adamopoulos IE, et al. The implication of vitamin D and autoimmunity: a comprehensive review. Clin Rev Allergy Immunol. 2013;45(2):217-26.

120) Sadeghi K, Wessner B, Laggner U, et al. Vitamin D3 down-regulates monocyte TLR expression and triggers hyporesponsiveness to pathogen-associated molecular patterns. Eur J Immunol. 2006;36(2):361-70.

121) Morandini AC, Chaves Souza PP, Ramos-Junior ES, et al. Toll-like receptor 2 knockdown modulates interleukin (IL)-6 and IL-8 but not stromal derived factor-1 (SDF-1/CXCL12) in human periodontal ligament and gingival fibroblasts. J Periodontol. 2013;84(4):535-44.

122) Zhang Y, Leung DY, Richers BN, et al. Vitamin D inhibits monocyte/macrophage proinflammatory cytokine production by targeting MAPK phosphatase-1. J Immunol. 2012;188(5):2127-35.

123) Kumar A, Negi G, Sharma SS. Neuroprotection by resveratrol in diabetic neuropathy: concepts & mechanisms. Curr Med Chem. 2013;20(36):4640-5.

124) Chung EY, Kim BH, Hong JT, et al. Resveratrol down-regulates interferon-γ-inducible inflammatory genes in macrophages: molecular mechanism via decreased STAT-1 activation. J Nutr Biochem. 2011;22(10):902-9.

125) Shindler KS, Ventura E, Dutt M, et al. Oral resveratrol reduces neuronal damage in a model of multiple sclerosis. J Neuroophthalmol. 2010;30(4):328-39.

126) Imler TJ Jr, Petro TM. Decreased severity of experimental autoimmune encephalomyelitis during resveratrol administration is associated with increased IL-17+IL-10+ T cells, CD4(-) IFN-gamma+ cells, and decreased macrophage IL-6 expression. Int Immunopharmacol. 2009 ;9(1):134-43.

127) Sato F, Martinez NE, Shahid M, et al. Resveratrol exacerbates both autoimmune and viral models of multiple sclerosis. Am J Pathol. 2013;183(5):1390-6.

128) Jia Y, Jing J, Bai Y, et al. Amelioration of experimental autoimmune encephalomyelitis by plumbagin through down-regulation of JAK-STAT and NF-κB signaling pathways. PLoS One. 2011;6(10):e27006.

129) Sandeep G, Dheeraj A, Sharma NK, et al. Effect of plumbagin free alcohol extract of Plumbago zeylanica Linn. root on reproductive system of female Wistar rats. Asian Pac J Trop Med. 2011;4(12):978-84.

130) Muthian G, Bright JJ. Quercetin, a flavonoid phytoestrogen, ameliorates experimental allergic encephalomyelitis by blocking IL-12 signaling through JAK-STAT pathway in T lymphocyte. J Clin Immunol. 2004;24(5):542-52.

Chapter 6D – Insulin-like growth factor

1) Steinman, G, Mankuta, D. Insulin-like growth factor and the etiology of autism. Med Hypotheses 2013;80(4):475-80.

2) Ozonoff, S, Young, GS, Carter, A, et al. Recurrence risk for autism spectrum disorders: a baby siblings research consortium study. Peds 2011;128:e488-95.

3) D'Ercole, AJ, Ye, P, Calikoglu, AS, et al. The role of the insulin-like growth factors in the central nervous system. Mol Neurobiol 1996;13:277-55.

4) Steinman, GD, Verni, C. Womb Mates: A modern guide to fertility and twinning. Baffin Books Publishing, New York, 2007.

5) Gluckman, PD, Pinal, CS. Regulation of fetal growth by the somatotrophic axis. J Nutr 2003;133(5):1741S-1746S.

6) Chellakooty, M, Skibsted, L, Skouby, SO, et al. Longitudinal study of serum placental GH in 455 normal pregnancies: correlation to gestational age, fetal gender, and weight. J Clin Endocrinol Metab 2002;87(6):2734-9.

7) Riikonen, R. Cerebrospinal fluid insulin-like growth factors IGF-1 and IGF-2 in infantile autism. Devel Med & Child Neuro 2006;48(9):751-5.

8) Sorem, KA, Siler-Khodr, TM. Placental IGF-1 in severe intrauterine growth retardation. J Maternal-Fetal Med 1998;7:1-7.

9) McMorris, FA, Mozell, RL, Carson, MJ, et al. Regulation of oligodendrocyte development and central nervous system myelination by insulin-like growth factors. In The role of insulin-like growth factors in the nervous system. MK Raizada, D LeRoith, eds., Annals of the New York Academy of Sciences, 1993, vol. 692, pp.321-34.

10) Zikopoulos, B, Barbas, H. Changes in prefrontal axons may disrupt the network in autism. J Neurosci 2010;30(44):14595-608.

11) Bondy, CA. Transient IGF-1 gene expression during maturation of functionally related central projection neurons. J Neurosci 1991;11(11):3442-55.

12) Al-Farsi, YM, Al-Sharbatim, MM, Waly, MI, et al. Effect of suboptimal breast-feeding practices: A case-control study. Nutrition 2012;28(7/8):2012.

13) Arends, N, Johnston, L, Hokken-Koelega, A, et al. Polymorphism in the IGF-I gene: Clinical relevance for short children born small for gestation age (SGA). J Clin Endocrin Metab 2002;87(6):2720-4.

14) Steinman, G, Breastfeeding as a possible deterrent to autism – a clinical perspective. Medical Hypotheses 2013;81:999-1001.

15) Purves, D, Augustine, GJ, Fitzpatrick, D. et al., editors. Neuroscience. 2nd edition. Sinauer Assoc., Sunderland, MA, 2001.

16) Roberts, TPL, Khan, AY, Rey, M, et al. MEG detection of delayed auditory evoked responses in autism spectrum disorders: Towards an imaging biomarker for autism. Autism Res. 2010;3(1):8-18.

17) D Purves, GJ Augustine, D Fitzpatrick, et al., eds. Neuroscience, 5th edition, Sinauer, Sunderland, MA, 2012, pp. 51-54, 477-558.

18) Rietveld, I. A polymorphism in the IGF-1 gene influences the age-related decline in circulating total IGF-1 levels. Europ J Endocrin 2003;148:171-5.

19) Steinman, G. Predicting autism at birth. Medical Hypotheses 2013;81:21-25.

20) Goldman, SA, Schanz, S, Windrem, MS, Stem cell-based strategies for treating pediatric disorders of myelin. Hum Mol Genetics 2008;17:R76-83.

21) Li, Y, Shelat, H, Geng, YJ. IGF-1 prevents oxidative stress-induced apoptosis in induced pluripotent stem cells which is mediated by microRNA-1. Biochem Biophy Res Comm 2012;426(4):615-9.

22) Boada, LD, Lara, PC, Alvarez-Leon, EE, et al. Serum levels of insulin-like growth factor-1 in relation to organochlorine pesticides exposure. Growth Horm IGF Res 2007;17(6):506-11.

23) Custodia, RJ, doCarmocutodia, VI, Scrideli, CA, et al. Impact of hypoxia on IGF-I, IGF-II, IGFBP-3, ALS, and IGFBP-1 regulation and on IGF1R gene expression in children. Growth Horm IGF Res 2012;22(5):186-91.

24) Geier, DA, King, PG, Sykes, LK, Geier, MR. A comprehensive review of mercury provoked autism. Indian J Med Res 2008;128:383-411.

25) Attias, Z, Werner, H, Vaisman, N. Folic acid and its metabolites modulate IGF-1 receptor gene expression in colon cancer cells in a p53-dependent manner. Endoc Relat Cancer 2006;13(2):571-81.

26) Lehti, V, Brown, AS, Gissler, M, et al. Autism spectrum disorders in IVF children: a national case-control study in Finland. Hum Reprod 2013;28(3):2013.

27) Gunnell, D, Miller, LL, Rogers, I, et al. Association of insulin-like growth factor-I and insulin-growth factor binding protein-3 with IQ among 8-to-9 year old children in the Avon Longitudinal study of parents and children. Ped 2005;116(5):e681-6.

28) Grandis, M, Nobbio, L, Abbruzzese, M, et al. Insulin treatment enhances expression of IGF-1 in sural nerves of diabetic patients. Muscle Nerv 2001;24(5):622-9.

29) Maile, LA, Xu, S, Cwyfan-Hughes, SC, et al. Active and inhibitory components of the insulin-like growth factor binding protein-3 protease system in adult serum, interstitial, and synovial fluid. Endocr 1998;139:4772-81.

30) Carro,E, Trejo, JL, Nunez A, Torres-Aleman, I. Brain repair and neruoprotection by serum insulin-like growth factor I. Mol Neurobiol 2003;27:153-62.

31) Lenninger, GM, Feldman, EI, Insulin-like growth factors in the treatment of neurological disease*in* IGF-I and IGF Binding Proteins, S Cianfarani, DR Clemmons, MO Savage, eds., Karger, Basel, 2005, pp.135-59.

32) Beck, KD, Powell-Braxton, I, Widmer, HR, et al. IGF1 gene disruption results in reduced brain size, CNS hypomyelination, and loss of hippocampal granule and striatal parvalbumin-containing neuronsl. Neuron 1995;14:717-30.

33) Zumkeller, W. The effect of insuin-like growth on brain Myelination and their potential therapeutic application in Myelination 91-101.

34) Sullivan, KA, Kim, B, Russell, JW, Feldman, EL. IGF-I in neuronal differentiation and neuroprotection *in* EE Muller, ed., IGFs in the nervous system. Springer-Verlag, Berlin, 1998, pp.28-46.

35) Herman, IP. Physics of the human body, Springer, Berlin, 2007, p.721.

36) Steinman, G, Mankuta, D, Breastfeeding as a possible deterrent to autism – a clinical perspective. Medical Hypotheses 2013;81:999-1001.

37) Hertz-Picciotto I, Delwiche L. The rise of autism and the role of age at diagnosis, Epidem. 2009;20(1):84-90.

Chapter 7A – Vaccination/MMR

1) Wakefield, A. J, Murch, S. H, Anthony, A., et al. RETRACTED: Ileal-lymphoid-nodular hyperplasia, non-specific colitis, and pervasive developmental disorder in children. The Lancet, 1998; 351(9103):637-41

2) http://www.phac-aspc.gc.ca/im/vs-sv/vs-faq01-eng.php

3) http://www.niaid.nih.gov/topics/vaccines/understanding/pages/whatvaccine.aspx

4) Afzal MA, Minor PD, Schild GC. Clinical safety issues of measles, mumps and rubella vaccines. World Health Organization. Bulletin of the World Health Organization 2000;78(2):199-204.

5) Whalen J, McKay B. Fifteen Years After Autism Panic, A Plague of Measles Erupts. The Wall Street Journal July 20, 2013:A1.

6) Ruebush M, Hawley L. COMLEX Level 1 Immunology and Microbiology Lecture Notes. Kaplan Medical 2011;393-394.

7) http://www.cdc.gov/vaccines/vpd-vac/measles/faqs-dis-vac-risks.htm

8) http://www.cdc.gov/vaccines/vac-gen/whatifstop.htm

9) Measles, MMR, and Autism: The confusion continues. The Lancet. 2000; 355: 1379.

10) http://www.immunizationinfo.org/vaccines/measles

11) http://www.cdc.gov/Mmwr/preview/mmwrhtml/00053391.htm

12) http://www.hpa.org.uk/web/HPAweb&HPAwebStandard/HPAweb_C/1195733835814

13) Daszak P, Purcell M, Lewin J, et al. Detection and comparative analysis of persistent measles virus infection in Crohn's disease by immunogold electron microscopy. Journal of Clinical Pathology 1997;50:299-304.

14) Napoli M. The possible link between MMR vaccine and autism—An interview with Barbara Loe Fisher. Health Facts 2000;25:2-3.

15) Bragesjo F, Hall berg M. Dilemmas of a Vitalizing Vaccine Market: Lessons from the MMR Vaccine/Autism Debate. Science in Context 2011;41:107-125

16) Ozonoff, S., Heung, K., Byrd, R., et al. The Onset of Autism: Patterns of Symptom Emergence in the First Years of Life. Autism Res. 2008;1(6):320–28.

17) Horton R. The lessons of MMR. The Lancet. 2004;363:748-749

18) Murray T. British fear MMR vaccine and autism link [Measles, mumps, and rubella vaccine]. Medical Post 1998;34(42):13

19) Offit, P. A. 2008. Autism's false prophets: bad science, risky medicine and the search for a cure. New York: Columbia University Press. P34-38

20) Flaherty, D. K. The vaccine-autism connection: a public health crisis caused by unethical medical practices and fraudulent science. The Annals of Pharmacotherapy, 2011;45:1302-04

21) Murray T. Spurious claims about vaccine lead to misconduct charges. Medical Post 2006; 42:49.

22) Baker, J. P. Mercury, vaccines and autism: one Controversy, three histories. American Journal of Public Health,2008;98(2):244-253.

23) D'Souza Y, Fombonne E, Ward BJ. No Evidence of Persisting Measles Virus in Peripheral Blood Mononuclear Cells From Children With Autism Spectrum Disorder. Pediatrics 2006; 118: 1164-1675.

24) Daszak P, Purcell M, Lewin J, et al. Detection and comparative analysis of persistent measles virus infection in Crohn's disease by immunogold electron microscopy. Journal of Clinical Pathology 1997; 50: 299-304.

25) Kawashima H, Mori T, Kashiwagi Y, et al. Detection and Sequencing of Measles Virus from Peripheral Mononuclear Cells from Patients with Inflammatory Bowel Disease and Autism. Digestive Diseases and Sciences 2000; 45: 4: 723-729.

26) Uhlmann V, Martin CM, Sheils O, et al. Potential viral pathogenic mechanism for new variant inflammatory bowel disease. Journal of Clinical Pathology: Molecular Pathology 2002; 55: 84-90.

27) Martin CM, Uhlmann V, Killalea A, et al. Detection of measles virus in children with ileo-colonic lymphoid nodular hyperplasia, enterocolitis and developmental disorder. Molecular Psychiatry 2002; 7: S47-S48.

28) Iizuka M, Chiba M, Yukawa M, et al. Immunohistochemical analysis of the distribution of measles related antigen in the intestinal mucosa in inflammatory bowel disease. Gut 2000; 46: 2: 163-169.

29) Hornig M, Briese T, Buie et al. Lack of Association between Measles Virus Vaccine and Autism with Enteropathy: A Case-Control Study. PLoS ONE 2008; 3(9): e3140. doi:10.1371/journal.pone.0003140.

30) Wing L, Potter D. The Epidemiology of Autistic Spectrum Disorders: Is the Prevalence Rising? Mental Retardation and Developmental Disabilities Research Reviews 2002; 8: 151-161.

31) Fombonne E, Chakrabarti S. No Evidence for A New Variant of Measles-Mumps-Rubella–Induced Autism. Pediatrics 2001; 108: e58.

32) Taylor B, Miller E, Lingam R, et al. Measles, mumps, and rubella vaccination and bowel problems or developmental regression in children with autism: population study. BMJ 2002; 324: 393-396.

33) Sandhu B, Steer C, Golding J, Emond A. The early stool patterns of young children with autistic spectrum disorder. Archives of Disease in Childhood 2009; 94: 497-500.

34) Taylor B, Miller E, Farrington CP, et al. Autism and measles, mumps and rubella vaccine: no epidemiological evidence for a causal association. The Lancet 1999; 353: 2026-2029.

35) Madsen KM, Hviid A, Vestergaard M et al. A Population-based study of Measles, Mumps, and Rubella Vaccination and Autism. NEJM 2002; 347: 19: 1477-1482.

36) Honda H, Shimizu Y, Rutter M. No effect of MMR withdrawal on the incidence of autism: a total population study. Journal of Child Psychology and Psychiatry 2005; 46: 6: 572-579.

37) https://catalogue.ic.nhs.uk/publications/public-health/immunisation/nhs-immu-stat-eng-2011-2012/nhs-immu-stat-eng-2011-12-rep.pdf

38) http://www.cdc.gov/mmwr/preview/mmwrhtml/mm6236a1.htm?s_cid=mm6236a1_e

39) http://www.cdc.gov/mmwr/preview/mmwrhtml/mm6135a1.htm?s_cid=mm6135a1_e%0d%0a

Chapter 7B - Thimerosal

1) Burbacher, B, Thomas M., Shen, D, et al. "Comparison of Blood and Brain Mercury Levels in Infant Monkeys Exposed to Methylmercury or Vaccines Containing Thimerosal." *Environmental Health Perspectives* (2005):

2) Zareba, Grazyna, Elsa Cernichiari, Rieko Hojo, Scott McNitt, Bernard Weiss, Moiz M. Mumtaz, Dennis E. Jones, and Thomas W. Clarkson. "Thimerosal Distribution and Metabolism in Neonatal Mice: Comparison with Methyl Mercury." *Journal of Applied Toxicology* 27.5 (2007): 511-18.

3) Clarkson, T. W., Vyas, J. B. and Ballatori, N. (2007), Mechanisms of mercury disposition in the body. Am. J. Ind. Med., 50: 757–764. doi: 10.1002/ajim.20476

4) Stajich, G, Lopez, G, Harry, S, Sexson, W. Iatrogenic Exposure To Mercury After Hepatitis B Vaccination In Preterm Infants The Journal Of Pediatrics –"Vaccines, Blood & Biologics." *Thimerosal in Vaccines*. 29 Sept. 2013.

5) Powell, H. M., and W. A. Jamieson. "MERTHIOLATE AS A GERMICIDE." *American Journal of Epidemiology* 13.1 (1930): 296`-310. *Oxford Journals*. Web. 8 June 2013.

6) Geier, D, Sykes, L, Geier,M. "A Review of Thimerosal (Merthiolate) and Its Ethylmercury Breakdown Product: Specific Historical Considerations Regarding Safety and Effectiveness." *Journal of Toxicology and Environmental Health, Part B* 10.8 (2007): 575-96. Print.

7) Baker, J. P. "Mercury, Vaccines, and Autism: One Controversy, Three Histories." *American Journal of Public Health* 98.2 (2008): 244-53.

8) Luch, Andreas. *Molecular, Clinical, and Environmental Toxicology*. Basel: Birkhäuser, 2009.

9) *Immunization Safety Review : Vaccines and Autism*. Washington, D.C.: National Academies, 2004.

10) U.S. Food and Drug Administration. *Thimerosal in Vaccines Questions and Answers*. N.p., n.d. Web. 13 Jan. 2014.

11) Fiore, Anthony E., et al., *Centers for Disease Control and Prevention*. Centers for Disease Control and Prevention, 29 Sept. 2013.

12) McMahon, AW., Iskander, JK, et al.. "Inactivated Influenza Vaccine (IIV) in Children." *Vaccine* 26.3 (2008): 427-29.

13) Roitt's Essential Immunology. Ivan M.Roitt - Peter J.Delves - Blackwell Science - 2001 "Methylmercury (MeHg) (CASRN 22967-92-6) | IRIS | US EPA." *EPA*. Environmental Protection Agency, 29 Sept. 2013.

14) Madsen, K. M., Lauritsen, MB,. Pedersen, CB, et al. "Thimerosal and the Occurrence of Autism: Negative Ecological Evidence From Danish Population-Based Data." *Pediatrics* 112.3 (2003): 604-06.

15) Burbacher, TM., Shen, DD, Liberato, N, et al. "Comparison of Blood and Brain Mercury Levels in Infant Monkeys Exposed to Methylmercury or Vaccines Containing Thimerosal." Environmental Health Perspectives (2005).

16) Withrow, SJ., Vail, DM. Withrow&MacEwen's Small Animal Clinical Oncology. St. Louis, MO: Saunders Elsevier, 2007.

17) "USGS Toxic Substances Hydrology Program." USGS Toxic Substances Hydrology Program. 29 Sept. 2013.

18) Sharpe MA, Livingston, AD, Baskin, DS. Thimerosal-derived ethylmercury is a mitochondrial toxin in human astrocytes: possible role of fenton chemistry in the oxidation and breakage of mtDNA. Journal of Toxicology. 2012;2012:12 pages.373-78

19) Campbell, NA., Williamson, B, Heyden, RJ. Biology: Exploring Life. Needham, MA: Pearson, 2004.

20) Green, Douglas R. Means to an End: Apoptosis and Other Cell Death Mechanisms. Cold Spring Harbor, NY: Cold Spring Harbor Laboratory, 2011.

21) Olczak, M., Duszczyk, M., Mierzejewski, P., et al. Lasting neuropathological changes in rat brain after intermittent neonatal administration of thimerosal. Folia Neuropathol. 2010;48:258–269.

22) Schmitt U, Tanimoto N, Seeliger M, et al. (2009) Detection of behavioral alterations and learning deficits in mice lacking synaptophysin. Neuroscience 162: 234–243.

23) Ceccatelli S, Daré, E, Moors M. Methylmercury-induced neurotoxicity and apoptosis. ChemBiol Interact.2010;188:301–308.

24) Liu S.I., Huang C.C., Huang C.J., et al. Thimerosal-induced apoptosis in human SCM1 gastric cancer cells, activation of p38 MAP kinase and caspase-3 pathways without involvement of [Ca2+]i elevation. Toxicol. Sci. 2007;100:109–117. doi: 10.1093/toxsci/kfm205.

25) Juurlink, BHJ. Response of glial cells to ischemia: Roles of reactive oxygen species and glutathione. Neuroscience and Biobehavioral Reviews. 1997;21:151–166.

26) Duszczyk-Budhathoki M, Olczak M, Lehner M, Majewska MD. Administration of thimerosal to infant rats increases overflow of glutamate and aspartate in the prefrontal cortex: protective role of dehydroepiandrosterone sulfate. Neurochemical Research.2012;37(2):436–447.

27) Sharpe, MA, Gist, TL, Baskin, DS. "B-Lymphocytes from a Population of Children with Autism Spectrum Disorder and Their Unaffected Siblings Exhibit Hypersensitivity to Thimerosal," Journal of Toxicology, vol. 2013, Article ID 801517, 11 pages, 2013. doi:10.1155/2013/801517

28) Wakefield AJ, et al. Ileal-lymphoid-nodular hyperplasia, non-specific colitis, and pervasive developmental disorders in children. The Lancet. 1998;351:637–641.

29) Smith M, Ellenberg S, Bell L, Rubin D. Media Coverage of the Measles-Mumps-Rubella Vaccine and Autism Controversy and Its Relationship to MMR Immunization Rates in the United States. Pediatrics. 2008;121(4):e836–43.

30) Harris, Gardiner (2 February 2010). "Journal Retracts 1998 Paper Linking Autism to Vaccines". The New York Times. Archived from the original on 1 December 2010. Retrieved 2011-01-06.

31) Blaxill M, Redwood L, Bernard S. Thimerosal and autism? A plausible hypothesis that should not be dismissed. Medical Hypotheses. 2004;62:788–794.

32) Offit PA. Vaccines and autism revisited—the Hannah poling case.The New England Journal of Medicine. 2008;358(20):2089–2091.

33) "Therapeutic Drug Levels, Toxic Levels, Steady State Concentration, Half-life." Therapeutic Drug Levels, Toxic Levels, Steady State Concentration, Half-life. 29 Sept. 2013.

34) Birth-18 Years & "Catch-up" Immunization Schedules. Centers for Disease Control and Prevention, 30 Sept. 2013.

35) Calvino FM, Parra CT. H. pylori and mitochondrial changes in epithelial cells. The role of oxidative stress. Rev EspEnferm Dig. 2010;102:41–50.

36) Patel RP, Cornwell, T, Darley-Usmar VM (1999). "The biochemistry of nitric oxide and peroxynitrite: implications for mitochondrial function". In Packer L, Cadenas E. Understanding the process of aging: the roles of mitochondria, free radicals, and antioxidants. New York, N.Y: Marcel Dekker. pp. 39–56.

37) Clayton R, Clark JB, Sharpe M. Cytochrome c release from rat brain mitochondria is proportional to the mitochondrial functional deficit: implications for apoptosis and neurodegenerative disease. Journal of Neurochemistry. 2005;92(4):840–849.

Chapter 8A – Genetic errors

1) Kanner L. Autistic disturbances of affective contact. Nervous Child. 1943;2:217-250.

2) Folstein S, Rutter M. Infantile autism: a genetic study of 21 twin pains. J Child Psychol Psychiatry. 1977;18(4):297-321.

3) Jorde LB, Hasstedt SJ, Ritvo ER et al. Complex segregation analysis of autism. Am J Hum Gene. 1991;49(5):932-938.

4) Hallmayer J, Cleveland S, Torres A, et al. Genetic heritability and shared environmental factors among twin pairs with autism. Arch Gen Psychiatry. 2011;68(11):1095-102.

5) Bailey A, LeCouteur A, Gottesman I, et al. Usiam as a strongly genetic disorder: evidence from a British twin study. J Psychol Med. 1995;25(1):63-77.

6) Steffenburg S, Gillberg C, Hellgren L, et al. A twin study of autism in Denmark, Finland, Iceland, Norway and Sweden. J Child Psychol Psychiatry. 1989;30(3):405-416.

7) Geschwind DH. Genetics of autism spectrum disorders. Trends in Cognitive Sciences. 2011;15:409-416.

8) McCarroll SA, Hyman SE. Progress in the genetics of polygenic brain disorders: significant new challenges for neurobiology. Neuron. 2013;3:578-587.

9) Sabeti P. Natural selection: uncovering mechanisms of evolutionary adaptation to infectious disease. Nature Education. 2008;1(1):13

10) State M. Genetics of Autism. Autism and Related Disorders Seminar. Yale University, New Haven, CT. 2010.

11) Schaefer BG, Mendeksohn NJ. Clinical genetics evaluation in identifying the etiology of autism spectrum disorders: 2013 guideline revisions. Genetics in Medicine. 2013;15:5:399-407.

12) Shao Y, Wolpert CM, Raiford KL, et al. Genomic screen and follow-up analysis for autistic disorder. Am J Med Genet. 2002;114:99–105.

13) Liu J, Nyholt DR, Magnussen P, et al. A genomewide screen for autism susceptibility loci. Am J Hum Genet. 2001;69:327–340.

14) Durand CM, Betancur C, Boeckers TM, et al. Mutations in the gene encoding the synaptic scaffolding protein SHANK3 are associated with autism spectrum disorders. Nat Genet. 2007;39(1):25-7.

15) Bozdagi O, Sakurai T, Papapetrou D, et al. Haploinsufficiency of the autism-associated Shank3 gene leads to deficits in synaptic function, social interaction, and social communication. Mol Autism. 2010;17;1(1):15.

16) Kopec CD, Real E, Kessels HW, Malinow R. GluR1 links structural and functional plasticity at excitatory synapses. J Neurosci. 2007;27:13706–13718.

17) Heilm KM, Schaaf CP. The genetics of autism spectrum disorders – a guide for clinicians. Current Psychiatric Reports. 2013;15(1):334.

18) Nagarajan RP, Hogart AR, Gwye Y, et al. Reduced MeCP2 expression is frequent in autism frontal cortex and correlates with aberrant MECP2 promoter methylation. Epigenetics. 2006;1(4):e1–11.

19) Singh J, Saxena A, Christodoulou J, Ravine D MECP2 genomic structure and function: insights from ENCODE. Nucleic Acids Res. 2008;36(19):6035–6047.

20) Hindorff LA, MacArthur J, Morales J et al. A Catalog of Published Genome-Wide Association Studies. Available at: www.genome.gov/gwastudies. Accessed January 6, 2014.

21) Wang K, Zhang H, Ma D, et al. Common genetic variants on 5p14.1 associate with autism spectrum disorders. Nature. 2009;459(7246):528-33.

22) Devlin B, Melhem N, Roeder K. Do common variants play a role in risk for autism? Evidence and theoretical musings. Brain Res. 2011;1380:78–84.

23) Psychiatric GWAS consortium coordinating committee. Genomewide association studies: history, rationale, and prospects for psychiatric disorders. AM J Psychiatry. 2009;166:540-556.

24) http://www.autismgenome.org. Accessed January 6, 2014.

25) International Human Genome Sequencing Consortium. Finishing the euchromatic sequence of the human genome. Nature. 2004;431:931-945.

26) Wetterstrand KA. DNA Sequencing Costs: Data from the NHGRI Genome Sequencing Program (GSP) Available at: www.genome.gov/sequencingcosts. Accessed January 6, 2014.

27) O'Roak BJ, Deriziotis P, Lee C, et al. Exome sequencing in sporadic autism spectrum disorders identifies severe de novo mutations. Nat Genet. 2011;43:585–9.

28) Sanders SJ, Murtha MT, Gupta AR, et al. De novo mutations revealed by whole-exome sequencing are strongly associated with autism. Nature. 2012;485:237–41.

29) O'Roak BJ, Vives L, Girirajan S, et al. Sporadic autism exomes reveal a highly interconnected protein network of de novo mutations. Nature. 2012;485:246–50.

30) Neale BM, Kou Y, Liu L, et al. Patterns and rates of exonic de novo mutations in autism spectrum disorders. Nature. 2012;485:242–5.

31) Iossifov I, Ronemus M, Levy D, et al. De novo gene disruptions in children on the autistic spectrum. Neuron. 2012;74:285–99.

32) Lingling Shi, Xu Zhang, Ryan Golhar, et al. Whole-genome sequencing in an autism multiplex family. Mol Autism. 2013;4:8.

33) Michaelson JJ, Shi Y, Gujral M, et al. Whole-Genome Sequencing in Autism Identifies Hot Spots for De Novo Germline Mutation. Cell. 2012;151(7):1431-1442.

34) Jiang YH, Yuen RK, Jin X, et al. Detection of Clinically Relevant Genetic Variants in Autism Spectrum Disorder by Whole-Genome Sequencing. Am J Hum Genet. 2013;93(2):249-263.

35) Hamdan FF, Daoud H, Rochefort D, et al. De novo mutations in FOXP1 in cases with intellectual disability, autism, and language impairment. Am J Hum Genet 2010;87:671–678.

36) Malhotra D, Sebat J. CNVs: Habringers of a rare variant solution in psychiatric genetics. Cell. 2012;148:6:1223-1241.

37) Schaefer GB, Mendelsohn N. Clinical genetics evaluation in identifying the etiology of autism spectrum disorders: 2013 guideline revisions. Genetics in Medicine. 2013:15(5):399-407.

38) Hallmayer J, Cleveland S, Torres A, et al. Genetic heritability and shared environmental factors among twin pairs with autism. Arch Gen Psychiatry. 2011; 68(11):1095-102.

39) Ronald A, Hoekstra RA. Autism spectrum disorders and autistic traits: a decade of new twin studies. Am J Med Genet B. 2011;156B: 255–274.

40) Nguyen AT, Rauch TA, Pfeifer GP. et al. Global methylation profiling of lymphoblastoid cell lines reveals epigenetic contributions to autism spectrum disorders and a novel autism candidate gene RORA, whose protein product is reduced in autistic brain. FASEB J. 2010;24(8):3036–3051.

41) Wong CC, Meaburn EL, Ronald A, et al. Methylomic analysis of monozygotic twins discordant for autism spectrum disorder and related behavioural traits. Mol Psychiatry. 2013;1-9.

42) Atladottir HO, Thorsen P, Ostergaard L, et al. Maternal infection requiring hospitalization during pregnancy and autism spectrum disorders. J Autism Dev Disord. 2010;40(12):1423–30.

43) Needleman, LA, McAllister, AK. The major histocompatibility complex and autism spectrum disorder. Devel Neurobio. 2012;72:1288–1301.

44) Volk HE, Kerin T, Lurmann F et al. Autism Spectrum Disorder: Interaction of Air Pollution with the MET Receptor Tyrosine Kinase Gene. Epidemiology. 2014;25(1):44-7.

45) Steinman G, Mankuta D. Insulin-like growth factor and the etiology of autism. Medical Hypotheses. 2013;475-480.

46) Ye P, Li L, Richards RG, et al. Myelination is altered in insulin-like growth factor-I null mutant mice. J Neurosci. 2002; 22(14):6041-51.

47) Riikonen, R. Cerebrospinal fluid insulin-like growth factors IGF-1 and IGF-2 in infantile autism. Devel Med & Child Neuro. 2006;48(9): 751-5.

48) Zikopoulos B, Barbas H. Changes in prefrontal axons may disrupt the network in autism. J. Neurosci. 2010; 30(44): 14596-609.

49) Arends N et al. Polymorphism in the IGF1 gene: clinical relevance for short children born small for gestational age (SGA). J Clin Endocrin Metab. 2002; 87(6):2720.

50) Pinto-Martin JA, Levy SE, Feldman JF, et al. Prevalence of autism spectrum disorder in adolescents born weighing <2000 grams. Pediatrics. 2011;128(4): 2010-846.

51) Bozdagi O, Tavassoli T, Buxbaum JD. Insulin-like growth factor-1 rescues synaptic and motor deficits in a mouse model of autism and developmental delay. Mol Autism. 2013;4:9.

52) Ellegren H. Characteristics, causes and evolutionary consequences of male-biased mutation. Proc Biol Sci. 2007;274(1606): –10.

53) Saha S, Barnett AG, Foldi C, et al. Advanced Paternal Age Is Associated with Impaired Neurocognitive Outcomes during Infancy and Childhood. PLoS Med. 2009; 6(3).

54) Durkin MS, Maenner MJ, Newschaffer CJ, et al. Advanced Parental Age and the Risk of Autism Spectrum Disorder. Am J Epidemiol. 2008; 168(11): 1268–1276.

55) Reichenberg A, Gross R, Weiser M, et al. Advancing paternal age and Autism. Arch Gen Psychiatry. 2006;63(9):1026-32.

56) http://www.cdc.gov/ncbddd/autism/data.html. Accessed January 6, 2014.

57) Betancur, C,Etiological heterogeneity in autism spectrum disorders: More than 100 genetic and genomic disorders and still counting. Brain Res 2011;1380:42-77.

Chapter 8B – Oxidative stress

1) Harvey, RA, Ferrier, DR. Biochemistry. 5th ed. Philadelphia: Wilkins, 2011.

2) Zimmerman, AW. Autism; Current Theories and Evidence. Baltimore, Maryland: Humana Press, 2008.

3) Bock, K. , Stauth, C, Stauth, F. Healing the new childhood epidemics: Autism, adhd, asthma, and allergies, the groundbreaking program for the 4-a disorders. New York: Ballantine Books, 2007.

4) Chauhan, A., Chauhan, V. "Oxidative Stress in Autism." PubMed. 3.171-181 (2006): Web. 26 Sep. 2013.

5) Ghezzo, A, Visconti, P, Mazzanti, I. "Oxidative Stress and Erythrocyte Membrane Alterations in Children with Autism: Correlation with Clinical Features." PLoS One. 8.6 (2013): Web. 26 Sep. 2013.

6) Goines , P, Paul Ashwood, and Judy Van de Water. "Autism Spectrum Disorders and the Immune System." Autism Society of America. 26 Sep 2013.

7) Harvey, Richard A. PhD, and Denise R. Ferrier. Biochemistry. 5th ed. Philadelphia: Wilkins, 2011.

8) "Tuberous Sclerosis."

9) "MECP2." Genetics Home Reference. 2013. http://ghr.nlm.nih.gov/gene/MECP2.

10) De Felice, C, C Signorini, S Leoncini, et al. "The role of oxidative stress in Rett syndrome: an overview." 26 Sep. 2013.

11) McLennan, Y, Polussa, J, Hagerman, R. "Fragile X Syndrome." Current Genomics; Bentham Science Publishers. (2011)

12) Pagano, G., Castello, G. "Oxidative stress and mitochondrial dysfunction in Down syndrome." (2012):

13) Wang , LW, Tancredi, DJ, Thomas, DW. "The prevalence of gastrointestinal problems in children across the United States with autism spectrum disorders from families with multiple affected members." 32.5 (2011):

Chapter 8C - Detoxification

1) Meguid, N. A., Dardir, A. A., Abdel-Raouf, E. R., & Hashish, A. Evaluation of oxidative stress in autism: defective antioxidant enzymes and increased lipid peroxidation. Biological trace element research, 2011:143(1), 58-65.

2) James, S. J., Rose, S., Melnyk, S., et al. Cellular and mitochondrial glutathione redox imbalance in lymphoblastoid cells derived from children with autism. The FASEB Journal, 2009;23(8), 2374-2383.

3) Al-Yafee, Y., Al-Ayadhi, L., Haq, S., & El-Ansary, A. Novel metabolic biomarkers related to sulfur-dependent detoxification pathways in autistic patients of Saudi Arabia. BMC neurology, 2011:11(1), 139.

4) Rose, S., Melnyk, S., Pavliv, O.,et al. Evidence of oxidative damage and inflammation associated with low glutathione redox status in the autism brain. Translational psychiatry,2012; 2(7): e134.

5) James, S. J., Cutler, P., Melnyk, S., et al. Metabolic biomarkers of increased oxidative stress and impaired methylation capacity in children with autism. The American journal of clinical nutrition, 2004;80(6): 1611-1617.

6) Melnyk, S., Fuchs, G. J., Schulz, E.,. Metabolic imbalance associated with methylation dysregulation and oxidative damage in children with autism. Journal of autism and developmental disorders, 2012;42(3): 367-377.

7) Gu, F., Chauhan, V., Kaur, K., et al. Alterations in mitochondrial DNA copy number and the activities of electron transport chain complexes and pyruvate dehydrogenase in the frontal cortex from subjects with autism. Translational psychiatry,2013; 3(9): e299.

8) Williams, T. A., Mars, A. E., Buyske,R. Risk of autistic disorder in affected offspring of mothers with a glutathione S-transferase P1 haplotype. Archives of pediatrics & adolescent medicine, 2007;161(4):356.

9) Gu, F., Chauhan, V., & Chauhan, A. Impaired synthesis and antioxidant defense of glutathione in the cerebellum of autistic subjects: Alterations in the activities and protein expression of glutathione-related enzymes. Free Radical Biology and Medicine,2013; 65: 488-496.

Chapter 9A – Diagnosis and prevention

1) Rutter, M. Diagnosis and Definition in Autism – a reappraisal of concepts and treatment, M. Rutter, E. Schopler, eds. Plenum Press, New York, 1978, pp.1-25.

2) Shcheglobitov, A, Shcheglovitova, O, Yazawa, M, et al. SHANK3 and IGF1 restore synaptic deficits in neurons from 22q13 deletion syndrome patients. Nature 2013;503(7475):267-71.

3) Buxbaum, J, Growth factor improves autism symptoms in mice. International Congress Human Genetics, 2011.

4) Bozdagi, O, Tavassoli, T, Buxbaum, JD. Insulin-like growth factor-1 rescues synaptic and motor deficits in mouse model of autism and developmental delay. Mol Autism 2013;4(1):9.

5) Tropea, D, Giacometti, E, Wilson, NR, et al. Partial reversal of Rett Syndrome-like symptoms in MeCP2 mutant mice. Proc Natl Acad Sci USA 2009;106(6):2029-34.

6) Field, T, Diego, M, Hernandez-Reif, DL, et al. Insulin and insulin-like growth

factor 1 (IGF-1) increased in preterm neonates. J Dev Behav Pediatr 2008;29(6): 463-6.

7) Steinman, G, Mankuta, D. Breastfeeding as a possible deterrent to autism – a clinical perspective. Med Hypoth 2013;81:999-1001.

8) Makkonen, I, Kokki, H, Kuikka, J, et al. Effects of fluoxetine treatment on striatal dopamine tranporter binding and cerebrospinal fluid insulin-like factor -1 in children with autism. Neuropediatrics 2011;42(5):207-9.

Chapter 9B – Stem cell therapy

1) Ramalho-Santos, M, Willenbring, H. On the Origin of the Term Stem Cell. Cell Stem Cell 2007;1(1):35-38.

2) Prindull, G. Prindull, B, Meulen, N. Haemotopoietic stem cells; CFUc in human cord blood. Acta Paediatr Scand. 1978;67(4): 413-6

3) Martin, GR. Isolation of a Pluripotent cell line from early mouse embryos cultured in medium conditions by teratocarcinoma stem cells. Proc Natl Aca Sci. 1981;78(12):7634-8

4) Lo, B, Parham, L. Ethical Issues in Stem Cell Research. Endocr Rev. 2009;30(3):204-213

5) Takahashi, K, Yamanaka, S. Induction of pluripotent stem cells from mouse embryonic and adult fibroblast cultures by defined factors. Cell. 2006;126(4):663-76

6) Yuan, S. et al, Bioengineered stem cells in neural development and neurodegeneration research. Ageing Research Reviews 2013;12:739-48

7) Vierbuchen, T. et al, Direct conversion of fibroblasts to functional neurons by defined factors. Nature 2010;463:1035-41

8) Han, D.W., et al, Direct reprogramming of fibroblasts into neural stem cells by defined factors. Cell Stem Cell 2012;10:465-72

9) American Psychiatric Association. Diagnostic and statistical manual of mental disorders (5th ed.). Arlington, VA: American Psychiatric Publishing. 2013.

10) Ebert, AD, Liang, P, Wu, JC. Induced pluripotent stem cells as a disease modeling and drug screening platform. J Cardiovasc Pharmacol. 2012;60(4):408-16.

11) Kim, K. et al. Cellular reprogramming: a novel tool for investigating autism spectrum disorders. Trends in Molecular Medicine. 2012;18:463-71

12) Yu, D., Marchetto, M. Therapeutic Translation of iPSCs for Treating Neurological Disease. Cell Stem Cell. 2013;12:678-88

13) Cocks, G, et al, The utility of patient specific induced pluripotent stem cells for the modeling of autistic spectrum disorders. Psychopharmacology. 2013.

14) Bailey, A, et al, Autism as a strongly genetic disorder: evidence from a British twin study. Psychol. Med. 1995;25:63-77

15) Steffenburg, S. et al, A twin study of autism in Denmark, Finland, Iceland, Norway and Sweden. J. Child Psychology. Psychiatry Allied Disciplines 1989;30:405-416

16) Griesi-Oliveira, K, Sunaga, DY, Alvizi, L, et al. Stem cells as a good tool to investigate dysregulated biological systems in autism spectrum disorders. Autism Research. 2013;6(5):354-61.

17) Ecker, C, Spooren, W, Murphy, D, et al. Developing new pharmacotherapies for autism. Journal of Internal Medicine. 2013;274(4):308-20.

18) Just, M, Cherkassky, VL, Keller, TA, et al. Functional and anatomical cortical underconnectivity in Autism: Evidence from an fMRI study of an executive function task and corpus callosum morphometry. Cerebral Cortex. 2007;17(4):951-61.

19) Ghosh, A, Michalon, A, Lindemann, L, et al., Drug discovery for autism spectrum disorder: challenges and opportunities. Nature Review Drug Discovery 2013;12(10):777-90

20) Depino, A. Peripheral and central inflammation in autism spectrum disorders. Mol. Cell. Neurosci. 2013;53:69-76.

21) Li, X, Chauhan, A, Sheikh, AM, et al. Elevated immune response in the brain of autistic patients. J Neuroimmunol 2009;207:111-16

22) Connolly, AM, Chez, M, Strief, EM, et al. Brain-derived neurotrophic factor and autoantibodies to neural antigens in sera of children with autistic spectrum disorders, Landau-Kleffner syndrome, and epilepsy. Biol Psychiatry 2006;59(4):354-63

23) Vojdani, A, O'Bryan, T, Green, JA, et al. Immune response to dietary proteins, gliadin and cerebellar peptides in children with autism. Nutr Neurosci. 2004;3:151-61

24) Cohly HH, Panja A. Immunological findings in autism. Int Rev Neurobiol. 2005;71:317-41

25) Casanova MF, van Kooten IA, Switala AE, et al. Minicolumnar abnormalities in autism. Acta Neuropathol. 2006;112(3):287-303

26) Folsom, TD, Fatemi, SH. The involvement of Reelin in neurodevelopmental disorders. Neuropharmacology. 2013;68:122-35

27) Siniscalco D, Bradstreet JJ, Antonucci N. Therapeutic role of hematopoietic stem cells in autism spectrum disorder-related inflammation. Front Immunol. 2013;4:140

28) Granick JL, Simon SI, Borjesson DL. Hematopoietic stem and progenitor cells as effectors in innate immunity. Bone Marrow. 2012;165107.

29) Chess S. Follow-up report on autism in congenital rubella. J Autism Child Schizophr. 1977;(1):69-81

30) Atladóttir, HO, Thorsen, P, Østergaard, L, et al. Maternal infection requiring hospitalization during pregnancy and autism spectrum disorders. J Autism Dev Disord. 2010;12:1423-30

31) Malkova, NV, Yu, CZ, Hsiao, EY, et al. Maternal immune activation yields offspring displaying mouse versions of the three core symptoms of autism. Brain Behav Immun. 2012;26(4):607-16

32) Hsiao, EY, McBride, SW, Chow, J, et al. Modeling an autism risk factor in mice leads to permanent immune dysregulation. Proc Natl Acad Sci U S A. 2012;109(31):12776-81

33) Park, DH, Borlongan, CV, Willing, AE, et al. Human umbilical cord blood cell grafts for brain ischemia. Cell Transplant. 2009;18(9):985-98

34) De Miguel, MP, Fuentes-Julián, S, Blázquez-Martínez, A, et al. Immunosuppressive properties of mesenchymal stem cells: advances and applications. Curr Mol Med. 2012;12(5):574-91

35) Shi, M, Liu, ZW, Wang, FS. Immunomodulatory properties and therapeutic application of mesenchymal stem cells. Clin Exp Immunol. 2011;164(1):1-8

36) Lv, YT, Zhang, Y, Liu, M, et al. Transplantation of human cord blood mononuclear cells and umbilical cord-derived mesenchymal stem cells in autism. J Transl Med. 2013;11(1):196

37) Sharma, A, Gokulchandran, N, Sane, H, et al. Autologous bone marrow mononuclear cell therapy for autism: an open label proof of concept study. Stem Cells Int. 2013:623875

38) Hashimoto, T, Sasaki, M, Fukumizu, M, et al. Single-photon emission computed tomography of the brain in autism: effect of the developmental level. Pediatr Neurol. 2000;23(5):416-20

39) Wright, DE, Wagers, AJ, Gulati, AP, et al. Physiological migration of hematopoietic stem and progenitor cells. Science. 2001;294(5548):1933-6

40) Arber, C. Li, M. Cortical interneuron from human pluripotent stem cells: prospects for neurological and psychiatric disease. Frontiers in Cellular Neuroscience. 2013;7:10.

41) Siniscalco, D. Sapone, A, Cirillo, A. et al. Autism Spectrum Disorders: Is Mesenchymal Stem Cell Personalized Therapy the Future. Journal of Biomedicine and Biotechnology. 2012;480289.

42) Mauron A. Autism, Stem cells and magical powder. Rev Med Suisse. 2012;8(354):1795.

43) Laron, Z. Insulin-like growth factor 1 (IGF-1): a growth hormone. Molecular Pathology 2001;54(5):311-6.

44) Wang, J, Tang, Y, Zhang, W, et al. Insulin-like growth factor-1 secreted by brain microvascular endothelial cells attenuates neuron injury upon ischemia. FEBS Journal 2013;280(15):3658-68

45) D'Ercole, A. Joseph, and Ping Ye. Expanding the mind: insulin-like growth factor I and brain development. Endocrinology 2008;149(12):5958-62.

46) Steinman, G, Mankuta, D. Insulin-like growth factor and the etiology of autism. Medical hypotheses 2013;80(4):475-80

CONCLUSIONS AND PROSPECTUS

1) Holzenberger, M, Dupont J, Ducos, B, et al. IGF-1 receptor regulates lifespan and resistance to oxidative stress in mice. Nature 2003;421(6919):182-7.

2) O'Roak, BJ, Vives, L, Fu, W, et al. Multiplex targeted sequencing identifies recurrently mutated genes in autism spectrum disorders. Science 2012;338(6114):1619-22.

3) Sykes, NH, Lamb, JA. Autism: the quest for the genes. Expert reviews in molecular medicine 2007;9.24:1-15.

4) Nordahl, CW, Braunschweig, D, Isosif, AM, et al. Maternal autoantibodies are associated with abnormal brain enlargement in a subgroup of children with autism spectrum disorder. Brain Behav Immun. 2013 May;30:61-5.

5) Ouyang, Q, Lizarraga, SB, Schmidt, M, et al. Christian Syndrome protein NHE6 modulates TrkB endosomal signaling required for neuronal circuit development. Neuron 2013;80(1):97-112.

6) Kanner L. Autistic disturbances of affective contact. *Nervous Child* **2**, 217-250 (1943).

7) Pelengaris, S, Khan, M. "Nature and Nuture in Oncogenesis" *in* The Molecular Biology of Cancer. Blackwell Publishing, Malden, MA, 2006, pp.61-87.

8) Martin, JJ, Schlote, W. Central nervous system lesions in disorders of amino-acid metabolism. A neuropathological study. J Neuro Sci 1972;15:49-76.

9) Dennis, M, Lockyer, L, Lazenby, AI, et al. Intelligence patterns among children with high-functioning autism, phenylketonuria, and childhood head injury. J Autism Dev Dis. 1999;29:5-17.

10) Pavone, L, Ruggieri, M. The problem of alternative therapies in autism *in* The Neurology of Autism, M. Coleman, ed. Oxford Univ Press, New York, 2005, pp.173-200.

INDEX

hypotheses, 7, 8, 11, 13, 104, 108, 120, 127, 143, 164, 246, 247, 248, 286, 322, 326, 329
Hypoxia, 4, 252

I

IGF, 127, 146, 247-254, 287, 290, 308, 311, 320, 321, 322
IL-6, 121, 126, 128, 318, 319
Infection, 5
Inflammation, 5, 297
influenza, 250, 301, 312, 329
Insulin-like growth factor, 5, 12, 127, 247, 248, 287

K

Kanner, 6, 277, 309, 313, 327
Koch, 8, 9

L

anguage, 65, 66, 67
lead, 4
Leaky gut, 5
limbic system, 103-107, 112, 117

M

macrocephaly, 282
macropathology, 4
maternal immune activation, 286, 319
MEG, 254
Mendel, 13
mercury, 5, 9, 12, 198-213, 253, 295
MET, 120-123, 128, 169, 172-175, 181, 286
methionine, 183-186, 292, 295-298, 306
methylmercury, 198-211
microarrays, 280
microglia, 105, 107, 297, 298
micropathology, 4
milk, 146, 162, 202, 250, 287, 311
Minamata, 198, 199, 200-203
minicolumns, 106
misoprostol, 163-167
mitochondria, 104, 105, 291-304
MMR, 13, 329
mother, 127, 128, 144, 146, 159, 163, 173, 185, 201, 202
MRI, 97, 105, 106, 110, 250, 309, 316
mutations, 5, 108, 123, 124, 127, 128, 281
myelin, 250-254, 309, 318, 322, 325
myelination, 5, 127, 250

N

National Institutes of Health, 13
neocortex, 104, 106
nerve, 4, 11, 97, 99, 112, 144, 145, 165, 199, 249, 250, 251, 284, 325
neuroimaging, 102
neurons, 101
neuropathologic, 7, 247, 325, 329
nitric oxide, 126, 298, 303, 304

O

obesity, 143-146, 177, 248
occurrence, 4
oligodendrocyte, 287, 322
omega-3 fatty acids, 202, 207, 208, 211, 213, 293
organophosphates, 168, 170, 173
oxidative stress, 5, 12, 171, 294, 306

P

pathogenesis, 102, 121, 123, 126, 127, 143, 175, 201
pesticides, 4, 12, 167, 170, 171
PET, 106, 110, 117, 316
placenta, 127, 128, 144, 199, 207, 211, 248, 250, 286, 287
pollutants, 4, 11, 12, 167-176, 202, 312, 328
polymorphism, 186, 250, 251, 252, 282, 287, 311
prefrontal cortex, 97, 106, 126, 127
pregnancy, 6, 11, 143-146, 159-176, 184, 185, 207-213, 248-250, 286, 302, 312, 319
prevalence, 103, 125, 128, 143-146, 167, 183, 200, 210, 278, 289, 294
public health, 146, 210
PUFA, 293
Purkinje, 99, 100, 105, 107, 318

R

radicals, 105, 291-307
receptor, 113, 114, 121, 125, 128, 171-173, 181, 248, 252, 253, 280, 283, 286
refrigerator, 4
Rett syndrome, 293, 294, 316, 326

S

schizophrenia, 283, 285, 309
serotonin, 10, 165
SHANK, 125, 128, 283
smoking, 167, 329
speech, 64-67

T

V

W

Pages – 376
Chapters – 42
References – 1069
Words – 175,767